# PSYCHOPATHOLOGY AND SOCIAL PREJUDICE

*Edited by Derek Hook & Gillian Eagle*

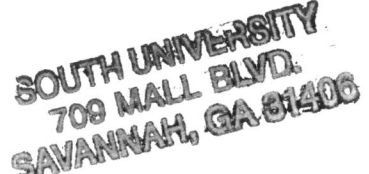

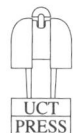

University of Cape Town Press

*Psychopathology and Social Prejudice*

First published 2002

© UCT Press 2002

PO Box 24309, Lansdowne 7779

ISBN 1 919 71367 0

This book is copyright under the Berne Convention. In terms of the Copyright Act, No. 98 of 1978, no part of this book may be reproduced or transmitted in any form or by any means, electronic or mechanical, including phorocopying, recording, or by any information storage and retrieval system, without permission in writing from the Publisher.

Copy editing: FPP Productions
Proofreading: FPP Productions
Indexing: G. M. Kettley
DTP: RHT desktop publishing cc, Durbanville
Cover design: Catherine Crookes
Printed and bound in South Africa by: Formsxpress, Cape Town

Set in Minion and Serif Gothic.

# Contents

Notes on contributors .................................................. iv
Acknowledgements ..................................................... vi

Introduction: A 'social psychology' of psychopathology (*Derek Hook*) ......... 1

**Section 1: Clinical problematics** ....................................... 19
1  Psychotherapy, discourse and the production of psychopathology
   (*Derek Hook*) .................................................... 20
2  Poised on the brink: The social construction of a new biological psychiatry
   (*Martin Terre Blanche*) ........................................... 55
3  The political conundrums of post-traumatic stress disorder (*Gillian Eagle*) .. 75
4  A critical re-reading of post-traumatic stress disorder from a cross-cultural/
   community perspective (*M. Brinton Lykes*) .......................... 92

**Section 2: Pathology as politics** ....................................... 109
5  Rewriting the body, reauthoring the expert: Reading the anorexic body
   (*S. Fuller & Derek Hook*) ......................................... 110
6  Avoiding the implicit repathologisation of male homosexuality: A politico-
   clinical direction for research (*Anthony Theuninck, Derek Hook &
   Vijé Franchi*) ..................................................... 124
7  'Race', ethnicity and the psychopathology of social identity
   (*George Ellison & Thea de Wet*) ................................... 139

**Section 3: South African pathologies** ................................... 151
8  Unsettling meanings of madness: Competing constructions of South
   African insanity (*Carol Long & Estelle Zietkiewicz*) ................. 152
9  Xenophobia: A new pathology for a New South Africa? (*Bronwyn Harris*) .. 169
10 Stigma in the social construction of sexually transmitted diseases
   (*Kopano Ratele & Tamara Shefer*) ................................. 185
11 Witches and watchers: Witchcraft beliefs and practices in South African
   rural communities of the Northern Province (*Teboho Lebakeng,
   Susan Sedumedi & Gillian Eagle*) ................................... 207

**Section 4: Philosophies of pathology** ................................... 221
12 Memory, madness and the market (*Erica Burman*) ................... 222
13 Rethinking normality through post-disciplinary practices (*Mark Smith*) ... 235
14 Norms, normativity and normalisation: Between the vital and the social
   (*Ulrike Kistner*) .................................................. 252

Index ................................................................. 264

# Notes on contributors

**Erica Burman** is Professor of Psychology and Women's Studies at the Manchester Metropolitan University. Her work spans feminist and critical engagements with therapeutic and research practices, and discussions of political subjectivities. She is author of *Deconstructing Developmental Psychology* (1994), and co-author of *Challenging Women: Psychology's Exclusions, Feminist Possibilities* (1995) and *Psychology Discourse Practice: From Regulation to Resistance* (1996).

**Thea de Wet** is Associate Professor of Anthropology in the Department of Development Studies at Rand Afrikaans University, Johannesburg. Her research interests include the health, development and social identity of children growing up in Soweto-Johannesburg.

**Gillian Eagle** is an Associate Professor in the Department of Psychology at the University of the Witwatersrand. She is a registered clinical psychologist and has completed a doctorate in the field of traumatic-stress studies and gender. She is interested in the interface between clinical psychology and critical social psychology and has consulted and published in the fields of gender policy, sexual violence, traumatic stress and integrative psychotherapy.

**George Ellison** is Assistant Director of the Social Science Research Unit at the Institute of Education, University of London. His research interests include the social construction of human diversity, social inequalities in health and the heritability of (dis)advantage.

**Vijé Franchi** is currently senior lecturer and researcher at the University of Lyon 2, and member of the Laboratoire d'IPSE, Université Paris X – Nanterre. Her research, community and clinical interventions have addressed issues related to the politics of intercultural identity among minority nationals, the mediation of 'racialised' conflict in organisations undergoing structural transformation, racism and self-articulated self-representation, and the primary prevention of risk behaviours among sociopolitically disadvantaged youth.

**S. Fuller** teaches in the Anthropology and Sociology Department at the University of British Columbia in Vancouver, Canada, and is the Chair of the Cultural and Media Studies Interdisciplinary Group at Green College, University of British Columbia.

**Bronwyn Harris** is a researcher at the Centre for the Study of Violence and Reconciliation. She is currently working on a large-scale research project on violence and transition in South Africa. She has an MA in psychology and is interested in the role of the media and social institutions in the perpetuation of inequality.

**Derek Hook** is a lecturer in the Department of Psychology at the University of the Witwatersrand, Johannesburg, South Africa. He is the co-editor of *Body Politics: Power, Knowledge and the Body in the Social Sciences* and of the multimedia CD-ROM package: *From Method to Madness: Five Years of Qualitative Enquiry*, which consists of academic papers, video and music clips, art images, interviews and student research material.

**Ulrike Kistner** is a research fellow at the Graduate School for the Humanities and Social Sciences at the University of the Witwatersrand. Her research and teaching interests include psychoanalysis and culture, the social and political conditions of the information age, the changing nature of the social tie and aspects of the history of medicine.

**Teboho Lebakeng** is a lecturer in sociology at the University of the North. He has written on various sociological topics including student politics and transformation of tertiary institutions. His current research interests are on the prospects and problems of Africanism for the social sciences and the humanities.

**Carol Long** is a clinical psychologist who lectures in the Department of Psychology at the University of the Witwatersrand. She has published on, and is interested in, post-modern theory.

**M. Brinton Lykes** is Professor and Chair of Psychology at the University of the Witwatersrand in Johannesburg, South Africa. She is an activist scholar and teacher. Her research explores the interstices of indigenous cultural beliefs and practices and those of Western psychology, with the aim of creating community-based responses to the effects of war and state-sponsored violence. She is the co-editor of *Myths about the Powerless: Contesting Social Inequalities* (1996), *Gender and Personality* (1985) and *Your Daughters Shall Prophesy: Feminist Alternatives in Theological Education* (1980), and co-author, with the Association of Maya Ixil Women – New Dawn, of *Voces e Imágenes: Mujeres Mayas Ixiles de Chajul/Voices and Images: Maya Ixil Women of Chajul* (2000).

**Kopano Ratele** lectures in the Department of Psychology at the University of the Western Cape. His areas of teaching are masculinity, social psychology, epistemology and research methods.

**Susan Sedumedi** is a lecturer in psychology at the University of the North. She teaches research methodology and social statistics to both undergraduate and graduate students. Her research interests include research for development and social change focusing on women, rural areas and AIDS, as well as student politics in institutions of higher learning.

**Tamara Shefer** is Director of Women and Gender Studies at the University of the Western Cape. Her major teaching areas are in epistemology, research methodology and discursive feminist psychology.

**Mark Smith** is a senior lecturer and Professor of Social Sciences in the Open University in the United Kingdom. His abiding interests are the philosophy of science, ecological issues and political theory. His recent books include *Social Science in Question: Towards a Postdisciplinary Framework* (1998), *Ecologism: Towards Ecological Citizenship* (1998), *Thinking through the Environment* (1999) and *Rethinking State Theory* (1999).

**Martin Terre Blanche** is a senior lecturer in the Department of Psychology at the University of South Africa, where he teaches research and community psychology. He has published on discourses of mental illness and is a founder member of the Research Group for the Study of Psychiatry in South Africa.

**Anthony Theuninck** completed his Masters of Arts at the University of the Witwatersrand, Johannesburg, South Africa. His chapter in this volume is based on his thesis: 'The traumatic impact of minority stressors on males self-identified as homosexual or bisexual'. He currently works as a researcher in the United Kingdom.

**Estelle Zietkiewicz** is a practising psychologist and a lecturer in the Department of Psychology at the University of the Witwatersrand. She is interested in the articulation of discursive epistemology and praxis, and is currently focusing on the political and performative potentials of discursive theory.

# Acknowledgements

There are a number of people whose work and involvement in this project ensured that it reached completion. Among these are Anthony Collins, whose reviews and structural advice proved particularly useful in the early stages of the preparation of this manuscript, Erica Burman, Ian Parker, Mark Smith, George Ellison and Brinton Lykes, whose participation lent the project an international flair, and Kenneth Wilson, whose early involvement proved vital.

# Introduction:
# A 'social psychology' of psychopathology

*Derek Hook*

Basically, this is a book about the social formation of psychopathology across different cultural, discursive and political contexts, many of which are particular to South Africa. Given the focus on the *social embodiment* of psychopathology, along with the particularly South African emphasis, the book is also, quite unavoidably, a text about *psychopathology's relationship to social prejudice*. Because of this, its focus falls directly in the area of overlap between two traditional (and typically separate) domains of psychology, i.e. social psychology and psychopathology. This focus defines the originality of the book's approach. It also means that the book lends itself strongly – as either a prescribed or recommended text – to tertiary courses in either subdomain of psychology. In fact, if one were to define a single overarching objective of this book, one might say it is an attempt to begin writing a rudimentary 'social psychology' of psychopathology, with particular application to South Africa. Clearly, this is a complex and multifaceted undertaking. It is also one that can be broken down into a series of smaller, interlocking agendas.

The first and perhaps most straightforward of these agendas is to facilitate the influx of new forms of theory and criticism into the discipline of psychology, both as it is practised within South Africa, and further afield. Consequently, one of the hallmarks of the book's approach is that it brings a far broader range of sociological, philosophical and multidisciplinary theory to the understanding of psychopathology than is often the case, particularly within psychology. This range of theory brings with it a range of opportunities that will enable both students and practitioners to critically re-evaluate and 'rethink' their notions of psychopathology. Although this multidisciplinary approach is spread throughout the book, its fourth section, **Philosophies of pathology**, is particularly focused on this objective of engaging with new critical theory.

The second of the book's basic agendas is to develop an awareness of how the socio-political and historical context of present-day South Africa produces its own unique varieties of 'pathology'. The vital idea here is that predominant forms of psychopathology in South Africa may vary from dominant forms in other parts of the world, not only in their prevalence, but also *in the very nature of their constitution*. South Africa may, in short, be able to produce its own unique forms of psychopathology, forms that – by virtue of the extent to which they are anchored in such a contingency of overlapping power relations – may be usefully put to work in demonstrating the overarching *political functioning* of pathology. The book's third section, **South African pathologies**, contains the chapters most relevant to this objective.

A third agenda lies with the connecting of discourses and conceptualisations of psychopathology to other forms of social prejudice, i.e. to other political mechanisms for producing 'the other'. The tactic here has been to encourage conventionalised forms of psychopathology to reassume their links to other 'social logics' of discrimination. The focus of the book here is therefore (as I have suggested above) not so much psychopathology *per se*, but rather *the social, cultural and discursive forces that so consistently construct difference* around those identity categories of race, sexuality, gender, ethnicity, nationalism and so on. The challenge here lies in thinking of variously realised forms of prejudice and certain conventionalised forms of psychopathology as, essentially, restatements of the same basic question, *that of the maintenance of diverse forms of social discrimination around a central political norm*, be that of whiteness, masculinity, heterosexuality, normality or sanity. It is for this reason that the book engages with those forms of 'deviance' and 'otherness' not necessarily considered typically psychopathological. **Pathology as politics**, the book's second section, includes a number of chapters that consider wider areas of 'deviance' and 'abnormality' than merely those contained in the notion of pathology.

As a fourth objective, the book hopes to provide the reader with a broad cross-section of critical vantage points able to unseat the notion of psychopathology as a decontextualised, individualistic, essentialist and organic category of 'sickness'. In fact, in this sense, the chapters of this book are more than a series of perspectives; they also comprise an extended argument about the necessarily *socio-political* and *constructed* nature of psychopathology.

What does it mean to say that psychopathology is socially constructed? Basically, it means that psychopathology does not just exist objectively 'out there', independently in the world, waiting to be discovered. It is not a discrete and innate entity inside the heads of isolated persons; rather, it operates as a discourse. In other words, psychopathology cannot be separated from the ways we speak of it, understand it and act upon it. In fact, these are the kinds of procedures, the ways of knowing, the ways of speaking that 'underwrite' what we refer to as psychopathology. They are the kinds of activities that, in many ways, constitute psychopathology's most fundamental reality. Without these social modes of speaking, action and knowledge, psychopathology – in the very specific and well-defined ways that we know it – would cease to exist. Such a constructionist approach does not mean that there may never be a biological underpinning or a set of physical correlates corresponding to a psychopathological state. It does, however, imply that as soon as we speak of psychopathology in a socially meaningful way and as soon as we are able to understand it in a way that produces knowledge, its discursive existence in a sense supersedes its physical existence. In other words, we will not reasonably be able to speak of, understand or attempt to cure the psychopathology in question outside of these 'rules of production'. So what we mean when we say that something is 'constructed' is that there is a series of rules governing how it may and may not be understood, thought, studied, practised and so forth. It is in this sense that a large part of the critical work this book wishes to undertake – as part of the objective of destabilising the notion of psychopathology as an essentialist, transhistorical category – will revolve around highlighting the constructedness of psychopathology and emphasising its contingence on a variety of social, historical, political and technological factors. This process of illuminating the constructed nature of the concept we know as 'psychology' is perhaps the single most strongly unifying feature of all the chapters in this book, supplying its basic underlying thematic cohesion.

Fifthly – and finally – the book hopes to do more than merely theorise, critique and deconstruct from afar. Rather, it hopes to critically inform in some meaningful way the difficult and thoroughly political process of *psychological intervention*. Given certain of the aims discussed above, this will no doubt prove a difficult task. Indeed, it would seem a large-enough undertaking to warrant a separate book altogether. Furthermore, if psychology, like psychopathology itself, is as much practice as knowledge, then the critical agendas of this book would be only half served by 'rethinking' psychopathology, without shedding some light on how clinical and counselling practices might be improved. It is therefore worthwhile briefly to flesh out these agendas.

## ■ Importing theory

The first section of the book, **Clinical problematics**, will discuss the issues involved in the attempt to implement a critical form of psychological practice. The drive to import new forms of theory and criticism into psychology was one of the prime motivations behind putting this text together. Why? Because it is becoming increasingly important for psychology to reflect upon its own insularity. As many critical psychologists would suggest, psychology has for too long been able to 'psychologise' away the political contexts of its practices and theories. Simply put, the more insular psychology is allowed to remain, the less easily it will be able to obscure the sociopolitical and discursive bases upon which much psychological work is founded, and which most psychological work inevitably reproduces.

Recourse to a multidisciplinary range of perspectives on a single subject, like that of psychopathology, typically enables us to fragment that subject and so open it up to a far greater degree of critical penetration. This is the reason behind both the book's unconventional focus on 'a social psychology of psychopathology' and its unusually diverse array of contributions. Such a cross-disciplinary approach makes for a very promising way of taking apart the very 'centralising nucleus' of a discipline from which its most basic assumptions, motivations and rationales emerge. What I have in mind here is the normally unquestioned *foundation* of a discipline: the one object of knowledge and practice that can never reasonably be brought into question from within the discipline itself. The implications of this would seem quite clear. Psychopathology itself may well be exactly this unquestioned foundation of the disciplinary structure of psychology, the keystone that is able to threaten the basic integrity and cohesion of the entire discipline if it were itself to be compromised.

What does this mean? Two things, broadly. Firstly, it means that the most effective way of establishing a critical perspective on what is arguably psychology's *prime object* is from *outside* of psychology itself (and preferably, if one were to extend the argument further, from a diverse range of perspectives that harbour no mutual loyalties). Secondly, if it is the case that psychopathology is the epistemic heart and basis of psychology, then this critical exercise will have ramifications far beyond the interrogation of psychopathology itself. It will constitute an integral part of a far wider critique of psychology as a whole, across the breadth of its various applied wings and subdisciplines.

The diversity of this book's range of engagements with psychopathology, like its use of a variety of disciplinary perspectives, is therefore intentional and is, in fact, a central component of its critical objectives. The tactic here has been to amass a heterogeneous variety of critiques and to 'cross-reference' the criticism of pathology across a wide range of critical theories and methods. In this sense, one might say that the objective of the book is to synchronise 'a broad sweep of critical voices', and its strategy to *overdetermine* the largely *underdetermined* notion of psychopathology. So while psychopathology is generally understood as being concerned with the manifest deviance from professional, statistical or socio-politically rooted sets of norms, it is here made to reassume relations to an array of different critical discourses and contexts, as will become apparent when we discuss the contents of the various chapters in more detail. Noteworthy here also is the fact that while the book focuses predominantly on *psycho*pathology, it will at times defer to the more generic term 'pathology'. This becomes particularly evident in the book's last section, **Philosophies of pathology**, which adopts a more abstract perspective on wider questions in the broader domain of the pathological in general. This movement between terms ('psychopathology' and 'pathology') is helpful in another way, for it opens up the discussions of this book to a wider audience, and helps in some way to despecialise psychopathology as the exclusive preserve of mental-health professionals.

## Discrete contexts, discrete pathologies

A further concern lies with developing an awareness of the specificity of *the South African context*, and how that context comes to pose a potentially *determining influence* upon what counts as 'pathological' within its parameters. Quite clearly, it would seem, there are unique historical, cultural, political and social factors at play within the South African environment that are perhaps less present, if present at all, elsewhere. So, although South African psychologists undoubtedly inherit a diagnostic structure from Anglo-American institutions and apply this structure to and in a local context, this does not invariably mean that certain distinctive and uniquely South African socio-political or cultural variables will not exceed the categories within this structure.

The 'soft' version of this attention to local conditions suggests that we need to be aware of the particular prevalence of certain disorders in South Africa. It would also suggest that we need to be particularly aware of the 'fit' of supposedly global diagnostic categories in South African situations. While attention to the efficacy (or danger) of such global diagnostic implementations within specific local contexts will be an important focus of this project – because 'teasing out' these issues will go a long way to suggesting how one might ultimately reformulate a *critical* clinical practice – it will certainly not exhaust the critical agendas of this book.

The 'harder' version of this attention to local conditions will extend the critical range of the book by suggesting not merely that different social circumstances yield very different forms of pathology, but that South African psychopathologies may vary, in vital and in fact *constitutive* ways, from those generic and seemingly predominantly Anglo-American and Eurocentric psychopathologies sketched in nosological compendiums such as the *Diagnostic and Statistical Manual of Mental Disorders* in its various editions. In this way, it becomes meaningful to speak of properly 'South

African pathologies', where distinctive socio-political, historical and cultural circumstances conspire to make it possible to 'bring into being' certain new pathologies that could not have ever emerged elsewhere. One should not see this as an impetus to relentlessly 'psychologise' an ever-growing realm of social problems. Instead, one should view it as a way of demonstrating the *social, cultural and historical contingency* of psychopathology.

Indeed, against universalising models that suggest that distinct pathologies could easily be cross-referenced across a series of different historical periods, this book will argue that pathology cannot reasonably be extracted from its socio-political and historical setting. Why? Because to do so would be to *dissipate the function of psychopathology*. Cutting psychopathology off from its political correlates, from the way it implicates, *and is implicated by*, the workings of certain structures of power, makes pathology properly *psycho*pathological – i.e. fixed within the exclusive 'interventional domains' of psychological and psychiatric experts (hence, one might argue, the motivation behind psychology's seemingly perpetual tendency towards making decontextualised, ahistorical and depoliticised generalisations about psychopathology). Extracted from the political field, psychopathology will lose both its shape (i.e. its highly specific and socially determined meaning that defines how it is understood and 'known' within a particular society at a particular time) *and* its function (i.e. its political utility, which refers to the sense of what it *does*, of why it is *useful* and of what it enables and/or disables within a social system). To ignore these questions is, for the assembled arguments of this book, to misunderstand precisely what is most fundamental about the workings of psychopathology. Furthermore, as we will see later, the removal of pathology from the political field also ignores the *responsibility* of certain socio-political structures *for* the emergence of particular pathologies. Furthermore, avoiding such issues leads to a limiting of treatment possibilities.

What we are calling for here is a greater awareness of socio-political factors *within* the realm of the psychopathological (i.e. of how the interests of power are served by the division of the pathological from the non-pathological) and of psychopathological factors within the realm of the political (i.e. of how the greater logic of this division may be usefully applied across different contexts by political forces). Simply put, the books aims at a calling into question of the psychopathological on the basis of the political; and of the political on the basis of (the social logic of) the pathological.

## A politics of normality

A strategic response to these imperatives to re-relate the political and the pathological – a response, that is to say, to the *'depoliticisation' of psychopathology* – is to suggest that conventionalised forms of psychopathology should be made to reassume their links to those multiple other forms of deviance and 'otherness' so traditionally prevalent within South African society. It is at this point where a focus on psychopathology *per se* needs to 'pull back' to accommodate a broader-based attention to the wider social realm of the '*ab*normal'. There is a vital qualification that needs to be made here. When we start dealing with the politics of psychopathology, which, seemingly, is one part of the larger domain of the 'abnormal', we must implicitly, if not directly, deal with the *politics of the normal*. Why? Because as the terms themselves suggest, *the* *abnormal is defined through the normal*; i.e. the psychopathological only becomes *conceivable, practicable and knowable* alongside the specification of the norm. Of course 'norms', i.e. that which comes to count as the average, the typical, the appropriate and the functional, are not themselves as 'normal' as we might consider them to be, not at least in the sense of universal, transhistorical or 'natural' sets of behavioural standards.

Norms are generated through elaborate processes and, for Foucault (1979) at least, are the outcome of the consistent cross-population comparison of individuals according to the basic minimum threshold value that should be attained in a certain field of endeavour, behaviour or performance. In Foucault's terms, the norms of modern society *differentiate, hierarchise, homogenise* and *exclude* groups and categories of people from a larger social mass. What is perhaps most important here, though, in terms of our present concerns, is that these actions of 'normalisation' continually define the 'external frontier of the abnormal' (Foucault, 1979: 183).

It is important to reiterate here that the norms that come to predominate within modern societies are not merely pre-existing social forms, customs or conventions that come to possess a certain social currency, and that reigning structures of power incidentally come to adopt and endorse. Rather, they *are*, from the very outset, the instruments of power; i.e. they are exactly the means through which social patterns of power become entrenched and habituated. The implementation of norms is a vital way through which individuals may be governed, influenced and even, in relative terms, controlled, beyond the reach of formalised and institutionalised rules, laws and prohibitions. From the perspective of power, the value of the norm is that it operates a 'micropenality' in which infractions too trivial to be granted legal status now became captured by power, and the slightest deviations from the norm become punishable. Furthermore, more extensive in effect than a simple binary opposition of permitted and forbidden, the norm brings into existence a far wider continuum of judgement. It is no longer good enough to be judged right or wrong, good or evil: the individual is now locked into a perpetual relationship with the standards set by the norm. In effect, then, it is through the establishment of a rigorous set of social norms that any nonconformist, any dissident or any other threat to a particular regime of normality becomes the object of curative or rehabilitative attentions.

Similarly, norms can be enforced successfully at the level of subjectivity, even though they have not been officially legislated or 'written into law', and can be applied in dispersed social groupings and environments where even fragmented populations can recognise and act to inhibit 'abnormal' practices, behaviours and suggestions. In this sense, then, one would agree with Foucault (1979) that such norms have effectively replaced the law.

What is particularly important here is that this political mechanism of producing 'the other' is able to operate as *an effect of identity*. It is exactly this quality that allows such political practices to be so internalised, direct, immediate and personalised. They become the discriminatory markers of identity such as whiteness (or blackness), masculinity (or femininity), heterosexuality (or homosexuality), European (or African), rationality (or madness), *normality (or abnormality)*. They work on the basis of an identity defined in terms of *like* (be this cultural, ethnic or national 'likeness') versus *other*. Each of these axes is marked by two loadings: one works on the basis of normalisation, idealisation and *naturalisation*; the other of problematisation, denigration and *pathologisation*. In this way, a politics of normality and a politics of abnormality are mutually reliant, working together on the basis of a powerful double coding, normalising so as to problematise and problematising so as to normalise.

This is not to say that such a politics of the normal works in a static, categorical or merely dichotomous way. There are always degrees of normality/abnormality: one can always be ostensibly closer to an idealised norm, just as one can always be somewhat more pathological. Speaking of a politics of the normal in this way makes it easier to understand the essentialising tendencies present in the above kinds of identity categorisation. The normalisation/pathologisation of various identity categories is always going to function more forcefully and is always going to have far more entrenched effects once sunk into essential 'nodes' of being. If essentialised in this way, such problematised qualities are going to be inescapable, universal across the species and everlasting. In this connection, it should be very clear why this book engages with a variety of forms of apparent social 'deviance' not considered typically psychopathological. Whether they occur on the level of psychological norms or on any adjoining level of an apparently essentialist component of identity, these various problematisations of the individual on the basis of the norm are not strictly divisible.

Moreover, and this is perhaps the most important aspect of the argument I am building here, an essential component of normalisation (i.e. the powerful mobilisation of the norm) is *the systematic creation, classification and control of anomalies in the social body* (Foucault, 1979). Here it is worth quoting Dreyfus and Rabinow at length:

> The spread of normalization operates through the creation of abnormalities [and deviancies] which it then must treat and reform. By identifying the anomalies ... the technologies [of normalisation] ... are in a perfect position to supervise and administer them. This effectively transforms into a technical problem – and thence into a field for expanding power – what might otherwise be construed as a failure of the whole system of operation. Political technologies advance by taking what is essentially a political problem, removing it from the realm of political discourse, and recasting it in the neutral language of science [or pathology] (1982: 196).

## The pathological and the political

What are the implications of this line of discussion? Firstly, if one agrees with Foucault's line of reasoning, one accepts the idea that the pathological – like the *ab*normal – is always at least partly political in nature. Grounded in social norms that have been brought into existence precisely by a given socio-political order, this much would seem inevitable. (The pathological would not have been thinkable *as pathological*, if we are to follow Foucault, without its political transformation from a problem of social control to that of discrete, individualised sickness and deviance.) Secondly, it means that the shape of the pathological, like that of normality itself, can change, because pathology is always mapped onto the political dynamics of a particular time and place. Quite clearly, and in very basic terms, what counts as pathological in one culture does not necessarily count as pathological in another, just as what constitutes a fundamental (and punishable) social deviance in one culture does not necessarily do so in another.

This is not to say that everything considered abnormal has necessary or immediate bearing on the pathological. And the two should not be conflated. Whereas reference to 'the pathological', and more specifically yet, 'the psychopathological', seems to imply the presence of a medico-clinical level of discourse (along with its institutional backing), 'the abnormal' – being that which represents a significant deviance from any basic social norm – would seem to suggest a far more inclusive realm of social phenomena. But what this suggests is that the pathological and the abnormal work on the basis of the same fundamental mechanism and the same fundamental logic, namely the relentless problematisation of the deviant, of that which threatens the norms of a given social order *to the ends of the ultimate strengthening and perpetuation of that order*.

Now, as I have made clear above, what is considered 'abnormal' is not always pathological, even though the pathological does seemingly always represent a particularly intensive (and discursively sophisticated) problematisation of the abnormal. Despite this distinction, this formal similarity across cases of abnormality and pathology, i.e. their joint priority of *problematising deviance*, provides considerable leverage for any argument that would assert *the social formation and embodiment of pathology*. Indeed, for the purposes of this argument, it is useful to emphasise the exchange between precisely these categories of the abnormal and the pathological. For a start, it might be argued that placing the *psycho*pathological in the broader terms of 'the abnormal' works, albeit in a limited way, to 'de-psychologise' the former, by removing it from the exclusive domain of clinical discourse and by making the implicit suggestion that the problem may be at root a socio-political one, rather than a necessarily intrapsychic or individualistic one.

A number of chapters in this book adopt this approach. Theuninck, Hook and Franchi's recouching of homosexuality *as a problem of a heterosexist discursive regime* rather than of an apparently 'deviant' individual sexuality is one case in point. Ratele and Shefer's de-essentialisation of patriarchal categories of female sexuality as misogynistic social constructions rather than innately problematic constituents of what it means to be a woman performs the same function. Ellison and De Wet's discussion of how racial categories may be either used in a straightforwardly racist fashion to denigrate and problematise individuals on one hand, or to call attention to the multiple ongoing forms of social inequity ignored by idealistic visions of a colour-blind society on the other, provides another example.

Similarly, using the wider terms of the abnormal and the deviant *within* the idiom of the psychopathological, i.e. *considering the psychopathological as that which fundamentally threatens the social order*, works to demonstrate what is at stake in the conversion of deviance to psychopathology. As touched upon by Eagle's, Harris' and Lykes' chapters, when social deviance is couched in the terms of pathology or, better still, *psychopathology*, then very real political questions of greater culpability and accountability are found to recede into the background. In different ways, both Eagle and Lykes illustrate how clinical conceptualisations of post-traumatic stress disorder can be applied so as to minimise the role of the socio-political context. In similar vein,

Harris' chapter foregrounds how the pseudo-clinical (and individually centred) notion of xeno*phobia* usefully deflects attention away from how the New South Africa has, much like the old, fostered a nationalism of insularity and prejudice. Indeed, the individualised locus of control implied by such a pseudo-clinical term works to suggest that xenophobia is a psychological problem of isolated individuals rather than the social prejudice of an entire nation.

To cautiously – and strategically – threaten the collapse of this distinction between the firmly psychopathological and the social or political basis of deviance certainly seems profitable, given our present objectives. In both fundamental and tentative ways, crossing these terms of reference – those of the psychopathological and the abnormal or deviant – enables us to set up a series of similarities that may not otherwise have been suspected. Maybe certain prescriptions of psychopathology are in fact at root nothing other than racism, heterosexism or misogyny, as various of the following chapters intimate. On the other hand, maybe certain forms of politics are quite ineffective, if not in fact even untenable, without the relentless pathologising, problematisation and 'othering' of those who seem to threaten the integrity of a given social order.

To make things slightly more concrete, one might make reference to recent South African political history. Apartheid, it seems, could not have functioned, or could not have functioned as effectively as it did, without the utilisation by those who applied it of a politics of normality conducted and perpetuated at the level of identity. A wide variety of different forms of deviance came into prominence under the apartheid regime. Certainly, as a regime built on the cornerstones of discrimination and prejudice, apartheid was particularly adept at 'pathologising' those deviancies from the racial, ethnic, gender and sexual-orientation norms it promoted and idealised. These axes of identity were thoroughly and deeply infused with power, so much so that apartheid's social logic was to prove resilient beyond the demise of explicitly institutionalised forms of racism. (Apartheid in this sense was not simply about infusing white-black interactions with a dramatic asymmetry of power – although this was no doubt its overwhelming focus – it was also about infusing a wide variety of person-to-person interactions with categorical power differentials.) Categorical means of differentiation and distinction, then, through the definition of the desirable norm and the undesirable deviant, appear to have formed an essential aspect of apartheid power, with politics overlaying and managing 'pathology', just as the pathological (or deviant) came to be a key term in the smooth functioning of apartheid power.

If we are able to take some of the logic at work within these social mechanisms of othering, discrimination and political control and apply them to the workings and functionality of psychopathology, then we will be well on our way to our critical goal of destabilising notions of psychopathology as exclusively individualistic, essentialist or organic forms of 'sickness'. Extracted from the exclusively clinical domain, the psychopathological will not be able to deny its links (and service) to the wider field of the political. In this way, we will also be well placed to understand just why essentialist notions come to gain so much currency, and come to be so substantially reaffirmed and reified in regimes that depend on a 'politics of normality'.

The converse is also true, however. If we are able to take some of this logic – i.e. the 'politics of normality' – at work within psychological conceptualisations and understandings of psychopathology and apply it to the macrolevel of straightforward (state) politics, we may well become sensitised to how such kinds of psychology come to be exploited by the interests of power. Hence, we may begin to speak of the 'political power of psychopathology', whereby a politics of normality, as practised upon the level of identity, becomes a crucial element in certain political regimes. The crucial link here is how certain kinds of psychology – i.e. how certain identity practices and proactive procedures of self-identification, 'de-identification', 'otherisation' and so on – become the political tools of large-scale political systems. (Two critical reading focuses will be important here. One will be a focus on the practices of otherisation, i.e. those processes whereby qualitative differences across subject positions are generated and emphasised so that the formation of even tentative identificatory bonds is barred, disabled or even totally prevented. The other will be a focus on processes of identification, in which those practices of likeness that emphasise similarity or sameness across subject positions come to constitute a basis for political discrimination and evaluation.)

Indeed, for a country like South Africa, whose history is so powerfully characterised by regimes of categorisation, discrimination and prejudice, it should come as no surprise that the production of 'otherness' and various assorted 'abnorms' became a virtually automatic and inherent practice of identity. So too the imperative to manufacture difference, and in slightly more formal and institutional contexts, varieties of pathology also. Indeed, race, gender, ethnicity and sexual orientation were all powerful anchoring-points both for the establishment of difference and, by the same token, for the perpetuation of that difference. What one might suggest here is a rephrasing of one of the outcomes this book aims at, namely that of unseating the notion of psychopathology as a decontextualised, individualistic, essentialist category *but on the level of those broader identity markers so instrumental to a more widespread, macro-politics of normality*. We might therefore propose an adjunct outcome, i.e. to unseat those traditional identity markers that have served for so long as vital pillars of power, those of nation, ethnicity, race, culture, gender, sexual orientation and so forth, and to do so by denying, where possible, their existence as decontextualised or essentialist capacities.

In this respect, as has been mentioned above, it is clear that this book engages with a range of forms of 'deviance' and 'otherness' not necessarily considered typically psychopathological. The reason why this is so should by now be abundantly clear: these are not separate spheres of purely political activity. For essentially this is what this book is about, not psychopathology *per se*, but those divisive applications of the notions of the normal and abnormal that, whether carried out on the levels of either medico-clinical or popular social discourse, aim to problematise particular categories of people as a way of entrenching social inequality.

Perhaps the single strongest unifying feature shared by all the chapters in this book is their authors' commitment to refuting essentialist notions of psychopathology and to showing up the constructed and contingent nature (contingent on history, place, culture, politics and material practices) of what we call 'the psychopathological'. This, and the book's last agenda, that of shedding some light on how the clinical and counselling applications of psychotherapy might be critiqued and, we hope, improved, are best dealt with together, by providing a brief 'walk through' of the contents of the book. Given the diversity, both in approach and content, of these chapters, such a walk through will prove an important way of binding together the disparate components of this overall project.

## An overview of the book

### Section 1: Clinical problematics

The book's first section includes a series of chapters that engage with what might be referred to as 'clinical technologies', i.e. those psychological treatment modalities (chiefly psychotherapy, psychiatry and their particular systems of diagnosis) at the interface of client/patient/community and the mental-health professional. The way these treatment schedules work and the way they conceive of psychopathology can pose a number of problems, such as treatment efficacy, ethics, politics and potential damage.

Adopting a close, critical and technicist approach to the therapeutic interchange, Hook's chapter, 'Psychotherapy, discourse and the production of psychopathology', builds an inductive argument as to how psychotherapy might be said to *discursively* produce psychopathology. By 'discourse' he refers to those systems of statements that are able to 'create' objects and to those regularising patterns of meaning that entail both textual and material elements that have real effects on the world on the levels of knowledge, subjectivity and action. His chapter poses a series of important questions to therapists about the interpellative, constructionist and authorial implications of the 'psychotherapeutic technology' they wield within the clinical arena. Ultimately, his warning is that therapists should rigorously problematise every facet of their therapeutic procedure that is even remotely able to position patients as psychopathological, because not to do so is to risk practising a form of therapy able to *discursively* generate psychopathology. Such a psychotherapy, as Hook suggests, would seem to be less than ethically viable.

If for Hook psychopathology is largely the constructed outcome of the activation of a concerted and directed technology of intervention, for Terre Blanche it is also constructed, but this time as the correlate of a bumbling and conflicted set of esoteric forms of rhetoric and practice. Terre Blanche's chapter, 'Poised on the brink: The social construction of a new biological psychiatry', provides an alternative history of psychiatry, one founded less on scientific refutation, studious experimentation, verificationism, empiricism and ethical accountability, and more on serendipity, dogma, insularity, infighting and error. (It is the latter that Terre Blanche seems to think plays the more formative role in what we come to think of as psychopathology.) Not only does this chapter have the effect of thoroughly de-essentialising and problematising psychopathology through its institutional bases, it also has the effect of questioning the factual nature, reliability and assumed ethics of psychiatry's supposed scientific status, which of course is precisely that element that most strongly grounds the ostensible legitimacy of any talk of pathology.

Extending the discussion of 'clinical problematics', although arguably at a more pragmatic level, Eagle's 'The political conundrums of post-traumatic stress disorder' challenges the political implications of the clinical diagnosis of post-traumatic stress disorder (PTSD). Taking apart, bit by bit, the ethical complications of this form of diagnosis, Eagle opens up wider debates in psychopathology more generally. For example, with PTSD it seems there can be little doubt that a disordered or violent social circumstance is the source of the 'psychopathology', a fact that leads to a relative absolving of the individual of 'causative responsibility' for his/her own condition. This is an important inversion of the individual with the social – both as a locus of causality and of accountability – and one that helpfully links PTSD to other forms of pathology with overtly political (and environmental) sources. Having demonstrated how exploitative the diagnosis of PTSD can be, Eagle closes by speaking of how certain 'scientific' and knowledge-producing initiatives need necessarily to be moderated by questions of ethical accountability. Her intimation is that the treatment imperative of humanism and the knowledge-producing drive of positivism should both be made secondary to an attempt to inject a powerful ethical and political conscience into the clinical project.

Critically engaging PTSD in the same way, but focusing more on effective strategies of research and intervention, Lykes' chapter, 'A critical re-reading of post-traumatic stress disorder from a cross-cultural/community perspective', hopes to break the epistemological 'set' of current normative uses of PTSD. Focusing on trauma as a cultural, historical and social phenomenon that cannot be isolated in a singular, individual psyche, Lykes emphasises its debilitating effects on what she refers to as 'social subjectivity'. A liberation psychologist, participatory action researcher and activist, Lykes is involved less in explicit forms of psychological intervention than in collaborative community involvements that centre around forms of meaning-making and memorial. The 'PhotoVoice' method her chapter describes is just such a collaboration, drawing on multiple discourses, from those of human-rights work, developmental theory and psychology, to the practices and indigenous knowledge systems of Mayan communities in which she is working. Lykes makes several contributions towards reconceptualising trauma and recovery. Firstly, in contrast to the traditional Western focus on individual identity, she claims that the therapist should emphasise that 'selfhood' is voiced and enacted through story and relationship as inherently social. Secondly, she appeals to psychologists to see beyond discourses of victimology in working with trauma. Lastly, and perhaps most importantly, she asserts that trauma, much like any supposed psychopathology, 'must be read within its social, cultural and political contexts over time, not as a ... static entity located and to be addressed within affected individuals'.

## Section 2: Pathology as politics

The second section of the book, which deals with psychopathology as a form and a domain of politics, begins with a chapter of interest to feminist criticism. Fuller and Hook's 'Rewriting the body, reauthoring the expert: Reading the anorexic body' presents the idea that psychopathology, or more specifically, anorexia nervosa, is in fact a form of resistance, rather than simply a capitulation to political forces of constraint and control. Their argument, under the influence of the work of the post-colonial theorists Spivak and Bhabha, is that the anorexic subject, like the colonised subject more generally, is able, through various forms of mimicry, to mock the power and authority of the coloniser. Whilst irrevocably still a product of the colonial, this mimicry possesses a uniquely subversive capacity particularly well suited to threatening those normalised knowledges and disciplinary powers that enforce the reiteration of norms in modern society. Not only do Fuller and Hook pose a new way of thinking about resistance, and perhaps more importantly, *agency*, in relationship to the discourses and norms of psychopathology, they also consider an adjunct form of practice to complement their theory, that of narrative therapy. They argue for this recourse to narrative therapy on the basis of Foucault's (1980) notion of the political and critical utility of discontinuous, subjugated and local knowledges. They also propose Epston and White's (1989) rethinking of therapy as a treatment schedule far less loaded with depoliticising and disempowering forms of discourse than many more rigid and overtly clinical models.

Dealing with the pragmatics of both applied-knowledge production and clinical activity, Theuninck, Hook and Franchi, in their chapter, 'Avoiding the implicit repathologisation of male homosexuality: A politico-clinical direction for research', negotiate the tension between *not* implicitly repathologising homosexuality (at either epistemic or clinical levels) on one hand, *and* drawing attention to the ways in which homosexual individuals are continually victimised and, in fact, damaged in heterosexist environments, on the other. Clearly focusing their attentions on heterosexist society as the source of pathologised constructions of homosexuality, and well aware of the traumatising effects of such a constant delegitimisation and marginalisation of identity, the authors propose a tentative reappropriation of aspects of an oppressive discourse of pathology as part of an empowering political project. More succinctly, the chapter questions whether or not gayness should, in a sense, be strategically 'repathologised', not so that it may again be stigmatised, but so that the damaging effects of being gay in a heterosexist environment may be properly recognised. The implication of such a move would be that individual pathology would be recast in predominantly social terms. In this way, individual psychological intervention and treatment may well remain, but the individual would be seen as the point of *damage* rather than as the implicit *cause* of the problem.

Ellison and De Wet's '"Race", ethnicity and the psychopathology of social identity', takes social-identity theory as the target of the authors' engagement with psychopathology. Social identities, they claim, 'come in all shapes and sizes' and are all socially constructed, which in turn shows up current psychosocial fault lines, as so dramatically evidenced in contemporary political discourse on 'equity' and 'diversity'. Contemporary discourses on social identity are thoroughly inculcated with the idiom of ethnicity, however, so much so that it becomes very difficult to separate the one from the other. This occurs to the extent that ethnic categorisation is now being used in much the same way that early formulations of 'race' were: to recognise the legitimacy of nation states and national identities. One of the most pronounced risks contemporary social scientists face in conducting social research is that 'In reproducing the hierarchical and xenophobic products of racial science by authenticating social identity through ethnic categorisation, and operationalising ethnicity through racialised categories, the psychopathological *appearance* of social identity is itself authenticated and essentialised'. The historical and contemporary injustices underlying the psychopathological manifestation of social identities as 'raced' and 'unraced' suggest that two potential solutions present themselves: the 'exnomination' of all social identities that remain 'raced'; *or* the 'renomination' of those that have become 'unraced'. The first involves eliminating 'colour consciousness' by adopting 'unraced' social identities across the board in a world that is genuinely, not just officially, 'colour-blind'. The second involves eliminating the unequal (dis)advantage of official 'colour-blindness', by adopting 'raced' social identities across the board in a world that is openly, but fairly, 'colour-conscious'.

### Section 3: South African pathologies

This section deals with that seemingly indigenous strain of psychopathologies unique, or largely specific, to South Africa. The intention of the section, as I suggested earlier, is not only to customise the book as particularly useful to South African practitioners, but is also to provide insights to psychologists working in other parts of the world from very different frames of reference. Long and Zietkiewicz's chapter, 'Unsettling meanings of madness: Competing constructions of South African insanity', engages with issues of the cultural 'rootedness' of psychopathology. Indeed, their claim is that rather than being an incidental element in the formation of psychopathology, culture makes for a very basic constituent, interacting with various biological, psychological and environmental components in determining the causes, manifestations and ultimate treatments of a given psychopathology. Their real concern, driven through a speculative engagement with the prospects of a more widespread practice of traditional healing in South Africa, is that of the discursive collision of biomedical and traditional taxonomies of pathology, at the intrasubjective level of the individual. Arguing from a firmly Foucauldian position, the authors present a vivid case study that powerfully dramatises the complexities of the interface of biomedical and traditional cultural discourses of 'madness'. Their hope is not only to gain some impetus for deconstructive criticism from this opposition, but also to critically inform therapeutic practice within the South African context. Their conclusion in this regard is that it is necessary to understand the narration of self of the person concerned – as well as the intersection of this with available discourses and power dynamics – if we are to attain any critical and clinical efficacy in interacting with the discursively constructed experiences of others.

Harris' 'Xenophobia: A new pathology for a New South Africa?' again explores an unconventional, or atypical, 'pathology'. Whilst xenophobia is certainly not a psychopathology in the traditional or applied sense, Harris' discussion of the contemporary phenomenon provides a fascinating application of how a 'social logic of pathology' may be transposed onto the most mundane representations of, and interactions with, the foreigner. The details of such discriminatory practices manifest on the smallest levels of appearance (skin tone, hair styles, clothing, vaccination marks and so on) and language (accent, pronunciation of certain words, understanding of colloquial meanings and so on). Reviewing popular media representations, Harris finds that foreigners in South Africa are recurrently criminalised and tainted in these depictions, and presented as contaminants to local society, fixed in metaphors such as those of disease, plague, flood and so on. Harris is also concerned with the psychological trappings of the term 'xenophobia'. The notion of xenophobia *as pathology* is strengthened, she claims, by the phonetic association of xeno*phobia* with the properly psychological conditions of a phobia. As an aberrant and extraordinary *psychological* condition, xenophobia is presented as something separate from the normal, healthy South African nation. The pathologisation (and psychologisation) of xenophobia hence effectively quarantines the phenomenon from the new, apparently tolerant and non-discriminatory South Africa of racial diversity. Harris' chapter therefore vividly shows how the terms and understandings of pathology may be used as political instruments. It also demonstrates the colonialising reach of pathologising conceptualisations, and explains exactly why they should be resisted.

The realm of sexuality has long since been recognised as a particularly powerful domain, both of general social prejudice and of the more specific problematisation of minority or 'deviant' categories of people. Ratele and Shefer's chapter, 'Stigma in the social construction of sexually transmitted diseases', shows just how apt this claim is. As they demonstrate, the social construction of sexually transmitted diseases (STDs), like that of HIV/AIDS, makes for something of a social mirror that powerfully reflects the current norms of a society. Perusing the relevant literature, Ratele and Shefer suggest that such constructions are emblematic not only of the moral configuration, social composition and racial boundaries of a given social grouping, but also, and perhaps even more importantly, of its attitude towards social marginality. This is made apparent in how STDs, again like HIV/AIDS, are so frequently seen as the exclusive preserve of one particularly problematised sector of society (hence notions of HIV/AIDS as an exclusively *gay*, or STDs as an exclusively *black*, problem). As Ratele and Shefer astutely observe, such categorical associations have historically functioned to fuel social prejudices, particularly, in the case of HIV/AIDS, that of homophobia. This mechanism is clearly evident in their own study, where the 'mentalities' of racism, sexism and misogyny are powerfully produced in the same way. Given this state of affairs, it would seem that discursive interventions would be as important as medical interventions in minimising the damaging effects of STDs, both socially and individually.

Another unconventional yet indigenous South African pathology is that which Lebakeng, Sedumedi and Eagle refer to as 'witchcraft-related anti-social practices' in their 'Witches and watchers: Witchcraft beliefs and practices in South African rural communities of the Northern Province'. It is important to note here that the pathology in question is that of the various forms of ostracisation, injury, violence and murder associated with witch-purging, *and not the belief in witchcraft itself.* Rather than relying on traditional (and individualised) psychological levels of explanation (i.e. interpersonal, biophysical or intrapsychic accounts of behaviour), the authors refer to questions of political disillusionment, racialised capitalism and transgenerational power relations as ways of building their analysis. It is on this basis that the authors suggest that the 'discourse of witchcraft thus becomes the framework within which many poor, struggling and competitive individuals express their frustration, disappointment, anger and disillusionment'. Witchcraft-related anti-social practices hence may be seen as 'a form of displacement derived inextricably from a situation of economic deprivation and underdevelopment'. A complex and multifaceted perspective of witchcraft-related anti-sociality is therefore substantiated without recourse to essentialised notions of either the individual psyche or absolute cultural difference. (Whereas the former is obviously a factor in clinical engagements with psychopathology, the latter is a dominant tendency in cross-cultural psychology and psychiatry.) In posing such a broad account, one that considers the roles of gendered power, socio-economic history, traditional belief structures, educational resources and even geographical placement, Lebakeng, Sedumedi and Eagle offer the bud of a multidisciplinary approach that could be used in engaging a far wider range of socially embedded pathologies.

## Section 4: Philosophies of pathology

In the sweep from the specific to the abstract, the applied to the general and the practised to the formulated, the book's last section deals with a number of broadly philosophical engagements with pathology. Burman's 'Memory, madness and the market' examines a rather unexpected discursive source – or relay – of 'madness', namely that of the images of popular culture in the mass media, while a second focus, implied by the first, is that of the social practices of remembering. Both these issues are examined in terms of how they intertwine with available forms of individuality and sociality. A proliferation of advertising's representations of madness has led, the author argues, to a greater socialisation of madness – which itself has given rise to further forms of individualisation – and, paradoxically as it may seem, to more opportunities to *repathologise* the individual at the expense of the social. Burman bases her discussion on three basic Foucauldian tenets, firstly that the limit-cases of pathology produce social norms, secondly that the talk of the vilified or abnormal actively constitutes these categories of person, and lastly that seemingly 'scientific' or 'natural' disciplinary practices actually perform culturally situated moral functions. In this way, she draws memorial practices, like the notion of memorial agency itself, into Foucault's disciplinary network. Put simply, we are, she claims, subject to powerful injunctions to remember (some things) and to forget (others). Questions of subjectivity and whether the individual or the socio-political system is more responsible for pathology are also touched on. Burman notes that models of memory can be seen as repositories of representations of subjectivity, especially so if we consider that models of memory and subjectivity share a commitment to some notion of experiential continuity. This makes for an interesting political question, namely how the subjective may be shaped through the memorial, if indeed the two are mutually constitutive. Burman also questions how certain 'moral lapses', like certain acts of violence and racism, may be exonerated either through reference to madness as illness, or through types of socially sanctioned forgetting. In closing, she highlights an interesting possibility. If individual and social memory are constructed in ways that institute certain responsibilities to/of subjectivity, then surely these subjects should be capable not only of remembering and forgetting, but also of changing, in important political ways?

Smith's 'Rethinking normality through post-disciplinary practices' wastes little time in making the crucial point that 'the plausibility of disciplinary narratives was achieved through the operationalisation of the distinction between the normal and the pathological'. This central 'fault line' between what is normal and what is not is the epistemological foundation for psychology and its various related disciplines. It is also the assumed starting point for a far wider range of knowledge-producing agendas. In this connection, Smith usefully dismantles the way(s) in which pathology works (both implicitly and explicitly) *as a form of knowledge*, which is a process seemingly far too frequently neglected in histories of the social sciences. His chapter in fact offers a sophisticated yet faithful handling of the Foucauldian notion of disciplinary power, and the disciplinary pursuit of knowledge – where, as Butchart summarises, 'methods of knowing the human [subject] … relate to it not as a means of discovery against an object waiting to be known, but as a productive power towards an object that is also its effect' (1998: x).

More directly still, the chapter also makes the assertion that 'in order to establish a plausible scientific approach, the disciplinary project had to construct a "political subject" that fitted the bill', the point here being that it was necessary to precipitously generate a subject so as to anchor and validate relevant research paradigms and forms of (disciplinary) knowledge production. This is a classic case of 'putting the cart before the horse', one that raises pressing epistemological issues and simultaneously exhibits the necessity of generating pathology as a necessary (yet after-the-fact) precondition and condition of the plausibility of a 'science' like that of psychology. In fact, by dealing with questions of scientific status at the same time as those of pathology, Smith succeeds in distancing, at each step, social-science procedures and knowledges from the surety of a secure and closed sense of scientific truth. The key points here are the author's arguments that 'social-scientific practices have been tied to power relations by translating cultural values into authoritative knowledge' and that 'the kinds of knowledge produced through social science operate through the normalising and pathologising of different kinds of behaviour and identities'.

The applied subject of Smith's chapter is also important. By following Foucault and drawing all the social sciences around the nucleus of criminality, Smith is able to make large-scale contentions about these forms of knowledge production more generally. The historical distance of the case he uses is effective also in that it draws incredulous responses despite the fact that this phenomenon (the production of criminality, delinquency and pathology) is structurally similar to the taxonomy and knowledge-producing systems still active within the social sciences. Moreover, by focusing on criminality, the erstwhile shadow of psychopathology, the author takes us on an excursion beyond the usual parameters of psychology, and hence seems able to drive his point – about the control and management of deviance – all the more effectively home.

In the spirit of self-critique, the book ends with a formidable theoretical challenge to much of its central social-constructionist ethos. Kistner's 'Norms, normativity and normalisation: Between the vital and the social' exposes a basic dilemma with regard to what has been a central motif throughout the book, namely the assertion of the fundamental social formation and/or embodiment of psychopathology. Importantly, Kistner's chapter (previously subtitled 'Notes on a missed controversy between Canguilhem and Foucault') is not partisan: it traces the fault line between two opposed epistemological and ontological conceptualisations of pathology without aligning itself necessarily with either. Foucault's influential notions of normalisation, biopower (the disciplining of the body) and biopolitics (the regulation of the population), are foregrounded as important ethical contributions to the 'problem of pathology'. Similarly, Canguilhem's ideas of the basic incommensurable nature of the vital and the social, along with his contestation of the expansion of notions of 'health', 'normality' and 'pathology' to the social body, are faithfully relayed. The terms of this debate are left unresolved, although the reader is left with the theoretical 'armaments' to take up either position. The attempt to import critique of *one's own critique* fits perfectly with the agendas of this book, as does posing an unresolved theoretical debate at its conclusion. (Both in fact seem important elements of how the content of this book may be taken up pedagogically: see below.) What this chapter does make clear is the extent to which Canguilhem's vitalist handling of pathology constitutes an obstacle and future challenge for those purely social, political or constructionist philosophies of pathology of the future.

# References

American Psychiatric Association (1994). *Diagnostic and Statistical Manual of Mental Disorders* (4th edn). Washington, DC: American Psychiatric Association.

Butchart, A. (1998). *The Anatomy of Power: European Constructions of the African Body.* London and New York: Zed Books.

Dreyfus, H. L. and Rabinow, P. (1982). *Michel Foucault beyond Structuralism and Hermeneutics.* New York: Harvester Wheatsheaf.

Epston, D. and White, M. (1989). *Literate Means to Therapeutic Ends.* Adelaide: Dulwich Centre Publishing.

Fernando, S. (1988). *Race and Culture in Psychiatry.* London: Croom Helm.

Foucault, M. (1979). *Discipline and Punish: The Birth of the Prison.* Harmondsworth: Penguin.

Foucault, M. (1980). *Power/Knowledge: Selected Interviews and Other Writings by Michel Foucault, 1972–1977.* New York: Pantheon.

# SECTION 1

# CLINICAL PROBLEMATICS

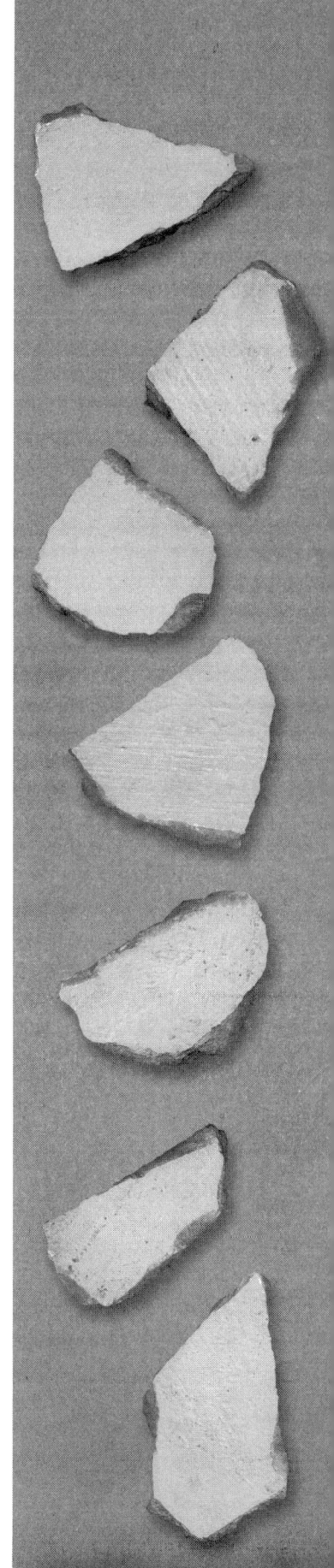

# Psychotherapy, discourse and the production of psychopathology

*Derek Hook*

## ■ Introduction

In recent decades, several critical strands of thought have argued that systems of knowledge do not simply *name* their objects of study, but in some sense *produce* them. In a similar vein, this chapter has its origins in the suspicion that psychotherapy is just as able to *produce* as to *detect* psychopathologies within its patients. To argue that psychotherapy has such a productive power is obviously to assert a serious ethical dilemma for clinical practice. If this production-detection distinction is as unstable, as immanently collapsible, as I will argue that in fact it is, then psychotherapy may be implicated in *generating the problems it has apparently been designed to treat*. In this case, psychotherapy would, theoretically at least, be just as capable of making patients psychopathological as healthy, and clinical involvement would, paradoxically, be more likely to induce 'psychopathology' than would avoidance of clinical treatment.

Basically, if this distinction between producing and detecting psychopathology is largely untenable within clinical psychotherapeutic practice, then what patients face in psychotherapy may be less an ameliorative or curative form of intervention than a cycle of *interpersonal problematisation* that works to generate psychological problems, such that the psychotherapeutic process itself is continually sustained and warranted. Rather than an altruistic treatment modality based on the over-riding (and humanistic) objective of achieving the optimum psychological adaptation of its patients, psychotherapy may in fact function primarily as a powerful and self-sustaining system of discourse, which, to paraphrase Said (1983), obeys the imperative to manufacture its material continually, and to continually expand a regime of control over what it constitutes as its special domain.

This chapter will engage with the contention that psychotherapy can indeed produce psychopathology, and will do so in two ways: firstly through a brief review of the relevant critical literature that in some way supports this notion, and secondly through an empirical study of the pathologising tendencies of *in vivo* psychotherapeutic practice. The conclusion will articulate the relationship between these two sources of critique.

## ■ 'Extra-therapeutic' pathologies

It is important to make several qualifications at this point. Firstly, to argue the collapse of this basic production-detection distinction is not to contend that the only psychopathologies dealt with within the psychotherapeutic realm have been generated by virtue of psychotherapeutic participation (although the suspicion is that a significant proportion has been). Similarly, to claim that psychotherapy is just as capable of producing as of detecting psychopathology is not to suggest that psychotherapeutic involvement never results in therapeutic or 'healing' effects. However, the fact that certain patients may affirm the beneficial outcomes of their therapeutic involvement in no way mitigates what I will argue is psychotherapy's ability to produce psychological problems. Indeed, certain sceptics might comment that it is psychotherapy's very ability to produce psychopathology that forms the precondition to the 'cures' it will ultimately aim to achieve.

It may be acknowledged that instances of psychopathology pre-exist entrance into psychotherapy. However, in this connection, it is important to note that the work of Foucault (1977) does suggest that in the modern disciplinary era, specific manifestations of pathology can in no simple way be divorced from the various technologies of power/knowledge that have in a sense 'brought them into being', and that thereafter take responsibility for studying and treating them. As an adjunct to this point, however, it may also be claimed that psychotherapy amplifies, cultivates, deepens or develops presenting problems, and that it 'psychopathologises' seemingly non-pathological concerns. Psychotherapeutic intervention might hence psychopathologically rewrite and re-represent certain aspects of a patient's life previously thought to be *entirely unproblematic*. Indeed, in terms of the therapeutic production of psychopathology, one could contend that areas of apparent psychological health are just as susceptible as those of prospective psychological difficulty, in terms of psychotherapy's ability to map pathologies upon the psychological life of its patients.

## ■ The discursive production of psychopathology

My second qualification is that, in arguing about psychotherapy's ability to produce psychopathology, I do not mean to suggest that therapists are having some kind of toxic psychological effect on their patients, and that exposure to this form of treatment will almost inevitably result in some kind of psychological damage to such patients. (There are those that *do* pursue this line of argument, however, most notably Masson (1993, 1994), but, in variations on this theme, also Cushman (1990) and Isack and Hook (1996).) Of course, to contend that psychotherapy is able to produce psychopathology certainly does mean that it has the potential to have damaging psychological effects on its patients. In this connection, it is vital to clarify that the argument I am making is about psychotherapy's *discursive* ability to produce psychopathology within patients as a function of the way in which it organises knowledge, as opposed to arguments that assert that it is the psychological mechanisms of therapy that cause harm. The former argument understands the very idea of pathology as being produced in psychotherapeutic practice, while the latter takes categories of pathology as given, and simply accuses psychotherapy of being implicated in causing them in specific patients.

Having made this clarification, it is important not to underestimate what is meant by 'the discursive'. Discourse here will be understood as entailing both textual *and material* elements that have real effects on the world, on the levels of *knowledge* (in both its formal, institutional and popular, common-sense capacities), *subjectivity* (with its correlating questions of identity and self-understanding) and *action* (implicit or explicit prescriptions to action or even regularised practice). To speak of *producing psychopathology* is hence to refer to a discursive function that entails powerful knowledge, subject and action effects.

A final qualification is important here. In speaking of psychopathology, I am using the term in a relatively loose sense, not exclusively in the sense of what might be taken to be a clinically coherent syndrome or disorder, but as a broad and inclusive category of psychological difficulties or disturbances, much in the sense of Szasz's (1961) notion of 'problems in living'. In short, the term is employed here in the sense of psychological or emotional concerns *as identified or recognised by a clinician as a reasonable and sufficient working focus of therapy* (cf. Szasz, 1961).

There is a variety of different arguments in the critical literature about how and in what ways psychotherapy might be said to be 'psychopathologising'. Both because aspects of the empirical analysis of psychotherapeutic practice that will follow in this chapter concur with aspects of the critical literature, and because such critiques make for a helpful introduction to the results of this analysis, it will be useful to provide a thumbnail sketch of relevant arguments in the literature before moving on to the empirical work.

# ■ Literature review

### 'Psychological reductionism' and victim-blaming

Holmes and Lindley (1989) suggest that psychotherapy may be used as a political instrument that diverts attention away from the structural socio-political conditions fostering human unhappiness and various other 'psychopathological' problems. Various political contexts (and causes) are, they claim, frequently psychotherapeutically reframed as problems stemming from within, and therefore becoming the responsibility of the individual. Both Pilgrim (1991) and Salmon (1991) have been vocal opponents of psychotherapy in this capacity, claiming that it has been politically evasive by reducing social structures to inner feelings and by overtly 'psychologising', *and pathologising*, human distress. The term that Pilgrim (1991, 1994) gives to this affirmation of the primacy of inner events – over and above the consideration of determining political or cultural contexts – is 'psychological reductionism'. Psychotherapy here, then, may be said to produce psychopathology, not by constituting the root cause of such 'problems in living', but by authoritatively reframing them within the aetiological ambit of *individual* psychology.

For Cross (1994), psychotherapy's powerful focus on the intrapsychic causation of problems, in conjunction with its lack of a concern with structurally ingrained inequalities of class, race, gender and economic deprivation, lead to implicitly asking its patients to 'adjust to the unjust'. Agreeing with this sentiment, Kaye (1999) argues that discourses that make the individual the locus of pathology also make the individual the unavoidable locus of moral responsibility. By placing the person in the subject position of the patient, the ownership of 'their' problem is effectively and essentially attributed to them; it is interiorised and 're-interiorised' in a way that is inseparable from their sense of self (Kaye, 1999). This discursive generation of a sense of the patient's responsibility for his/her own problems or of a deficit within the patient means that the patient becomes locked in an insidious form of victim-blaming. As Gergen (1991) has asserted, this form of giving responsibility taken in conjunction with a therapeutic language of deficiency can be iatrogenic, leading to 'a spiral of infirmity' where the patient's sense of efficacy is gradually eroded by participation in psychotherapy.

It is not difficult to imagine the broader implications of the depoliticising and individualising tendencies of psychotherapy. As Salmon (1991) notes, such an overvaluing of human agency and such an understating of the role of material conditions can lead to the situation where real powerlessness is converted into personal inadequacy and blameworthiness, and where socio-political advantage comes to be seen as inner strength. The logical extension of these arguments is that therapy, as Spinelli (1994) puts it, can be a means of suppressing social dissent and of advocating social conformity. Hurvitz suggests that 'psychotherapy creates powerful support for the established order – it challenges, labels, manipulates, rejects or co-opts those who attempt to change the society' (in Kaye, 1999: 27). In this way, psychotherapy pathologises 'deviants' in line with certain socio-moral-political imperatives of the day.

By implicitly safeguarding the status quo and conveying and spreading dominant moral and political values (as some would suggest was its function within the apartheid state (cf. Dawes, 1985)), psychotherapy may hence be thought of as pathologising in the sense that it reproduces socio-political asymmetries of power and relentlessly problematises marginalised and minority groups. In this vein, Cecchin asks: 'Can anyone do effective therapy without becoming an instrument of social control, without participating [in] and contributing ... to the construction or the maintenance of a dominant discourse of oppression?' (in Kaye, 1999: ix).

This conversion of socio-political factors into the syndromes of individual psychopathology is damaging not only in the discursive but also in the psychological sense. A good case in point of how psychotherapy both reproduces socio-political arrangements of power and correspondingly damages disenfranchised patients is provided in critical feminist accounts. Bernardez (1988), for one, argues that rather than challenging conditions seemingly oppressive to female patients, the most common reaction by therapists to female patients was and is, firstly, to discourage and disapprove of behaviours that did not conform with traditional gender-role prescriptions and, secondly, to disparage and inhibit expressions of anger, 'negative' affects and aggressive behaviours not expected of women. Subsequently, both Bernardez (1988) and Nugent (1994), like Braude (1988), assert that therapy contributes to a socialisation of women towards dependency and disempowerment and away from autonomy and personal agency. Chesler, in *Women and Madness* (1972), similarly argues that psychotherapeutic treatments typically blind their female patients to oppression by conceptualising their unhappiness and anger as personal pathology, and by keeping them from exploring, understanding and resolving conflicts produced by social determinants.

## The 'Therapeutic State'

Cushman (1990, 1991, 1992) extends these arguments at an arguably more fundamental level by affirming Foucault's (1977) formulation that the social sciences developed at the same time as the emergence of the isolated, individual self and the modern state's need to control it through study and calculated manipulation. On this basis, he argues that the products of the social sciences, psychology and psychotherapy 'have often worked to the advantage of the state by helping to construct selves that are the subjects of control and develop techniques that are the means of control' (Cushman, 1990: 600). For Cushman (1990), the varieties of self manifesting over time and across culture indicate not only that selves are constructed, but that they can be routinely *shaped*. This, says Cushman, is the business of psychologists, who have an immensely powerful political function to play in constructing and reconstructing selves that reproduce the current socio-political forms and structures of our world: 'those who are accorded the right to define, describe, understand, and heal the self are in a powerful, prescriptive position. They can determine what constitutes health and pathology, proper and improper behaviour ... . All social activity is thus defined, described, and controlled by those who are experts of the self' (Cushman, 1991: 218).

For Cushman (1990, 1991) psychotherapy may be thought of as pathologising not only in the sense that it constructs problems in living as *psychopathological*, but also in the sense that it contributes to the positive maintenance and cultivation of the normal (and ideal) self. While this positive promotion of certain 'ideal' values of self may not sound particularly pathologising *per se*, one needs to bear in mind that this self is a culturally and historically variable construct that provides a benchmark against which deviance may be made visible, i.e. brought into recognised existence. The function of such an ideal concept of the self is to displace as problematic virtually every actual person to which it is compared.

To follow Foucault (1977), the pathologising potential of psychotherapy is therefore underwritten by the fact that it no longer works in the mutually exclusive evaluative categories of good/bad, right/wrong, but instead brings into play a far more extensive continuum of values through the mediation of the norm. In other words, one's relation to the norm is not categorical, but is instead always one of degree, which means that one can never be fully normal, or conversely, completely free of problems.

There are two important implications stemming from this contention. The first is that, if Isack and Hook (1996) are correct, everyone at some stage in their lives may conceivably be construed as being in need of psychotherapeutic assistance. Secondly, psychotherapy can never really be absolutely value free or politically neutral. This is because in its assessments and evaluations of patients it is so fundamentally reliant on the specific socio-cultural norms on which its definitions of normality, deviance and pathology are based (cf. Rose, 1991, 1995). In other words, given that the standards of reasonable, adaptive and normal behaviour and social adjustment are, by definition, normative – i.e. generated from current socio-cultural values, standards and discourses – then the curative, or *normalising*, work of psychotherapy must necessarily reflect the popular or dominant socio-political values of the day.

In a complementary way, Cushman (1992) notes that psychotherapists are doctors of 'the psychological interior', with the cultural justification and the technological means to intrapsychic penetration. To this, and with overtones of Szasz (1961, 1973, 1993), Cushman adds that the state's attempts to control a population of self-contained individuals has provided psychology with a rationale for existing as an independent discipline. Szasz similarly asserts that the 'Therapeutic State' is an appropriate name for the 'new political order in which the state uses psychiatrists and psychologists, hospitals, clinics and psychotherapeutic interventions rather than policemen and prisons, to coerce, transform and rehabilitate miscreants' (1993: 799).

## Psychotherapies of damage

This form of normalisation that both critics, like their forerunner, Foucault (1977), see as so implicit an objective of psychotherapy, has thoroughly damaging effects. For Cushman, this damage results because, as I touched on above, and as Ingelby (1985) warns, psychotherapy is not limited to just policing dominant norms and values, but actively contributes to the generation of such norms. This means that patients of psychotherapy that fall short of these norms are caught in a vicious circle in which, as Sampson (1981, 1992) describes, psychotherapy attempts to treat them by reinforcing those very qualities that have caused the problem in the first place. In other words, such normalising means of treatment typically implicate exactly the values, discourses and understandings that have been so fundamental in constituting the problem in the first place, so that the supposed 'cure' may therefore simply cause further damage.

With reference to the ideals of what he considers to be the self-responsible, self-contained and individualised self, Cushman defines the damage caused by psychotherapy in the following way:

> [B]y outwardly adhering to the practices of an objective technology and the ideology of self-contained individualism and the bounded self ... [psychotherapy] perpetuates the social problems that caused the patient's wounds in the first place. This paradoxical situation undermines the ... work of the therapy because it is unempathic (the therapist is choosing adherence to an ideology over the needs of the patient), harmful (it inflicts on patients the discourse by which they have previously been harmed), and ultimately counterproductive for our society as a whole (it reproduces the present power hierarchy and economic structure that have caused our present suffering) (1990: 607).

Szasz (1974) states the damage of such normalising treatments in slightly more polemical terms when he defines psychotherapy as a potentially persecutory instrument, both inegalitarian and coercive, through which 'deviants' like drug-takers, homosexuals, schizophrenics and single parents would be defined, labelled and stigmatised. To him (1961, 1973), mental illness and, by extrapolation, certain varieties of psychopathology, are myths validated only on the basis of fallacious borrowings from the medical model. (The medical model, in brief, proposes that it is useful to think of abnormal behaviour as disease and, accordingly, abnormal actions as the result of mental illness, psychological disorder and/or psychopathology.) For Szasz (1973), this is not only a fallacious comparison, it is one with serious ethical problems. If it is the case that, strictly speaking, there is no such thing as mental illness, that 'Minds can be "sick" only in the sense that jokes are "sick" or economies are "sick"' (Szasz, 1961: 275), then psychotherapy has granted itself an illegitimate series of warrants for making psychological evaluations, prescribing 'treatments' and implementing interventions that are illegitimate, undeserved and potentially harmful (Szasz, 1961).

Szasz (1961) is intent on reminding us that psychiatric/psychological treatments are suffused with serious, implicit, moral value-judgements: to him, such interventions embody a 'moral-discursive formation', to use Kaye's phrase (1999), prescribing what is socially normative and, just as importantly, what is *not*. So sure, in fact, is Szasz of the unethical and damaging qualities of these forms of intervention, that he suggests that the concept of mental illness has come to replace the concept of witchcraft. Such discourses of psychopathology to him 'have the same moral implications and political consequences as did the belief in witchcraft and the social actions to which it led' (Szasz, 1961: 24). Within the terms of this comparison, diagnoses of psychopathology (no matter how informal or implicit) ascribe certain roles to the 'pathological' patient, roles thoroughly infused with connotations of the sick, bad, stupid or wrong roles that scapegoat and categorise so-called 'pathological' people, setting them apart as inferior and depriving them of a wide array of rights and civil liberties (Szasz, 1973).

Both substantiating and anchoring Szasz's arguments, Dreyfus and Rabinow (1982) refer to Foucault (1977) in observing that social technologies typically advance by taking what are essentially political problems (i.e. problems of social control) and recasting them as technical problems for the sole attention of discrete and qualified experts, like psychologists. It is in this way that such problems are removed from the domain of political discourse and rearmed in the neutral language of science or its associated disciplines, despite the fact that fundamental political objectives (such as the normalisation of deviant members of society) are still served (Dreyfus and Rabinow, 1982). It is also in this way that such 'technologies' assert the need for the autonomy and relative sovereignty of their experts within the fields of their technical expertise.

### Diagnostic power

In slightly less controversial terms, Hare-Mustin and Marecek (1997) also call attention to the discursive and diagnostic power of psychotherapy and, more particularly, its potential to label, which has led some to label the therapy session as the 'power hour'. This 'power to give a name' constitutes, as Brown (1990) comments, an integral part of psychotherapy and a 'pathologising gravity' within it that, overtly or implicitly, attends the full duration of the therapeutic process. Hare-Mustin and Marecek (1997) warn that although the formulation of a diagnosis is generally reliant on a categorised list of symptoms – typically contained in a manual like the *Diagnostic and Statistical Manual of Mental Disorders* (American Psychiatric Association, 1994) – the decision as to which disorder suitably characterises the patient resides with the individual psychotherapist.

Harper (1994) highlights the subjectivity of therapists' diagnoses and emphasises how the use of empirical and contingent accounting in explaining diagnoses affords mental-health professionals a wide (and frequently unreasonable) latitude in dealing with challenges to diagnoses. The subjective dimension of diagnosis is problematised further by Brown's (1990) warning that the elasticity of certain disorders and syndromes, with such seemingly ubiquitous and generalisable symptoms (notably those of borderline personality disorder), means that they could conceivably be attached to almost anyone. Parker *et al.* (1995) add to this debate when they suggest that diagnostic criteria could be said to be *justificatory arguments* rather than objective signs. Frequently, they claim (1995), diagnoses are rhetorical constructions assembled from ambiguous and ambivalent interview responses. In this way, rather than simply 'recognising' psychological disorder, psychotherapists could be said to be 'bringing forth' or constructing psychopathology.

More than being merely subject to personal biases (implicit or explicit), forms of diagnosis within psychotherapy are sometimes a function of race/gender pairings between therapist and patient (DeVaris, 1994). Indeed, in results supported by Hare-Mustin and Marecek (1997) and Brown (1990), DeVaris (1994) reported that white therapists generally rated their black patients as psychologically more impaired than did black therapists for the same patients. These findings of the influence of racism upon diagnostic procedures parallel those of what Brown (1990) has called 'diagnostic sexism'.

Extending this line of argument, Gergen asks how it is that people in other cultures and times managed without the concept of depression, yet contemporary psychologists detect depression in all corners of society (even in infants), to the extent that today over six million Americans 'require' Prozac (1994: 414). He warns that it is the healing experts, like psychotherapists, who are in the privileged, and largely uncontested, position of operating and controlling the discourses of pathology (Gergen, 1992). Voicing a similar concern is Albee, who notes that the first volume of the *Diagnostic and Statistical Manual of Mental Disorders* (DSM-I) of the American Psychiatric Association,

> ... published in 1952, listed 60 types and subtypes of mental illness. Sixteen years later, DSM II more than doubled the number of disorders. The number of disorders grew to more than 200 with DSM III in 1980. The current guide ... includes tobacco dependence, developmental disorders and sexual dysfunctions, school learning problems, and adolescent rebellion disorders ... . The decision in 1973 by the American Psychiatric Association to remove 'homosexuality' from its list of mental disorders lowered overnight by many millions the total number of Americans considered mentally ill ... . The decision by the National Association for Retarded Citizens to make a 70 IQ rather than an 80 IQ the cutoff point for defining mental retardation reduced by millions the number of retarded Americans (1990: 372).

## The expanding jurisdiction of the psychotherapist

As Hare-Mustin and Marecek (1997) warn, the proliferation of categories of psychopathology means that as more 'aberrant' behaviours come to be in need of 'remedy', so more behaviour is brought under critical scrutiny and the regulation of clinical experts. The discursive production of psychopathology through the conventionalisation and spread of diagnostic labels enables psychotherapy to extend its domain of intervention and ever further legitimate the terms and nature of its practice. As Isack and Hook (1996) assert, psychotherapy's creation of a proliferation of psychopathologies, along with its implicit promises of 'treatment', 'cure' and psychological 'health', functions to cement and colonise a population of psychological 'illnesses' that then become *its* responsibility to deal with. In this way, psychotherapy works like a powerful discourse that is *self-* rather than *patient-*serving, and that capitalises off whatever pathologies or problems it finds (or situates) within its patients as the continued and continuing reasons for the necessity of its practice (Isack and Hook, 1996).

The obvious extension of Isack and Hook's argument would be that there is almost never a therapeutic interaction without the impulsion to unearth psychopathology or detect some disturbance or dysfunction within the patient, because these are the nodal points which authenticate current, and necessitate future, psychotherapeutic interventions. Isack and Hook (1996) even insist that psychotherapists have a staunch and active economic imperative to find psychopathologies within patients, a suspicion supported by Parker's (1998) claim that being able to find and treat psychopathology is crucial to the identity and salaries of psychologists.

On the more specific level of the actual and technical practice of psychotherapy, Isack and Hook (1996) warn of the discursive, language-based powers at the disposal of the psychotherapist. Extending earlier claims about the diagnostic power at the disposal of psychotherapists, Isack and Hook (1996) assert that psychotherapists have access to a technical language consisting of a 'psychotherapeutic discourse' of specialist terms and forms of jargon. This specialist language provides therapists with access to a wide range of rhetorical devices that not only make their diagnoses difficult to refute, but also empower and drive their interpretive and prescriptive abilities. In short, what is being referred to here is the discursive ability of the psychotherapist, who, being in the privileged possession of specialised technical knowledge and its concomitant technical vocabulary, can produce pronouncements, descriptions and interpretations that are representative of vested institutional power and at the same time are extremely difficult to question or refute (Fillingham, 1993). Indeed, this specialist language grants therapists privileged access to certain concepts and explanations, and to precise and guarded bodies of knowledge. The resultant discursive power enables qualified experts to make declarations and assessments of their patients with stronger claims of 'truth' than unqualified persons. Because of this, therapists are able to make assessments and hypotheses about patients' problems that are more 'definitive' than are the patients' own hypotheses about themselves.

The use of such a language of technical expertise and control, inaccessible to the layperson, not only enables psychotherapists to make pronouncements about people and intervene in their lives, it also enables them to call into being new psychological problems, new forms of treatment and new forms of intervention that extend their warrants of control and surveillance. Rose (1991) notes that these specific discursive abilities do not simply mystify domination and legitimate power, they also work to make new sectors of reality thinkable and practicable.

### The systematic generation of pathology

Foucault (1977) maintains that curative or therapeutic practices like those of psychotherapy take as their paradoxical goal *the generation and spreading* of the abnormalities that they in theory simply apprehend and treat. To Foucault, curative and therapeutic practices are integral to the systematic creation, classification and control of anomalies within a given social body. Both Foucault's *The History of Sexuality* (1978) and *Discipline and Punish* (1977), as Dreyfus and Rabinow (1982) note, show examples of how the appearance of certain curative/rehabilitative institutions was contemporaneous with the proliferation of the very anomalies – the delinquent, the sexual pervert and so on – that such technologies of power/knowledge had seemingly been designed to eliminate.

This systematic creation of anomalies is ensured by the fact that these curative/therapeutic procedures function as discursive systems of knowledge and understanding that are increasingly reified throughout modern (Western) society. This systematic creation is further ensured by the fact that these procedures maintain, as an integral component of their functioning, a high degree of failure. Such failure rates paradoxically come to be cited as the reason to further develop the sophistication and jurisdiction of these discrete technologies of cure and rehabilitation. According to both Foucault (1977) and Cushman (1992), the goal of psychotherapeutic practice is not to actually erase psychopathology or psychological distress, but rather to assimilate these problems into greater tactics of observation, measurement, control and subjection, such that greater schedules of control and surveillance can be distributed ever more widely throughout society. In this way, relentless programmes of self-problematisation across the concerns of individual sexuality, psychology and emotion, where individuals vocalise their smallest and most secret transgressions in a variety of confessional situations, take their place as the satellite procedures of state control, i.e. as autonomous localities of power corresponding to the overall disciplinary project of modern regimes of control.

Just as the threat of criminal activity gives the police an excuse to patrol the whole of society, so the threats of psychological disturbance, psychopathology, perversity, deviance and illness sanction the interventionist powers of mental-health experts over society. As prisons are for Foucault (1977) 'factories for producing criminals', so the psychotherapeutic arena is a veritable greenhouse for the production of psychopathology. It is here that Said's comment that a discourse is 'a regime of control over what it constitutes as its special domain' (1983: 214) appears to have its greatest applicability to the current argument. Similarly, his notion that a discourse is a 'self-sustaining system which obeys the imperative to manufacture its material continually' (Said, 1983: 214) seems an especially incisive characterisation at this juncture of psychotherapy's ability to produce psychopathology in its patients.

## ■ Empirical study

### Methodology

The arguments I have discussed above present a useful theoretical backdrop to the analytical work to follow. This work takes a far more specific and empirically grounded approach to the problem at hand, and maintains a particularly strong focus on how the discursive production of psychopathology is *technically* managed within psychotherapy. The argument from this point onwards will hence be a deductive one that will assemble a variety of clinical examples drawn from a larger study on the functioning of power at the micro-, face-to-face level of psychotherapy (Hook, 1999).

This study analysed 250 pages of published transcriptions of therapeutic dialogue using a constructionist revision of Glaser and Strauss' (1967) grounded-theory method of analysis (cf. Pidgeon, 1996; Pidgeon and Henwood, 1996). The grounded-theory method provided a 'data representation language', i.e. an open-ended indexing system that enabled me to work systematically through a basic body of data, generating codes referring both to low-level concepts and more abstract categories (Pidgeon, 1996). Likewise, the constructionist aspect of the grounded-theory method enabled me to draw on discursive forms of analysis, to utilise elements of this method in a deconstructive way, to insert new discourses into old systems of meaning and ultimately to remain vigilant regarding the *constructed* rather than the *transparent* nature of analysed protocols (cf. Pidgeon, 1996).

The results of this study suggested that the psychotherapeutic production of psychopathology was achieved in no one single way, and was instead to be found at the confluence of a number of therapeutic functions. Accordingly, this presentation will critically describe several aligned therapeutic functions, and will ultimately offer a ten-point argument that brings together the relevant 'faculties' of psychotherapy that so efficaciously enable it to produce psychopathology.

### 'Therapeutic listening'

As became clear at the outset of the analysis, perhaps one of the most obvious psychotherapeutic functions to be 'performed' upon the patient by the therapist is the basic act of *listening*. Despite at first bearing some similarity to the more passive function of 'hearing', therapeutic listening appeared, within the analysis, *as a purposeful and goal-driven form of action* strongly characterised by purpose and intent. Comparative analysis suggested that psychotherapists, like priests, counsellors and doctors, were professional listeners, typically involved in more than a purely passive and facilitative activity when 'listening'. The performance of therapeutic listening appeared to be intrinsically tied to certain strategic objectives. Upon close scrutiny, and with the correlation of attending activities and therapeutic goals, it became clear that therapeutic listening frequently functioned as an auditory form of inspection, assessment and examination. Therapeutic listening, in short, was a form of monitoring, observing and inspecting patients, i.e. an eliciting form of auditory surveillance strategically designed to draw out and develop patient disclosures.

Accordingly, despite the 'even-hovering' appearance of therapeutic listening, this phenomenon functioned as a strongly directing and focusing activity that filtered and hierarchised incoming data into categories of varying importance. Cross-sectional comparisons across the data pool yielded a variety of similarly motivated questions posed by therapists in early sessions, suggesting that therapists were listening more intently to certain aspects of patients' narratives than others (e.g. 'Would you like to tell me about your problem? ... When did this start? ... Have you any idea what's causing this problem? ... How about your childhood?'). Similarly, clear evidence of diagnostic and aetiological 'priorities in listening' (along with high premiums on patient disclosure regarding interpersonal relations and emotional states) was traced by mapping and grouping types of therapists' questions within early sessions (e.g. 'How did that make you feel? ... Do you remember? ... How do you feel now? ... What about your husband? ... How did your mother make you feel?'). Furthermore, therapists' interruptions of material deemed less relevant or unimportant to the therapeutic value of sessions likewise functioned as indices of the directing and focusing functioning of therapeutic listening (e.g. 'But maybe we should focus on what's at hand ... But how did you feel about that? ... Do you feel that that has relevance here?').

Like the doctor's gaze, which yields knowledge and prescriptions of intervention from the visual analysis of the injured body – i.e. which imposes discourse upon perception, as Bryson (1993) puts it – so the attentive ear of the psychotherapist brought with it certain values, understandings and knowledges to be implemented within the therapeutic setting. Although these professional knowledges, values and clinical norms remained for the better part *unspoken* by the therapists, they were omnipresent in *how the clinicians practised their listening*. On a pragmatic note, of course, the necessity of these impositions is clear: they are the frameworks of understanding, the platforms of assessment, through which the therapist engages the case and establishes from this a coherent and realistic basis of intervention.

### Eliciting disclosure

The 'force' of therapeutic listening was enhanced in a variety of ways. The concentrated performance of an *interested* and *attentive* presence was, for example, an important factor. By acting as an 'emotional sounding board', by 'communicating presence' and providing tacit indications of acknowledgement, encouragement and support, this 'listening functioning' of the clinician was able to elicit deeper and more personal forms of disclosure. This was particularly the case when such listening was used in conjunction with the provision of an authenticating environment and the diligent 'tracking' and non-verbal reflection of emotions. These authenticating variables, once paired off with implicit forms of support, unconditional acknowledgement and the camaraderie of the 'working bond' of the relationship, made for a strong sense of trust, which in turn was an essential factor in 'soliciting' the most private and shameful disclosures.

A variety of 'frame elements' was also apparently at play here, such as patients' expectations of the necessity of their own expository and disclosing role in therapy. Particularly important here was the apparent assumption by patients that beneficial therapeutic work would be possible only proportionate to the degree to which they were willing to *honestly* disclose the most intimate and secretive details of their personal lives. The 'clinical gravity' of the therapeutic situation was also an apparent factor, for the very presence of a professionally qualified expert in psychology who was being paid to attend to the patient appeared to have played a role in insidiously 'soliciting' their disclosure. The combination of these various techniques and frame elements proved extremely successful in eliciting not only intimate personal expositions, but also in encouraging various patient 'confessions' – of 'sinful', 'wrongful' personal feelings or desires, and of deviant or 'unacceptable' wishes, habits and peculiarities. Given the clinical setting, these were obviously not 'confessions' in the religious sense of the term. They were, however, powerful emotional admissions of deviant or shameful intentions/acts offered up to a psychological expert who was seen as being able to properly make sense of and/or treat such 'problems'. The regularity of this phenomenon across protocols was both striking and difficult to account for, as was the seemingly *automatic* nature of this 'confession-making'. Indeed, this unfailing tendency of patients to disclose their most deviant or shameful acts, and to then implicitly relate them to current norms or standards of right/wrong or normal/abnormal, soon came to represent something of an explanatory crisis to me in the course of my research.

### 'Externalising conscience'

Part of the frequency of this phenomenon seemed to lie in the fact that patients generally assumed (often quite explicitly so) that the therapeutic environment was an evaluative space, a place where their normality would implicitly be assessed (e.g. 'I know this isn't normal, doctor ... This isn't right, is it? ... I hope you don't think I'm strange, doctor ... That's not normal is it? ... You don't think there's something wrong with me do you?'). Often this assumption accounted for patients' anxieties about entering psychotherapy, and therapists often needed to expend a good deal of effort trying to persuade patients to the contrary. Whatever the case may have been (and I should emphasise at this point that the good therapist was certainly able to 'function-alise' various frame elements, such as patient expectation, as part of the therapeutic work), it soon became apparent that these confessional forms of 'externalising conscience' were a powerful characterising feature of what was generally deemed effective psychotherapy. Ultimately, the only reasonable hypothesis that I could come up with, within the frame of the data itself, was that one of the prime functions of eliciting personal disclosure, through various combinations of technique and context, *was precisely to displace a form of normative self-evaluation within patients.*

Importantly, though, this was never an explicitly coercive function, i.e. the results of my analysis did not suggest that therapists *directly* forced or demanded confession from their patients. In fact, the active dialogical input of therapists suggested quite the opposite, as is indicated by the interchange that follows:

> *(The female patient describes to the therapist a dream in which a woman had made sexual advances to her.)*
> Th. ... she was making a pass at you.
> Pt. Oh, oh yes. Oh, I wouldn't think of it ... nothing like that.
> Th. What about your ideas about homosexuality?
> Pt. Well, I ... it disgusts me. I think it's an awful thing ... .
> Th. ... you haven't any idea as to what the reasons for it are?
> Pt. No ... . Is it ever normal, doctor?
> Th. Well in puberty ... children of the same sex often experiment sexually with each other.
> Pt. Until they don't ... until they know better, is that it, doctor? (Wolberg, 1977: 1072).

Here is another similar example:

> Pt. ... this girl I told you ... of ... lives with this doctor. He hasn't married her ... why he hasn't married her, I don't know. He's free to do so; he's been divorced and she's divorced, and why they should live in sin when they don't have to, that's something

> I can't understand ... and there's about a 23 year age difference .... This old man ... old, I mean, real old – 65, 66 – that's old doctor, when you're 50 or so ... don't you think so? ... I wonder what woman wouldn't want to be married, instead of living that way.
>
> *Th.* There are some.
>
> *Pt.* Really?
>
> *Th.* I believe so (Wolberg, 1977: 1082).

Clearly, in these cases the therapist cannot be blamed for explicitly impressing a 'normal' viewpoint on the patient – indeed, the therapist's *active* influence often tends to overtly discourage and *interrogate* such views of 'normality', to apparently offer liberal rather than conservative norms. Despite this, the displacement of normative evaluation remains a strong and arguably essential function of psychotherapy, as substantiated by the number of times it was identified in the analysed data, and by the ways that patients so repeatedly tested their evaluative assessments against the opinions of the clinical expert (e.g. '... is that it, doctor? ... is this normal? ... I know it's wrong ... I know this isn't normal ... Do other people do this?'). This is a difficult contradiction to overcome, except for the fact that the displacement of normative self-evaluation might not proceed simply explicitly, directly or exclusively from the therapist. This point will be discussed in further detail as we proceed; given the regularity and the seeming strength of this phenomenon, however, I can nonetheless assert the first strand of my argument, namely that *psychotherapy functions to elicit, with impressive regularity, and through non-directed or explicit means, a powerful gravity toward normative self-evaluations on the part of its patients*. Put differently, I would suggest that psychotherapy institutes a form of reality testing that works to continually consolidate a set of norms.

As is apparent in the above example, however, and as is borne out in the results of the analysis more generally, such self-evaluative procedures occurred not only *indirectly* through the 'inactive influence' of the psychotherapist, but also on the apparent basis of the patient's *own initiative,* sometimes in response to the therapist's apparently non-judgemental attitude. Indeed, what the data suggested was that the 'surveillance' of therapeutic listening, together with patients' understandings and expectations of the role of the clinical professional, seemingly displaced *within patients* an implicit leaning towards normative values and standards. The effect of this displacement was that it was really the patients who ultimately situated *themselves* relative to social and moral values. To the first strand of the argument I can therefore now add a second: *this gravity toward self-evaluation quickly becomes an automatic function within psychotherapy, occurring largely on the basis of the patient's own initiative and responsibility.*

## Self-attendance; 'therapeutic talking'; patient 'subjectivisation'

If listening was one of the most basic therapeutic functions performed by the therapist, then talking was certainly one of the most basic therapeutic functions performed by patients. Cross-protocol comparison across the data pool revealed a relatively unexpected result concerning this 'therapeutic talking' of patients: although frequently *apparently* disordered and rambling, it was ultimately a very cohesive and directed activity, unified by a number of strongly characterising and structuring features. The first such feature of this 'talking' was that it was powerfully 'egocentric' and self-focused.

At its most basic, the therapeutic talk of patients was that of a personal story or personal narrative, of which they were both author and protagonist. In this way, such narratives were marked by a fundamental self-attention, a strong 'I' foundation and pivot. Indeed, a central component of this self-attending 'talking' was the provision of a reflexive attitude that, while often vague at first, soon grew in strength. This self-focus was in many ways the outcome, again, of the 'inactive intervention' of therapists, who, through explicit refutation of typical conversational structures, and through their strong prioritisation of patient subjectivity, came to discretely promote and encourage this self-attending orientation.

Inappropriate questions, personal enquiries and overly result-based queries were gradually extinguished by the therapists' avoidance of providing answers, or by their 'bouncing back' of patients' questions in the form of personal probes. Both of these tactics resulted in the encouragement of a strict personal focus for the patients. As therapy progressed, therapists 'slimmed down' their contributions to a bare minimum and enforced a guarded and tactical form of detachment, such that the therapeutic narrative came very close to approximating the therapeutic monologue of the self-monitoring patient. This combination of continual redirection and strategic disinvestment made patients increasingly self-reflexive and independent. Patient self-awareness was further encouraged by therapists' encouragement of patients' subjectivity. In fact, at each point of the therapeutic narrative, the 'egocentricity' of the patients' narratives was supported and reinforced, so that the focus on the self and the self's problems was soon the vastly predominant, and speaking relatively, *only* real concern within the patients' narratives.

The use of prescribed or generic answers/responses along the lines of 'this must be difficult for you' likewise served to keep the personal involvement of the therapist to an absolute and clinical minimum, while simultaneously facilitating the narrative emergence of the *subjective, personal life* of the patient. The reuse of large segments of the patients' descriptions and of their own words and terms of understanding similarly ensured that each therapeutic narrative was, at times, essentially a monologue, i.e. the narrative of *one* voice, that of the *subjective patient's*, even if it was repeated, re-emphasised, or extended by the therapist in ways that structured or directed the session. Take the following example, in which the therapist explicitly directs the patient towards a self-monitoring and (emotionally) self-aware form of narrative:

> Pt. ... I've had some disappointments. There's no question about that ... . I took an interest in helping crippled children ... . Normal children hurt little children, you know, that aren't up ... . And these little children are protected. So, I mean, that really doesn't hurt me too much. I feel badly about it, but I don't think that has anything to do with ... what's happening to me.
> Th. There are other things?
> Pt. It goes further.
> Th. It goes further? *It involves your own feelings about yourself?* (Wolberg, 1977: 1052; my emphasis).

As evidenced in the above extract, the accessing and reinforcement of subjectivity also generally occurred through therapists' continual querying of the personal opinions of patients. Typical of this tactic was a therapist's redirected retort to direct questions, like: 'But what do *you* think?' Or, more simply: 'Do *you* have any idea what causes these feelings?' (Wolberg, 1977: 1050; my emphasis). The patient's comment: 'It's how I feel about myself that really counts' (Wolberg, 1977: 1081) provides evidence of this kind of therapeutic effect, as does the comment: 'Ever since I've been coming to see you, I've been giving more thought to myself than I've ever done in my whole life' (Wolberg, 1977: 1079). A useful adjunct here was the emphasis of the words used to reference the patient, e.g. the vocal italicisation of the patient's name and of mentions of 'you': 'But how do *you* feel?'; 'And then what did *you* do?'

The placement of such a premium on the development of patient subjectivity and reflexivity was a strong and unremitting pattern throughout therapeutic protocols. The patient's *self* increasingly became a level of awareness and a surface of intervention that needed to be prioritised; more than this, it became the vessel through which therapists could repeatedly appeal to the patients' agency, to *their* own personal prerogative – and responsibility – to change. This was a fact that led me to conclude – and this is the third strand of the developing argument – *that an essential factor of therapeutic involvement is the powerful foregrounding of patient subjectivity and agency as fundamental bases from which psychological problems needed to be approached*. In short, *instrumental to psychotherapy is the systematic assertion, within patients, of practices of personal reflexivity*.

### Speaking the role of therapist: therapeutic questioning

An interesting correlate to the therapeutic objective of patient 'subjectivisation' was that of encouraging the development of an 'auto-therapeutic' narrative on the part of patients. By virtue of the above-mentioned clinical minimisation of the personal or conversational input of the psychotherapists, the patients frequently appeared to take up both (patient and therapist) roles in the dialogue, thus becoming both authors and evaluators of their own dialogue. Take for example the comparison between the questions a patient asks her psychotherapist in their second session, and a comment she makes in her ninth session, respectively:

> Pt. I would like you to tell me what is wrong, doctor … (Wolberg, 1977: 1050).

> Pt. My big problem … is what I do to myself because I feel no good (Wolberg, 1977: 1098).

Such a shift in the focus of the therapeutic narrative and the locus of attention and responsibility is, typically, viewed as evidence of therapeutic progress. Similar longitudinal comparisons across protocols suggested that patients' narratives increasingly mimicked the form of the therapists' vocal contributions. Taking on the speaking function of the therapists, not only in content, but in structure and impetus, the patients, almost without fail, started to 'speak their roles' and conduct the facilitative, explorative and 'knowing about self' therapeutic functions autonomously and verbally. Streamlined through the excision of superfluous detail, the avoidance of therapist-directed questioning and the adoption of accurately aimed self-examination and scrutiny, the 'talks' of patients in late stages of therapy came increasingly to be 'auto-therapeutic', i.e. to perform their therapeutic lessons:

> *(The patient is speaking of a previously dysfunctional relationship that she is now out of.)*
> Pt. Do you see? He will keep on dabbling with the women … I say 'Yes, all right, I'll be here; all right, I'll see you.' And as soon as I say it, I *know* I shouldn't have said it. I know I'm wrong. I know I'm being too soft, too easy about things …. Do you understand? … You see? I say 'Yes' or 'All right, I'll do it', and if I say I will, I'll do it, no matter what. But I shouldn't. I should be very careful of what I answer and what I say …. There'll be a lot of opportunities, but I must watch out not to start anything with someone – well, a man who isn't deserving: and I'm not going to get involved, no matter what demands are made (Wolberg, 1977: 1098).

In the above example, the patient in fact even appears to be *instructing the therapist* by continually querying whether he follows *her* self-instructions. This adoption of the narrative structure previously lent by the therapists frequently ensured that patients were able to motivate and guide their own treatments with a relative amount of independence; similarly, patients often, at this point, began to lead their own narratives with questions of a self-probing nature, e.g. 'I don't know why that is …'; 'I wonder why I feel that way …' (Wolberg, 1977: 354). Also, patients often came to provide self-assessments, self-recommendations and personal suggestions of reparative behaviour, as in the following extract:

> *(The patient is speaking here of the prospect of doing an antiques course, an idea that she initiated and that she feels might 'do her some good'.)*
> Pt. It's just something that will help me to build up a different impression of myself. I've got to do that … because things are no good the way they have been. That's why I thought I'd go ahead with studying, to build myself up to feel different (Wolberg, 1977: 1088).

A similar example of the patient taking on therapist functions is seen in the 'therapeutic corrections', i.e. the verbal amendments made by patients to their own narratives. Dysfunctional trends and directions within their typical narratives (like excessive acquiescence, for example, as in the earlier extract) were gradually, systematically eliminated and became the subject of patients' reflexive criticisms, where they were able to identify such recently highlighted 'dysfunctions' and vocally check their 'mistakes'. Hence we can assert the fourth strand of the developing argument: *the apparent effect of this form of patient narrative was the 'installing' of a therapeutic subject position through which a relentless and seemingly automatic habit of self-problematisation (and self-correction) was instituted in an internal and subjective manner.* The fifth strand of the argument is that *this therapeutic subject position appeared to be so firmly and durably entrenched at the level of individual and personal subjectivity as to exert its influence beyond the parameters of the therapeutic setting.*

Another core function of the psychotherapeutic arena was the therapists' tactical use of questioning to ensure the continual outflow of patient disclosure. Indeed, cross-protocol comparisons quickly revealed what I had suspected, that therapeutic questioning (along with a variety of associated techniques like prompting, redirecting, reflecting and echoing sentiments) often clustered around the querying of relational, personal, historical, symptomological and emotional details. Each of these areas represented a strong potential location point for indications of psychopathology. The use of unbroken sequences of related questions and the building up of a 'momentum of enquiry', for example, were not only inevitably successful in invoking disclosure around these relevant 'location points', they also yielded, almost without exception, potential 'nodes of pathology', i.e. working focus or problem areas that the therapists could continue to probe for further evidence of psychopathology. This tactic was particularly useful with resistant patients: take for example the following extract from a therapist's first session with a new patient (note the therapist's leading question):

Th. Would you like to tell me about your problem?
Pt. (*rapidly and angrily*) The first thing I'm going to tell you is that I am against psychotherapy completely.
Th. Why?
Pt. Because of my past experience. I'm coming here against my will.
Th. I see.
Pt. Definitely against my will.
Th. Can you tell me about that?
(*Patient relates anecdote about unsuccessful psychotherapeutic experience.*)
Th. Well it does sound like you had some ungratifying responses.
Pt. The first doctor wasn't really a psychotherapist ….
Th. How long did you go to him?
Pt. Just a few times … it wasn't doing me any good.
Th. What was the reason for going to him in the first place?
Pt. I was kicked out of school.
Th. College? (Wolberg, 1977: 460).

This tactic was also useful where no discernible problems seemed to be evident:

Th. Are you completely satisfied with your present life and adjustment?
Pt. Yes.
Th. It's very gratifying to be so well satisfied. Understandably you wouldn't want any treatment if there is nothing wrong.
Pt. No.
Th. Your mother thinks you ought to get treatment. I wonder why?
Pt. I don't know.
Th. Maybe you're angry that she sent you here if you don't need treatment.
Pt. I'm not angry.
Th. Mm hmmmm. (*pause*) But there must be some area in which you aren't completely happy.
Pt. Well … . (*pause*)
Th. Are you satisfied with the way everything is going in every area of your life?
Pt. (*pause*) No, not exactly.
Th. Mm hmmm. (*pause*)

*Pt.* It's that I don't go out much, not much, I don't go out with boys ... (Wolberg, 1977: 463).

In the last extract, the therapist comes very close to using the patient's very resistance to the process as, in fact, the motivating reason for why she should be there, and manages this through the questioning of her prospective anger. Here a sequence of questions was compounded with the use of a rhetorical trick – which forced the patient into admitting that there may have been at least one thing wrong with her life. Indeed, few people would be able to claim that they are satisfied with 'the way everything is going in every area of [their] life'.

Questioning techniques such as this added significantly to the therapists' ability to *construct* rather than merely *discover* psychopathology. In fact, rhetorical tricks seem 'par for the course' in the therapeutic attempt to 'unearth' psychopathology within its patients. Indirect or oblique patterns of enquiry, for example, were effective in preventing patients from guarding against developing aspects of the information they imparted. In probing for aetiological and diagnostic information, therapists would typically avoid asking 'point-blank' questions with yes/no answers that would risk incidentally cueing patients in on what *not* to say. The question 'Do you dream a lot or a little?' was, for example, preferred by Wolberg (1977) to the more direct 'Do you dream?' The latter was seen as risking betraying an assumption of abnormality that may have prejudiced the patient's reply.

In attempting to ascertain accurate symptomological details, therapists very seldom asked outright or blunt questions, but approached the characterisation of problem areas far more obliquely, picking up on *certain trends and tendencies already mentioned by the patients*. The question 'Was there ever a period when you felt happy?' (Wolberg, 1977: 1045), for example, was an effective means both of tacitly asserting a presenting 'problem' and of 'closing down' the patient's ability to avoid discussing what the therapist later construed as a state of depression. Various other forms of indirection, such as that of peripheral questioning and of juxtaposing placid and provocative enquiries (or obvious and investigative questions), were frequently used in conjunction with the tactical reconstruction of patients' own words. All of these techniques 'opened up' the therapeutic dialogue, made it easier for the patients to converse freely, and provided questions that were immanently more answerable than directed queries that risked being prescriptive, e.g. 'Do you feel suicidal?' By the same token, however, the use of these techniques also made it far harder for patients to guard against providing the kinds of answers that could be reconstructed as potential indications of psychopathology. Frequently, indeed, by selectively reconstructing a patient's own words, a psychotherapist appeared to be playing less the role of a detached and observant scientist than that of a clever attorney able to twist witnesses' words into evidence to be used against them.

Presented in the absence of a set of 'control' questions through which contrary representations and depictions may be actively sought – by which seemingly pathogenic qualities may be refuted and denied – such forms of therapeutic questioning ran the risk of directly soliciting the kinds of accounts the therapists wanted to hear. In this respect, I found it difficult to determine whether psychotherapy was a probing process of discovery or a 'calling into being'; a balanced testing of psychopathology, or a selective collection of the basic 'building blocks' from which the therapists gain the necessary 'corroborating evidence' to build a picture of pathology. More concerning yet, the 'problem-centric' nature of these lines of enquiry could not but beg the question of whether the therapists *could ever fail to find what they were looking for.* We may therefore assert the sixth basic strand of this argument: *therapists have at their disposal a variety of rhetorical and questioning abilities that, along with their ability to reconstruct patients' own accounts, provides them with a broad constructive latitude with which to generate certain 'nodes of psychopathology'.* The seventh strand of the argument is that *the 'problem-centric' nature of the process, together with the tactical and technical abilities afforded the therapists in order to 'discover' psychopathology, lacks a balancing set of controls to the extent that the psychotherapeutic search for pathology frequently resembles a scenario that works on the principle that if the therapists look hard enough, they will find what they are looking for.*

## The co-construction of therapeutic accounts

The possibility that therapists exercised certain constructive powers within the therapeutic arena came to represent an important analytical focus for me. Indeed, despite having asserted earlier that a patient's therapeutic narrative was at times essentially that of a monologue, contributed to and supported by the therapist's redirected and structuring use of the patient's *own* therapeutic voice, I feel that it is important to point out that the therapeutic narrative also frequently took the form of a *dialogue*, in the true sense of being made up of, and constructed by, *two* voices.

Despite the fact that therapists attempted to cultivate the development of autonomous, reflexive 'self-dialogues' within patients, they never lost their directing function within the therapeutic interaction. The therapists' use of unfinished or trailing sentences, for example, was frequently leading, not only in terms of directing the patients' exposition, but also in terms of suggesting *what* they may say. Indeed, sometimes words were offered by the therapists that were then picked up and used by the patients, as in this specific example:

> *Pt.* ... instead of building me up, you see, which would have been a wonderful thing for me, because I never had any opportunities, until I married him .... And, well, he always ... (*pause*)
> *Th.* He always minimized ...
> *Pt.* Minimized my ability, my thinking capabilities (Wolberg, 1977: 1078).

At other times, emotional descriptions were made stronger, or were 'resited' within the 'subjective subject' of the patient:

> *Pt.* ... I crossed myself up with this man .... Three and a half years I went with him ... and he hasn't called me up in three months ....
> *Th.* You resented the fact ... (Wolberg, 1977: 1066).

> *Pt.* I'm afraid of being hurt.
> *Th.* You're afraid of being hurt. Rejected? (Wolberg, 1977: 1067).

Whether it was through the offering up of a pin-pointing emotional term that carried a weight of resonance with it, and which the patient then went on to adopt, or whether it was the case of the therapist's introduction of a new term, with a different weighting of meaning altogether (as in the case of 'resent' and 'rejected'), either way the therapist appeared to play an active role in co-constructing the meaning of the therapeutic narrative. Although generally accurate in a reflective manner, such comments nonetheless effectively narrowed down what the patient could say, and 'streamed' the therapeutic narrative toward a certain destination of meaning.

### Interpellations of meaning and emotion

The use of probing, pin-pointing or narrative-generating words or half sentences involved an important interpellative function, in the sense that it 'hailed' patients or called them to answer or complete them, in ways that they could not resist or, perhaps more accurately, decline to answer (cf. Althusser, 1971). (It is important here to briefly distinguish the notion of construction from that of interpellation. Whereas construction, for the purposes of this chapter, refers to the discursive generation of *meaning*, interpellation refers to the tactical *positioning* of the subject by virtue of which *he/she* is made to actively adopt and extend the influence of power *over him-/herself*. So whereas the notion of construction prioritises the production of *discursive meaning* as an outcome of power, interpellation prioritises certain subject positions, certain roles and their attendant *behaviours* as the outcome of largely irrefutable forms of influence and suggestion.)

More than simply co-constructing patients' therapeutic narratives, then, psychotherapists could be said to have played a part in *interpellating* the meanings of patients' therapeutic narratives by making compelling and largely irrefutable contributions to the development of these accounts of self. Indeed, despite the fact that some latitude was granted patients in exactly how they picked up on such contributions, the point is that, practically speaking, within the therapeutic encounter, they *had* to be picked up on, answered and integrated within the patients' developing sense of self. This was not simply a case of the therapists 'putting words into someone's mouth', because the patients could, and at times did, refute such meanings. It was, however, a case of the therapists bringing meaning into the sessions that, once introduced, could not be simply ignored, removed, 'undone' or 'voided'. The patients had in some ways to 'take these up', to confront them, to take them into account and/or integrate them within the context of the present therapeutic narrative and in the context of their own developing self-awareness, even if that were to mean apparently rejecting them.

Such interpellative comments were introduced in a number of ways. The use of an 'echoing voice', of reflection and of forms of synopsis and summary all played a role in delineating and narrowing the therapeutic narrative. Such a 'narrowing' also occurred through the reinflection of meanings, and through 'checks' of meaning ('Am I understanding you rightly when you say …?'; 'So you were angry to hear that …'). This interpellation tended to occur most effectively once it had taken the form of hypothesising about the patient's motives and emotions, e.g. 'You acted in that way so that …'; 'That must have made you feel …'. The general 'murkiness' of emotions, their overlapping qualities, their lack of clear-cut distinction and the way they lend themselves to distortion over time made them easy targets for the interpellative powers of the psychotherapist. Take for instance the struggle of emotional meaning contained in the following extract:

> (Speaking of the man that a friend of the patient recently married, the therapist asks):
> Th. Does he appeal to you at all?
> Pt. To be married to? No.
> Th. Not at all?
> Pt. Well, he's nice. I like him, I respect him, but for marriage, no.
> Th. There's no jealousy at all?
> Pt. No, not at all.
> Th. No envy of this woman?
> Pt. No, no. Why, did you feel there might have been?
> Th. Well, I don't know. I'm just thinking about that dream … .
> Pt. Well, I … (patient goes on to discuss past bitterness with the aforementioned friend).

Certainly, a fundamental factor in the therapist's 'warrant' to make emotional attributions in the extract above was the very ambiguity and instability of emotions once retrospectively reconstructed. This example is useful in another way also: it makes clear the extent to which therapists in general maintained a powerful authorial privilege in the therapeutic narrative. (In fact, this would seem to be implicit to psychotherapy in general, given the assumption that therapists are able to detect meanings and emotions in patients' narratives that may in fact remain hidden to patients themselves.) This authorial privilege is clearly evidenced in the above example, when, despite her own repeated denials, the patient eventually asks the therapist whether *he* thought she may have in fact been jealous despite her feelings to the contrary. The important point here is that such interpellations may be thought of as having an impact on the level of *patient subjectivity*, on the ways and means by which patients continue to gain self-understanding and on the dispositions to behave and act that stem from such 'therapeutic' realisations.

The interpellative powers of the psychotherapist also appeared to include the capacity for a form of emotional influence. Typically, reflective statements ('That must have been very difficult for you'; 'You find that very difficult to accept …'), like 'cueing' prompts ('Uh-huh'; 'Go on'; 'Take your time'), while generally accorded an empathetic value in the literature, appeared to possess a more complex interventional value in the analysis. Analysing such reflective comments not merely on the basis of their clinical meaning, but on the linguistic basis *of the action of language in use*, I found that such responses were a strong way of *enforcing emotional experiences within patients*. A key tactic in this regard was the use of pin-pointing emotional terms that refined the patients' given meaning and that were unconditional and direct in their identification of strong labels for evidenced emotions. Such terms were often stronger and more extreme in degree than the words the patients were using, so as to highlight, in an unremitting way, the power of underlying emotions, to ostensibly therapeutic ends.

As an example of this, when a patient stated that she was left without support after her husband and sister died, the therapist retorted, probingly, that she felt 'totally isolated' and 'alone'. Similarly, when a patient said she felt empty and without hope after a certain unfortunate event, the therapist distilled this meaning by 'reflecting' that she felt 'devastated'. More than supporting a growing emotional reality of meaning, this kind of reflection/repetition/reinflection possessed a rhetorical 'irrefutability'. Like rhetorical questions that require no answer and are directed primarily at making an effect, rhetorical statements of this sort kept the patients' 'manoeuvring room' to a minimum, and effectively closed down the patients' ability to differently position themselves in relation to the reality of the developing therapeutic narrative.

In this way, more than simply being vehicles of empathy or reflection, these kinds of statements had an accentuating and emphasising function that furthered meaning and amplified it in the direction pursued by the therapist, whether that was of facilitating catharsis, pursuing the 'corrective emotional experience' or attaining revealing personal insight. In a sense, then, it is true to say that therapists were able to 'make their patients cry', to steer them, where deemed clinically effective, into provocative emotional terrains, and to elicit strong, actual, *in vivo* emotional responses. Take for example the following extract, in which the therapist 'built the patient up' with reflective comments, and then pin-pointed a lack in her life with the focused and tactical use of questioning:

> *Pt.* ... I've been going a long time with these people .... You know how it is .... And I feel as if I'm neglecting them if I don't call them and say, 'How are you?' ... Isn't it awful?
> *Th.* It must be kind of tough for you.
> *Pt.* It is. It really is. You see what I mean. And that's about all there is to it.
> *Th.* Do you think you need a few new interests?
> *Pt.* Well, there's no question ....
> *Th.* Have you ever done anything – hobbies, art, anything?
> *Pt.* No, all I've ever done ... is work at our book business. You see what I mean? ... Well you know ... you do that for 22 years, and then I finally got out of it ... I couldn't stand it any more.
> *Th.* Apparently it was more than you could stand.
> *Pt.* That's why I got out of it. (*cries*)
> *Th.* You've suffered a great deal (Wolberg, 1977: 1053).

The therapist here has made use of a kind of unrelenting reflection, a confrontation of the patient with the powerful emotional reality of the presenting problem. It is this special focusing that appears to have 'broken the wall' for the patient and brought a formidable level of emotion to the fore. Basically, then, the therapist is instrumental in both the construction *and the interpellation* of the patient's therapeutic narrative. The psychotherapist is participant both in the discursive production of certain meanings within the therapy session and in the active positioning of the patient in relationship to the 'irrefutability' of a variety of co-constructed meanings, emotional values and experiences.

### Therapeutic 'role-induction'

A further apparent means of interpellation that therapists had at their disposal was that of therapeutic 'role-induction', i.e. the ability to ensure that patients adopted appropriate 'patient roles' and responsibilities in the clinical setting. In fact, such a role-induction appeared to have underscored many of my earlier observations, particularly with reference to the typical willingness and appropriateness of patients' participations (and investments) in psychotherapy. The extent to which patients seemed so active, so 'obedient' and in fact *proactive* in their therapeutic treatment, particularly following the first few sessions of treatment, the extent to which they seemed to independently and almost enthusiastically 'take up' the patient role, made for an intriguing analytical challenge for me.

The notion of interpellation again proved helpful here, particularly in the sense of a *role interpellation*, in which the therapists would, in multiple ways, position their patients *as patients* by never interacting with them in any way that might exceed the patient-doctor relationship. (One might argue that psychodynamic forms of psychotherapy, with their strong emphasis on the professional detachment of clinicians and on the therapist's qualities of anonymity, neutrality and personal distance, operate such forms of role interpellation implicitly and intrinsically by virtue of the basic structure of the form of intervention.) The notion of such a form of interpellation, namely role-induction, enabled me to account for the readiness and appropriateness with which the majority of patients took to the patient role. Similarly, it helped explain how patients seemed to so naturally structure their therapeutic narratives around self-attending and problem-centred focuses (not to mention the readiness and frankness of the often personally compromising disclosures made by patients within treatment). Furthermore, this notion of role-induction also helped explain how a variety of frame elements (and other contingencies, like patients' assumptions and expectations of the therapeutic process) could be so vitally mobilised by therapists as *functional aspects* of the therapeutic work.

This role-induction hypothesis was arrived at by a variety of cross-sectional comparisons of type-type role behaviours across the progress of psychotherapy. To use a familiar example, the concerted performance of *'therapeutic listening'* by the psychotherapist was typically enough to elicit, and be accompanied and matched by, the appropriate therapeutic response of *personal disclosure* on the part of a patient. Similarly, the therapist's role of *authoritative interpreter* was typically enough to elicit, and be matched by, the appropriate role of *attentive learner* on the part of the patient, just as the patient's role of *expositor* was marked, conditioned and elicited by the therapist's role of *empathetic facilitator*, and so on. Just as therapeutic constructions of meaning were contributed to by both 'partners' of a dialogue, and were hence indivisibly mutual, so the acting of appropriate therapeutic roles, while largely initiated and controlled by the therapist, as similarly mutual, 'interlocked', interdependent and mutually constructive. Basically, such pairing relationships, such role-inductions, where each aspect of the therapist's clinical function elicited suitable, *reactive* role-appropriate behaviour on the patient's part, were strongly characterising features of the therapeutic interaction.

We can therefore assert the eighth strand of the developing argument: therapists exercised not only an important authorial privilege in leading, amplifying and co-constructing patients' therapeutic narratives, *they also exercised an important interpellative function by virtue of which they were able to irrefutably position patients in relation to a given set of therapeutic meanings, emotions and roles. Role-induction appeared to be the most basic of these various forms of interpellation.*

## Constructing ailments

The interpellative capacity with which therapists were able to use words, emotions and roles within psychotherapy seemed most apparent in their attempts to probe for, and then solidify, psychological problems *within* patients. A brief example illustrates how the therapist was able to place the attribution of emotional disturbance within the patient's narrative. Here the probe for emotions capitalised on current feelings exhibited by the patient, and, in fact, the apparent anger of the resistant patient was very nearly transformed into the emerging surface of a larger presenting problem:

> Pt. Dr ... sent me here for these headaches. He thinks it might be mental. I really don't think it was necessary for me to come.
> Th. Do you believe it's mental?
> Pt. Good Lord, No! I think I need something that will ease this pain, I've been told a million different things of what's wrong.
> Th. Perhaps you are right. It may be entirely physical. What examinations have you had?
> Pt. *(Patient details the many consultations that he has had, maintaining his position that his problem is physiological.)*
> Th. Then it perhaps made you angry to come here?
> Pt. I was angry. Not now though. Do you think you can help this headache?
> Th. I'm not sure; but if you tell me about the trouble from the beginning, I might be able to help you with any emotional factors that can stir up a headache.
> Pt. How can that do it? I know I have been emotional about it (Wolberg, 1977: 398).

Noteworthy here is the way in which the therapist has asserted an emotional problem, if not as the fundamental complaint, then as undeniably attached to, or as having intrinsically surrounded the presenting complaint. Basically, then, the therapist leaves the patient with very little room to escape his expert attentions and suggestions. Despite the fact that there is sometimes quite plainly resistance to these emotional attributions, expressed through doubt and refutation, the patient nonetheless ends up 'picking up' the threads of language placed within the therapeutic narrative by the therapist and absorbing them into their self-explanations. Be it through agreement or even denial and refutation, the strategic situation of certain hypotheses or questions about emotional disturbance (on the part of the therapist) places these assertions squarely as dominant features of the therapeutic narrative with which the patient has to engage on a subjective level.

Important in the following extract is the distinction between physical and emotional symptoms that ultimately appears to be collapsed by the therapist's interpellative probing of emotional forms of disturbance. Interesting also is the number of times that the patient refutes the therapist's emotional attributions, and the struggle that occurs over such an attribution of feelings and emotional difficulties. Indeed, these appeared to be key stakes in the development of the therapeutic narrative, and in the struggle for authorship that infrequently accompanied its development:

*Pt.* But how can stomach trouble be caused by the mind?

*Th.* The brain is connected to every organ in the body, and when a person is disturbed, it is understandable that the disturbance or worry or conflict can get into every organ of the body ... .

*Pt.* But there's nothing wrong with my mind. I'm not worried about anything except this pain and how to get rid of it.

*Th.* Perhaps that's right. As a matter of fact you may have something really wrong with your stomach ... .

*Pt.* Do *you* think there is nothing wrong with my stomach?

*Th.* There must be something wrong; otherwise you wouldn't have any pain. The question is whether the cause of the pain is emotional, or organic, or both. Frankly I don't know which it is, since I'm not too acquainted with your condition. But from your account nothing organic has been found. And you've had good doctors. Dr ... is a good doctor; he's conservative, and he sent you to me, which shows he feels there is at least the possibility of an emotional factor.

*Pt.* But what could it be, if it isn't my stomach?

*Th.* You mean what would the emotional factors be if your stomach trouble was not organic?

*Pt.* Yes.

*Th.* That's why you were referred to me. Perhaps we might be able to find out. You know emotional trouble can give you a bigger bellyache than physical trouble ... . Apparently you can't accept this fact as applying to you. Maybe you think it is disgraceful to have emotional problems?

*Pt.* ... Well, maybe it's so, but I don't, can't see, how. Wouldn't I know if there was something wrong with my mind ...?

*Th.* With your emotions you mean? ...

*Pt.* ... do you think *you* can help me?

*Th.* If you have an emotional problem that is causing this trouble, yes, that is if you really want to be helped ... but you are still not convinced. Why don't you think things over, and, if you'd like to give this a try – with an open mind I mean – call me and we'll get started.

*Pt.* I get pain over here. (*points to his abdomen*) ... it drives me practically out of my mind.

*Th.* You know, a person with even a real organic problem ... can get very upset. And his emotional tension can in turn stir up trouble for him ... . So you see, emotional trouble, worry and tension can upset your stomach (Wolberg, 1977: 466–7).

Probing of this sort, while clinically valid both as a way of surfacing material that the patient would otherwise avoid and as a means of approaching more pressing problems than those first identified by the patient, creates an interpellative net of emotional ailments that the patient cannot escape from. Therapists are lent this interpellative 'net' of ailments by virtue of the ubiquity of feelings, and by their ability to characterise certain emotions as extreme for their context, when in fact they may be relatively reasonable. As suggested earlier, propositions of emotionality lack comparative frames of reference, just as they lack accurate measures of degree. In this way, extending the eighth general proposition of my building argument and introducing its ninth strand, we may assert that *therapists have what may be considered 'an interpellative net of emotional ailments', a powerful latitude in identifying and fixing the strength and appropriateness of feelings within patients, and in ascertaining the 'pathology' within such feelings.*

## Declarative powers

The constructive and interpellative capacities of the psychotherapist were substantiated by a more crude instructive or *declarative* power that was difficult at first to ascertain, precisely because it functioned so implicitly. Attempting to generate an explanation for why there was such a (relative) lack of resistance among patients to therapists' interpretations, directions and suggestions within the psychotherapy, I turned to examine exactly how the therapists *themselves* bolstered and validated their contributions to the therapeutic narrative. The answer, as provided by therapists themselves, proved to be fairly easily forthcoming:

> Th. ... as we begin to talk about your problems, things will become more obvious to me than to you. This is because I can be more objective than you. You live too close to your problems to be objective about them. Second, I'm trained to do psychotherapy and can see the problems better (Wolberg, 1977: 1050).

Basically, therapists' contributions to the therapy were authoritative and loaded with the weight of a qualified and professional sense of 'psychological expertise', factors that they themselves did not typically seek to minimise. The contributions of therapists hence functioned, particularly from the perspective of the patient hopeful for a cure, in a *definitive* or *prescriptive* rather than a descriptive or hypothetical manner. In this way, even the slightest indications and suggestions of the therapist carried an implicit instructive force, despite frequently being voiced in the indefinite sense:

> Pt. ... I'm being forced to see those old friends who are bores and whom I don't want to see. What can I do?
> Th. It may be that you have to take a stand with some of your friends (Wolberg, 1977: 1053).

Never informal (i.e. personal), never unconditionally direct, these guarded therapeutic suggestions never took the form of advice or prescription, while implicitly managing to fulfil this function nevertheless. Indeed, this form of instructing was overwhelmingly managed by implication, not so much by *what* was said, but by *how* it was said. The following extract contains the therapist's notes on tone and inflection, given in square brackets:

> Pt. ... it all seems so hopeless.
> Th. Particularly when you give, give, give, and nothing happens. [*implying indirectly that she gives materially to make up for a lack of substance within herself*]
> Pt. I always enjoy doing things for people.
> Th. I guess you do. (*pause*) [*this is said a little ironically*]
> Pt. Why, is that wrong ...? [*the patient picks up the irony of my tone*]

>    *Th.* Why should it be wrong?
>    *Pt.* I don't know.
>    *Th.* Let me ask you this, do *you* enjoy having people do things for *you*? (Wolberg, 1977: 1062).

Evidence of the instructive force of therapists' contributions was particularly noticeable in comments made by patients:

>    *Pt.* Yes, doctor, I see what you mean (Wolberg, 1977: 1063).

>    *Pt.* Yes, I can see. I can see how what you've told me is true (Wolberg, 1977: 1088).

>    *Pt.* Yes, and then I felt, well Dr. Wolberg says no, that sort of thing is just poison for me, and why do I want anything that isn't good? (Wolberg, 1977: 1089).

The instructive power of the therapist is clearly evoked in the following passage (the patient's part of the dialogue has been omitted to foreground the therapist's instructive role):

> (*Speaking of the patient's always giving, never receiving pattern of interaction*):
> *Th.* You really feel you haven't been on the receiving end? You've been on the giving end.... To be on the receiving end, you'll have to think enough of yourself so that you feel you can deserve receiving.... The best way is through good relations with people. Perhaps you minimize a lot of things that you have about yourself.... Well it isn't too late to change.... It's important for you to be discriminating, even if you wait.... Another experience that tears you down will be very hard to bear.... You've already gone through enough, except for that one interlude in your life.... If it comes again you have to be ready for it. You can't expect to be ready if you have a bad opinion of yourself. If you correct the bad opinion of yourself, when someone worthy comes along, you'll be able to accept the situation.... There is one thing you may have to watch for when you meet a worthwhile person. In the face of this man's apparent good qualities, you may say to yourself, 'Well, gosh, he'll never see anything in *me*. Why should I get myself messed up over him? If he sees something in me, it's because he just wants sex, or because he wants to take advantage of me, or something like that; it isn't likely that he respects me for myself.' And after that, you won't give him a chance; you'll just run like a deer. Now you've got to build up this estimate of yourself, if things are to be different. We have a fairly good idea of the origin of this bad estimate of yourself in your early upbringing. But this has produced in you an extremely insidious situation in which you keep on despising yourself, in which you feel you have no inherent qualities, in which you feel that you can only be loved for what you can do for people, and not for yourself. Now these patterns keep messing you all up ... (Wolberg, 1977: 1080).

In this lengthy extract, the therapist 'tells how it is', and provides a summarising and definitive assessment of the patient's typical patterns of interaction, rooted in the patient's early determining history. This is more than a description or a general likeness, it is *the* conclusive, clinical distillation of the patient's problem. By virtue of his expertise and qualifications, his clinical experience and knowledge, the offerings of the psychotherapist, whether interpretations, hypotheses, tacit suggestions or confrontations, carried powerful and prescriptive claims of truth. Quite simply put, the therapists generally had a privileged vantage on the truth of the patients' psychological lives; they were in possession of a more accurate and effective psychological knowledge of patients than patients themselves were. So we can state the tenth and final strand of the argument: *there is, practically speaking, no higher authority within psychotherapy on the psychological life (and prospective psychopathology) of the patients than the psychotherapists themselves, whose therapeutic contributions typically function, on the part of the patients, as definitive and prescriptive rather than descriptive or hypothetical.*

## ■ Synthesis and conclusion

The foregoing argument asserted a series of basic, interlocking deductions. It claimed that psychotherapy constituted something of an evaluative space that was successful in drawing out largely automatic, self-initiating and self-responsible forms of self-evaluation from patients. These functions were lent momentum by the systematic assertion of the subjectivity and agency of patients, and by the therapeutic development of practices of personal reflexivity on their part. This 'subjectivisation' of patients was attached to another psychotherapeutic function: the ability to install persistent and durable 'therapeutic subject positions', i.e. self-problematising and self-correcting tendencies within patients that, typically, appeared to outlast the therapeutic encounter. Therapists also exercised an important authorial privilege in leading, developing, amplifying and co-constructing patients' therapeutic meanings, emotions and role-appropriate behaviours. Taking this one step further, therapists also had at their disposal a variety of rhetorical and questioning abilities. These abilities, taken in conjunction with the therapeutic ability to reconstruct the therapeutic narratives of patients, provided psychotherapists with a broad constructive latitude with which they were able to discursively generate psychopathology within patients' accounts of themselves.

Attached to this capability, therapists appeared to maintain what may be considered 'an interpellative net of emotional ailments', i.e. the discretionary power to ascertain the latent 'pathology' within emotions. More than just playing a role in co-constructing patients' therapeutic meanings, emotions and roles, therapists also possessed a powerful interpellative function, by which such meanings, emotions and roles were definitely imposed upon patients in a manner difficult to effectively refute. Further solidifying this interpellative power was the instructive or declarative force of therapists' therapeutic pronouncements, which, from the perspective of patients, often appeared to function as definitive and prescriptive rather merely descriptive or hypothetical. Lastly, and as a way of pulling together the critical impetus of these collected arguments, the 'problem-centric' nature of the process, along with the tactical and technical abilities afforded therapists in order to 'discover' psychopathology, ultimately lacked a balancing set of controls or a means of effective opposition, a fact plainly advanced in the assertion that there was, practically speaking, no higher authority within the psychotherapy on the psychological life (and prospective psychopathology) of the patients than the psychotherapists themselves.

There were a number of arguments within the foregoing critical literature that the results of the above study did not explicitly affirm. The study did not have sufficient basis to assert that psychotherapy necessarily reproduced dominant socio-political asymmetries of power, that it operated as a satellite institution for broadly articulated state interests or that it necessarily implemented forms of 'psychological reductionism' within its patients (although one might speculate that with a different analytical framework, such results may have been more forthcoming). Similarly, this study was unable to provide explicit support for contentions that psychotherapy damages patients through: 1) overt forms of victim-blaming, 2) the perpetuation of certain ideological discourses (or unrealistic, ideal social norms), 3) the substantiation of stigmatising diagnostic labels, or 4) functioning as a prescriptive moral-discursive formation. This apparent lack of support should, however, not be taken as necessarily contesting or 'disproving' these arguments. Rather, it should, perhaps more appropriately, be contextualised with reference to the limitations of a study whose micropolitical, face-to-face level of analysis was not necessarily suitable for the testing of larger-scale socio-political arguments about the functioning of power in the psychotherapeutic realm more generally.

There were, however, a variety of themes from the critical literature that this study *did* resonate with. Firstly, the fact that psychotherapy succeeded with such regularity in constituting an 'evaluative space' and eliciting normative self-evaluations on the part of patients certainly did suggest that psychotherapy was a normalising intervention, particularly in the sense of *a self-problematising technology designed to bring the self into question on the basis of dominant socio-political norms*. The upshot of this was, as I mentioned earlier, that one can never be too normal, or absolutely free of potential psychological maladaptation. Accordingly, the results of the study certainly did support the contention of Isack and Hook (1996) that everyone, at some time, may be construed as in need of psychotherapeutic assistance and as potentially psychopathological. In fact, the results extended this argument by suggesting that, once the patient is within psychotherapy, it is almost inevitable that some node of pathology will be 'discovered', whether or not this might represent a necessary or even realistic basis for intervention.

The critical notion that psychotherapy 'interiorises' problems, which then become the individual responsibility of patients, was similarly supported by the study. Indeed, the inordinate focus on patient egocentricity, reflexivity, subjectivity and agency certainly supported these suggestions, as did the fact that self-evaluative procedures became so quickly the automatic functions of the patient's own initiative. More than just this, the results of the study suggested that psychotherapy often installed a permanent self-problematising voice within patients through the cultivation of a 'therapeutic subject position', in which the patients increasingly internalised the role and speaking voice of the psychotherapist.

Likewise, the study did affirm that psychotherapy exudes a 'pathologising gravity'. There seemed little doubt that psychotherapists possessed various constructive, rhetorical and questioning abilities through which convincing indications and suggestions of psycopathology could quite easily be reconstructed out of patients' therapeutic narratives. In short, psychotherapists maintained an authorial privilege in the development of therapeutic narratives, a broad constructive latitude with which to generate certain 'nodes of psychopathology' within patients. The study hence definitely supported the contention of Parker *et al.* (1995) that broadly diagnostic or problem-ascertaining activities on the part of therapists could be said to be more 'justificatory arguments' than merely 'objective signs'. Similarly, the idea that therapists have access to a 'psychotherapeutic discourse' of specialist terms and rhetorical devices that are both difficult to refute and intrinsically instructive, or prescriptive, was unequivocally supported by the results of the study. This makes one question the extent to which psychopathology may be said to exist independently, or wholly outside of, such psychotherapeutic forms of discourse.

Furthermore, Gergen's (1992) idea that psychotherapists control the discourses of psychopathology in a privileged and largely uncontested way was empirically substantiated by the results of the study. Less directly, but importantly nonetheless, Szasz's (1961, 1973) critique of psychiatry's/psychology's adoption of the medical model was also, albeit obliquely, supported by the study. The fact that emotions, along with a variety of seemingly everyday problems, came to be framed as lying within the jurisdiction of specialist and professional pseudo-medical (psychotherapeutic) practices certainly reiterated his suspicions that psychology/psychiatry makes illegitimate claims and advances of 'psychopathology' over that which should not necessarily be seen as problematic or as even in fact necessarily *psychological*. Indeed, the fact that therapists had at their disposal an 'interpellative net of emotional ailments' through which feelings could basically be 'psychopathologised' and centred as the fundamental rationale for ongoing psychotherapeutic intervention most certainly reproduced the basic logic of Szasz's critique.

## Psychotherapeutic technology

One might therefore suggest, on the basis of the links between the critical literature and the current study described above, that there are alternative grids of analysis to that of *curative effect* through which one might gauge the workings of 'therapeutic efficacy'. Indeed, on the basis of these links, one may affirm with some confidence the notion, asserted by Foucault (1977) and Rose (1991, 1995), that psychotherapeutic intervention may be likened to a *technology*, in the sense of a set of applied skills, techniques, strategies and specialised forms of knowledge and language used conjointly as part of a systematic goal of control. In fact, in this way, one might recode the workings and efficacy of psychotherapy not with reference to a vocabulary of therapeutic healing or to a register of amelioration and benefit, but instead with reference to a powerful therapeutic *technology* of attempted change, control and influence.

No doubt such a conceptualisation may not sit well with many practitioners, perhaps principally because of its anti-humanist overtones. Indeed, this conceptualisation has a mechanistic and almost behaviourist ring to it, which suggests that psychotherapy is a procedure where 'certain buttons are pushed' and certain therapeutic outcomes are routinely, and reliably, obtained as a result. Assuredly, this is a 'technicist' take on psychotherapy, one that has adopted a refined *technical focus* to understanding precisely those aspects of therapeutic interaction typically considered most therapeutically efficacious. The pragmatic adopted here is the belief that to understand how power functions within psychotherapy, one needs to look exactly at those operations of greatest therapeutic impact. It is at precisely these points of therapeutic efficacy where we will find the resources of psychotherapy's power, those resources that drive and enable its psychopathologising potential. These are the points of psychotherapy where, by the same token, 'ground-breaking' clinical work is managed, where the therapist-patient power differential is at its most asymmetrical, and where the possibility of clinical breakthrough is matched by the technological ascendancy of the therapist. It is here where clinical and political power coincide almost completely, if in fact they may be considered discernible at all.

On this basis, one might surmise that psychotherapy is a highly technological and power-ridden process that attains its clinical efficacy exactly by virtue of the wide power differential it embodies, and by its technological sophistication that mobilises applied skills, techniques and strategies and specialised forms of knowledge and language. Building on this argument, one might suggest that psychopathology is the *raison d'etre* of psychotherapy, its prime object and its means of sustenance. It is that which acts as the motivating rationale that both validates and warrants psychotherapy and enables and extends the ongoing perpetuation of its practice.

Here we are reminded of the abovementioned assertions of the 'problem-centric' nature and structure of the psychotherapeutic process. Here too we are reminded of similar assertions that the technical and tactical abilities afforded therapists to 'discover' psychopathology appear to lack an adequate basis of refutation from which patients may contest or resist such productive efforts. It is both the case, then, that psychotherapists have a dazzling array of instruments and resources with which to 'call psychopathology into being', and that this productive capacity is fundamentally inequitable. If we are to believe those critics like Isack and Hook (1996) and Parker and Hook (forthcoming) who claim that psychotherapy entails a staunch and active economic imperative to uncover and substantiate psychopathology, then this combination of technological prowess with such a psychopathology-seeking imperative poses a substantial ethical dilemma. If it is the case that psychotherapy, like the individual psychotherapist, has enormous investments of career and identity in this entity, then it may well be, as suggested earlier by Isack and Hook (1996), that there is never a therapeutic interaction without an attendant gravity, or even in fact a *compulsion*, to unearth, substantiate and treat psychopathology.

Rather than a *precondition* of psychotherapy, psychopathology may be a *function of psychotherapy*, an outcome of a psychotherapeutic interchange designed and structured to engender psychopathology, to relentlessly seek it out, and to discursively substantiate it and its various approximating forms. In fact, it may well be the case, to apply Said's (1983) maxim, that psychotherapy is a discourse that manufactures its material (of psychopathology) continually, so as to continually expand its regime of control over that which it constitutes as its special domain. If it is the case that a great deal of the formidable technology of psychotherapy is weighted towards the detection, substantiation and foreclosure of pathology, then psychotherapy comes dangerously close to being an iatrogenic process. Further yet, if it is the case that the gravity to discover psychopathology within psychotherapy is at times so overbearingly strong that the therapist cannot fail *but* to uncover some suitable 'problem in living', some suitable 'working focus' for the therapy, then psychotherapy is *a constitutively iatrogenic form of treatment*. And this is the ethical conundrum and the question of paramount importance for all of those engaged in the discipline and practice of the psy-sciences: if psychotherapy is iatrogenic in this sense, then how can it continue to be thought of as an ethically viable activity?

Given that psychopathology is the very basis of psychotherapy's existence, the necessary, apparent 'precondition' and 'working focus' of ongoing treatment, it should come as no surprise that psychotherapy can, and in fact *does*, produce psychopathology. What, by contrast, *should* come as a surprise is that there are ever-presenting forms of psychopathology that are *not* called into being, that are not given form, substance and a practicable 'interventional reality' by so formidable a technology.

# ■ References

Albee, G. W. (1990). The futility of psychotherapy. *Journal of Mind and Behaviour*, 11 (3–4), 369–84.
Althusser, L. (1971). *Lenin and Philosophy and Other Essays*. New York: Monthly Review Press.
American Psychiatric Association (1994). *Diagnostic and Statistical Manual of Mental Disorders* (4th edn). Washington, DC: American Psychiatric Association.
Bernardez, T. (1988). Gender based countertransference of female therapists in the psychotherapy of women. In M. Braude (ed.), *Women, Power and Therapy*, pp. 25–40. New York: Harrington Park Press.
Braude, M. (1988). *Women, Power and Therapy*. New York: Harrington Park Press.
Brown, P. (1990). The name game: Toward a sociology of diagnosis. *Journal of Mind and Behaviour*, 11 (3–4), 385–406.
Bryson, N. (1993). House of wax. In R. Krauss (ed.), *Cindy Sherman 1975–1993*, pp. 4–23. New York: Rizzoli International.
Burman, E. and Parker, I. (eds) (1993). *Discourse Analytic Research: Repertoires and Readings of Texts in Action*. London: Routledge.
Burr, V. (1996). *An Introduction to Social Constructionism*. London: Routledge.
Chesler, P. (1972). *Women and Madness*. San Diego: Harcourt Brace Jovanich.
Cross, J. (1994). Politics and family therapy. *Dulwich Centre Newsletter*, 1, 7–10.
Cushman, P. (1990). Towards a historically situated psychology. *American Psychologist*, 45 (5), 599–611.
Cushman, P. (1991). Ideology obscured political uses of the self in Daniel Stern's infant. *American Psychologist*, 46 (3), 206–19.
Cushman, P. (1992). Psychotherapy to 1992: A historically situated interpretation. In D. K. Freedheim (ed.), *History of Psychotherapy: A Century of Change*, pp. 21–63. Washington, DC: American Psychological Association.
Dawes, A. (1985). Politics and mental health: The position of clinical psychology in South Africa. *South African Journal of Psychology*, 15, 55–61.
DeVaris, J. (1994). The dynamics of power in psychotherapy. *Psychotherapy*, 12 (4), 588–93.
Dreyfus, H. L. and Rabinow, P. (1982). *Michel Foucault beyond Structuralism and Hermeneutics*. New York: Harvester Wheatsheaf.
Fillingham, L. A. (1993). *Foucault*. New York: Writers and Readers Publishing.
Foucault, M. (1977). *Discipline and Punish: The Birth of the Prison*. Harmondsworth: Penguin.
Foucault, M. (1978). *The History of Sexuality: An Introduction*, Vol. 1. London: Random House.
Gergen, K. J. (1991). *The Saturated Self: Dilemmas of Identity in Contemporary Life*. New York: Basic Books.

Gergen, K. J. (1992). Towards a postmodern psychology. In S. Kvale (ed.), *Psychology and Postmodernism*, pp. 17–30. London: Sage.
Gergen, K. J. (1994). Exploring the postmodern perils or potentials? *American Psychologist*, 49 (5), 412–16.
Glaser, B. G. (1992). *Basics of Grounded Theory Analysis.* Mill Valley: CA Sociology Press.
Glaser, B. G. and Strauss, A. L. (1967). *The Discovery of Grounded Theory Strategies for Qualitative Research.* Chicago: Aldine.
Hare-Mustin, R. T. and Marecek, J. (1997). Abnormal and clinical psychology: The politics of madness. In D. Fox and I. Prilleltensky (eds), *Critical Psychology: An Introduction*, pp. 104–20. London: Sage.
Harper, D. J. (1994). The professional construction of paranoia and the discursive use of diagnostic criteria. *British Journal of Medical Psychology*, 67, 131–43.
Holmes, J. and Lindley, R. (1989). *The Values of Psychotherapy.* Oxford: Oxford University Press.
Hook, D. (1999). Power in psychodynamic psychotherapy. Unpublished masters thesis, University of the Witwatersrand.
Ingelby, D. (1985). Professionals as socializers. *Research in Law, Deviance, and Social Control*, 7, 79–109.
Isack, S. and Hook, D. (1996). The psychological imperialism of psychotherapy. *Changes International Journal of Psychology and Psychotherapy*, 14 (4), 306–13.
Kaye, J. (1999). Toward a non-regulative praxis. In I. Parker (ed.), *Deconstructing Psychotherapy*, pp. 19–38. London: Sage.
Layder, D. (1993). *New Strategies in Social Research.* Cambridge: Polity Press.
Masson, J. (1993). *Against Therapy.* London: Harper Collins.
Masson, J. (1994). The tyranny of psychotherapy. In W. Dryden and C. Feltham (eds), *Psychotherapy and its Discontents*, pp. 7–28. Buckingham and Philadelphia: Open University Press.
Nugent, C. D. (1994). Blaming the victims: Silencing women sexually exploited by psychotherapists. *Journal of Mind and Behaviour*, 15 (1–2), 113–38.
Parker, I. (1998). Against psychotherapy. *Sunday Times* (UK), September 20, p. 16.
Parker, I., Georgaca, E., Harper, D., McLaughlin, T. and Stowell-Smith, M. (1995). *Deconstructing Psychopathology.* London: Sage.
Parker, I. and Hook, D. (forthcoming). Deconstruction, psychotherapy and dialectics. *South African Journal of Psychology.*
Pidgeon, N. (1996). Grounded theory: Theoretical background. In J. T. E. Richardson (ed.), *Handbook of Qualitative Research for Psychology and the Social Sciences*, pp. 75–85. Leicester: BPS Press.
Pidgeon, N. and Henwood, K. (1996) Grounded theory: Practical implementation. In J. T. E. Richardson (ed.), *Handbook of Qualitative Research for Psychology and the Social Sciences*, pp. 86–101. Leicester: BPS Press.
Pilgrim, D. (1991). Psychotherapy and social blinkers. *The Psychologist*, 2, 52–5.
Pilgrim, D. (1994). Psychotherapy and political evasions. In W. Dryden and C. Feltham (eds), *Psychotherapy and its Discontents*, pp. 225–42. Buckingham and Philadelphia: Open University Press.
Potter, J. and Wetherell, M. (1987). *Discourse and Social Psychology: Beyond Attitudes and Behaviour.* London: Sage.
Richer, P. (1992). An introduction to postmodern psychology. In S. Kvale (ed.), *Psychology and Postmodernism*, pp. 31–74. London: Sage.
Rose, N. (1991). *Governing the Soul: The Shaping of the Private Self.* London and New York: Routledge.
Rose, N. (1995). *Inventing Our Selves.* London and New York: Routledge.
Said, E. (1983). *The World, the Text and the Critic.* Cambridge, Mass.: Harvard University Press.
Salmon, P. (1991). Psychotherapy and the wider world. *The Psychologist*, 2, 50–1.
Sampson, E. E. (1981). Cognitive psychology as ideology. *American Psychologist*, 36 (7), 730–43.

Sampson, E. E. (1992). The deconstruction of self. In J. Shotter and K. J. Gergen (eds), *Texts of Identity*, pp. 1–19. London: Routledge.
Spinelli, E. (1994). *Demystifying Therapy.* London: Constable.
Strauss, A. L. and Corbin, J. M. (1990). *Basics of Qualitative Research: Grounded Theory Procedures and Techniques.* Newbury Park: Sage.
Strauss, A. L. and Corbin, J. M. (1997). *Grounded Theory in Practice.* London: Sage.
Szasz, T. S. (1961). *The Myth of Mental Illness.* New York: Harpar.
Szasz, T. S. (1973). *The Second Sin.* New York: Routledge and Kegan Paul.
Szasz, T. S. (1974). *The Ethics of Psychoanalysis.* London: Routledge and Kegan Paul.
Szasz, T. S. (1979). *The Myth of Psychotherapy.* London: Oxford University Press.
Szasz, T. S. (1993). Curing, coercing, and claims-making: A reply to critics. *British Journal of Psychiatry,* 162, 797–800.
Wolberg, L. R. (1977). *The Technique of Psychotherapy.* New York, San Francisco, London: Grune and Stratton.

# Poised on the brink: The social construction of a new biological psychiatry

*Martin Terre Blanche*

You know the difference between a real science and a pseudo-science? A real science recognises and accepts its own history without feeling attacked (Foucault, in Martin, 1988: 12).

## ■ Introduction

If it is the case that what counts as 'the truth' about psychopathology is always the effect of specific kinds of institutional and discursive practices, as Foucault (1980) suggests, then the histories of such institutional and discursive practices would seem vital and clear-cut targets for the destabilisation of essentialist notions of psychopathology. Psychiatry, of course, counts as one of the most formidable ensembles of institutional and discursive practices in Western modernity, at least within the terms of the definition and treatment of psychopathology. The historical destabilisation of psychiatry, its values and its understandings of psychopathology seem, perhaps surprisingly, to require the expenditure of fairly modest deconstructive energies. In fact, some of the most effective forms of criticism at hand exist in an almost 'ready-made' way in the internal history of the discipline. Some of these less-than-illustrious representations of psychiatry come to a head around the growing prospects of a new dominance within the discipline, i.e. the development of 'the new biological psychiatry'.

Resorting to what, following Foucault (1980), may be loosely termed a 'critical history', this chapter will recount not so much the reconstructed *and representable* public face of psychiatry's history, but will instead present an account of psychiatry's unstable, discontinuous, serendipitous and bumbling development, a history characterised by exclusions, infighting, arbitrary discoveries and a particularly notable lack of 'scientificity'. The hoped-for outcome of these efforts is to produce a very different 'surface of emergence' from which psychopathology became knowable, speakable and practicable in the modern world.

## ■ The new biologism

It is common knowledge that the past three decades have seen the rebirth in psychiatry of an enthusiasm for somatic explanations and the pharmacological management of mental disorders. The first of the new drug treatments came on the market in the late 1950s, and by the mid-1970s 25% of National Health Service prescriptions in Britain were for psychiatric medications (Rose, 1986a). By the early 1980s, faced with the apparent success of drug therapies, academic psychiatry had fully embraced a new biological orthodoxy.

Light describes how 'within a short time the leading departments of psychiatry left their imitators and camp followers behind as they forged a new professional identity around advances in biopsychiatry' (1982: 43), while Cockerham, writing at about the same time, states: 'Bolstered by recent biochemical discoveries, a current view in psychiatry is that the discipline is entering a new era, possibly making psychiatry one of the most scientifically precise of all medical specialties and ending its traditional dependence upon subjective judgements of and insights into the human mind' (1981: 79–80). A review (Pincus *et al.*, 1993) of research articles published in the two leading American journals of general psychiatry, *The American Journal of Psychiatry* and *Archives of General Psychiatry*, showed that by the early 1990s, Clinical Psychobiology had become the largest content category (25%), having risen sharply from 14.4% in 1969–70, while Social Science (12.8% to 10.2%) and Psychosocial Treatments (3.1% to 3.6%) remained more or less static.

Even psychiatrists who are not positively inclined towards biopsychiatry acknowledge its increasing predominance. Arthur Kleinman, an anthropologically orientated psychiatrist, portrays the 1980s as a 'period of biological revanchism in psychiatry – when many psychiatrists seem[ed] to believe that understanding the biological basis of mental disorders is, if not around the corner, at most two or three streets away, and that such knowledge will be all the clinician needs to know to treat patients with schizophrenia and depression' (1988: xi). He goes on to speak of how psychiatry 'has been overtaken in the 1980s with a fervour for biological explanations' (1988: 1) and complains that 'academic psychiatry aims to become a version of high-technology internal medicine' (1988: 140). The 1990s, designated the 'decade of the brain' in psychiatry (Wallace, 1997), has been dominated by biological research and therapy, and there is widespread agreement that there has been a rapid expansion in understanding of the neurochemistry of the brain (Meador-Woodruff and Watson, 1997). Even at the start of the decade, the American Psychiatric Association (APA) president already felt unsettled by 'continuing excellent but unbalancing advances in brain biology' (Hartmann, 1992: 1137). In fact, as early as the mid-1960s, Alexander and Sheldon complained of the rising new biologism:

> The role of the devil now has been taken over by brain chemistry. No longer a devil but a *deus ex machina*, a disturbed brain chemistry rather than the person's own life experiences, is responsible for mental illness. Whatever the cause of faulty brain chemistry may be, the new conviction is that the disturbed mind can now be cured by drugs and that the patient himself as a person no longer needs to try to understand the source of his troubles and master them by improved self-knowledge (1966: 14).

These authors for the most part seem to assume that scientific advances constitute the driving force that has catapulted biopsychiatry into its currently 'unbalancing' pre-eminence. This is typical of 'insider' accounts of the development of science. Insiders tend to place much emphasis on the way in which scientific progress occurs through a process of verification, with incorrect theories replaced by correct ones on the basis of empirical evidence. Thomas Kuhn, whose *Structure of Scientific*

*Revolutions* has been enormously influential in casting doubt on such views, describes them as follows:

> If science is the constellation of facts, theories, and methods collected in current texts, then scientists are the men who, successfully or not, have striven to contribute one or another element to that particular constellation. Scientific development becomes the piecemeal process by which these items have been added, singly or in combination, to the ever-growing stockpile that constitutes scientific technique and knowledge. And history of science becomes the discipline that chronicles both these successive increments and the obstacles which have inhibited their accumulation (1962: 1–2).

The kind of historiography that Kuhn seeks to debunk has been labelled 'Whig history', after a phrase used by the British historian Herbert Butterfield to satirise the tendency of some English constitutional historians to portray their field in terms of the continued broadening of human rights resulting from the struggle between forward-looking liberals and backward-looking conservatives (Brush, 1974). In medicine, Mishler *et al.* describe Whig histories as follows:

> Many discussions of the history of medicine center ... on the history of ideas or on the history of people and events; they view medicine ... as the evolution and advance of important concepts and theories or as the product of key discoveries by researchers .... These approaches tend to stay within medicine; in them its development is isolated from significant social forces outside the profession. Their implication is that the way medicine developed is the only way in which it could have developed, and – 'should' replacing 'could' – that medicine has been a constant advance of 'better' theory and practice (1981: 244–5).

Since Kuhn, many philosophers, sociologists and historians of science have been active in criticising such justificatory histories, and substituting more 'accurate' accounts of their own (cf. Woodward, 1986; and for psychiatry, Alldridge, 1990; MacDonald, 1990; Miller, 1986; Scull, 1991; Vandermeersch, 1991), but perhaps more interesting and logically prior to identifying the forces that 'really' shape science is simply describing the rhetorical and other devices used by scientists themselves to construct the unfolding of their disciplines (Gilbert and Mulkay, 1984). Doing just that, Scull describes the general form of Whig histories in psychiatry as follows:

> Psychiatric history was here cast as a morality tale, a movement from the dark period when lunacy was not seen as a condition requiring medical treatment, through a drawn-out struggle in which the steady application of rational-scientific principles by people of good will produced halting and irregular but unmistakable evidence of progress towards humane and effective treatments for those afflicted with the various forms of mental alienation – a process supposedly culminating in our present state of grace (1991: 240).

In this chapter, I aim to appraise the ways in which biologically oriented psychiatrists view the past and future of their profession. To distinguish the biopsychiatric movement that has flourished since the late 1950s from previous periods of biological

dominance in psychiatry, I label it the New Biological Psychiatry (NBP), and identify three distinctive features of its emerging historiography:
1. Scientific discovery is viewed as the primary mechanism of historical progression.
2. Psychiatry is presented as having only recently emerged from a period of superstition.
3. The NBP has strongly millenarian overtones.

The first characteristic is shared with science and medicine in general, while the second and third appear to be specific to the NBP. The chapter concludes with a consideration of the prospects for a new anti-biopsychiatry.

## ■ 'Specific questions of fact': the logic of scientific discovery in psychiatry

In a lecture at London's Maudsley hospital, later reprinted in *Psychological Medicine* and provocatively titled 'Biological psychiatry: Is there any other kind?' Samuel Guze (1989), senior professor at a leading American medical school, spelled out the credo of the New Biological Psychiatry, i.e. that all good psychiatry is necessarily biological. He states that 'Psychiatry is a branch of medicine, which in turn is a form of applied biology. It follows, therefore, that biological science, broadly defined, is the foundation of medical science and hence of medical practice' (1989: 319). Political, religious and philosophical objections to this kind of reductionism are easily dismissed because they are not scientific and, in any case, can themselves be reduced to biology. 'I believe', said Guze, 'that continuing debate about the biological basis of psychiatry is derived much more from philosophical, ideological and political concerns than from scientific ones .... We will increasingly be thinking and discussing specific questions of fact and their interpretation rather than argue about ideological matters as substitutes for scientific discourse' (1989: 322). So in the minds of some biopsychiatrists at least, philosophy is lumped together with the presumably equally subjective and wordy enterprises of religion, ideology, politics and psychology, and opposed to the 'specific questions of fact' that make up the realm of science.

This is Whig history at its best, and if it differs from scientific and psychiatric historiography in general, it does so, perhaps, only in degree. In essence, the story remains a tributary of the main medico-scientific tale in which enlightened doctor-scientists gradually, through the painstaking accumulation of facts, overcome the forces of intolerance and superstition. Classics of psychiatric historiography such as Zilboorg and Henry (1941) and Alexander and Sheldon (1966) give dramatic accounts of that great, mythical, upward sweep of humanism and science with which psychiatry has always wished to align itself. The New Biological Psychiatry simply believes even more firmly that an adherence to medical and scientific principles can guarantee for the discipline an ever-upward trajectory from past to future. The word 'progress' leaps out at one from the pages of biopsychiatric texts; it is used no fewer than five times on the first page of Trimble's (1988) authoritative handbook of biological psychiatry.

The irony is that biological psychiatry, perhaps more so than most branches of medicine, has progressed not through rational enquiry and evolutionary growth, but as a result of serendipitous discoveries. Below is an incomplete discussion of somatic treatments that, by common consent, were arrived at serendipitously.

**Electroconvulsive treatment** was introduced by Cerletti and Bini on the apparently mistaken theoretical grounds that psychosis and epileptic convulsions are mutually exclusive. Only when the treatment failed with schizophrenic patients, did they extend their trails to include those with affective disorders.

Cade (who afterwards styled himself as 'a little known psychiatrist with no research training') stumbled on **lithium** treatment for mania in the course of testing his theory that manic patients are intoxicated by an excess of naturally occurring substances (such as lithium) in the body. On observing lithium's sedative effects, Cade reversed his theory, now speculating that mania is caused by a lithium *deficiency*. However, this theory appears also to have been wrong, and as with electroshock, 'the mode whereby it exerts its effects in psychiatry remains unknown' (Kiloh *et al.*, 1988: 69). Colp (1989) tells another version of the story, namely that Cade thought mania was caused by an excess of natural metabolites (such as urea and uric acid), and that since lithium had been used in medical conditions in which these metabolites were elevated, he speculated that it might also help for mania. It was only when he injected guinea-pigs with lithium that he noticed that it produced drowsiness and might for that reason be useful in mania. Cade himself said he wanted to see if uric acid would *enhance* the toxicity of urea, which he had injected into guinea-pigs, apparently with the purpose of bringing about convulsions in the course of research on epilepsy: 'The great difficulty was the insolubility of uric acid in water, so the most soluble urate was chosen – the lithium salt' (1949: 350).

**Chlorpromazine** (CPZ), the first major anti-psychotic, was first synthesised in 1883 by a chemist analysing chemical dyes, rediscovered in 1937 in the course of searching for a synthetic anti-histamine to counteract allergic shock, tested in 1944 as an anti-malarial drug, and in 1951 as a tranquilliser for surgical patients (where it was thought to induce 'artificial hibernation') (Johnson, 1990). In 1952, Jean Delay and Pierre Deniker reported that CPZ affected mood, thinking processes and behaviour in psychotics. It was consequently tried first on manic, and later on agitated schizophrenic patients. **Iproniazid**, the first of the monoamine oxidase inhibitors, was initially used in the treatment of tuberculosis, where it was noticed to have mood-elevating properties. **Imipramine**, on the other hand, being an analogue of chlorpromazine, was on theoretical grounds expected to have value as an anti-psychotic, and only when its clinical effects were found to be different from chlorpromazine was it tried on depressed patients. Moprobamate (**Miltown**), the first of the now notorious minor tranquillisers such as Librium and Valium, was stumbled upon in the course of animal-testing for new anti-bacterial drugs, where it was observed to relieve tension. And so on.

Of course, attempts at linking the history of biological psychiatry to the logic of scientific enquiry differ in sophistication. Kiloh *et al.*'s (1988) historical introduction to their standard text on physical treatments in psychiatry is possibly the most detailed account yet given by biopsychiatrists of the historical development of their discipline. Their technique is first to describe with great candour the various inhumane and senseless treatments that have been the province of biopsychiatry, and then to point out how each became discredited through rational scientific research.

So their readers learn how 'the most pervasive and dangerous aetiological invention of the twentieth century' (Kiloh et al., 1988: 6), focal infection, and its treatment by the removal of teeth, tonsils, reproductive organs, etc. reigned supreme until Kopeloff and Kirby demonstrated in a controlled study that more of the controls survived. Similarly, the insulin-therapy vogue held sway, we are told, until Ackner and his colleagues published their double-blind controlled trial which showed that insulin coma was no more effective than barbiturate-induced coma. Acetylcholine treatment was long administered to schizophrenic and later neurotic patients, but fortunately Pare and others eventually carried out controlled trials in which they demonstrated that equal numbers improved on active treatment and placebo. Carbon dioxide was used in neuroses, anxiety states and hysteria with initial positive results, but 'it was left to Hawkings and Tibbets ... to conduct a clinical trial' (Kiloh et al., 1988: 10), in which they demonstrated equal efficacy for inhalations of compressed air.

Another example of this kind of presentation is Colp's version of how chlorpromazine got to be an accepted drug: 'In 1964, a double-blind study by the National Institute of Mental Health, which compared the clinical effects of placebos, chlorpromazine, and two other antipsychotics, when each was administered to hospitalised patients, scientifically demonstrated the effectiveness of the antipsychotics and established guidelines for the future clinical evaluation of psychoactive drugs' (1989: 2141). However, Johnson (1990) has shown that the drug came to be used on a massive scale *before* any controlled studies had been done. Moreover, in their review, Wyatt et al. (1996) could find only nine studies that had ever been done comparing first-hospitalisation schizophrenic patients given anti-psychotic medications with a control group given other treatments. Even among these studies, many were not carefully controlled, and only two of the nine 'found that patients initially given anti-psychotic medications did significantly better than those given nonsomatic treatments' (Wyatt et al., 1996: 362).

Kiloh et al. (1988) admit that scientific refutation was not always immediately followed by the clinical abandonment of a treatment (as for instance with the treatment of hard-to-eradicate focal infection), and that treatments may also have been abandoned simply because more convenient or apparently better ones came along (as in the case of insulin-coma treatment, which got overtaken by reserpine and chlorpromazine). However, the overall implication is that it was primarily rational scientific research that had weeded out useless and harmful treatments.

This dressing up of the facts encourages practising psychiatrists to assume that convincing scientific refutation of the efficacy of any currently used treatment or theory will soon enough result in its abandonment by the psychiatric establishment. This is so not only for 'true believers', but also for those such as Charlton (1990) who are highly critical of the New Biological Psychiatry. Charlton believes that biological psychiatry is poised on the brink of a paradigm crisis, i.e. 'when inconsistencies begin to build up, when good predictions are not forthcoming: when, in other words, things are not working as well as they used to' (1990: 6). While inevitably there will be inconsistencies and failed predictions in the biopsychiatric literature, there is little evidence that this is leading to a loss of nerve.

An example is Mellon's (1989) review of genetic-linkage studies in bipolar disorder. Once the great hope of biopsychiatric research, linkage studies have increasingly run into difficulties, leading Mellon to conclude that 'after 20 years and approximately 30 studies, the status of the bipolar linkage field has not changed much' (1989: 155) and that 'lack of replication in the field has contributed to a growing skepticism about the usefulness and reliability of the linkage study approach in psychiatric illness' (1989: 154). However, despite these devastating conclusions, Mellon does not hesitate to add: 'Yet it still holds great promise for answering basic questions of etiology and diagnosis' (1989: 155).

Similarly, Murray et al. suggest, from their review of the biology of schizophrenia, that 'the reader may conclude that the neurochemical findings we have reviewed represent a meagre reward for 25 years of effort' and that the last decade has seen nothing more than 'modest progress in understanding the biology of schizophrenia' (1988: 176). Nevertheless, they remain hopeful that the apparent confusion in the theorising about the neurochemistry of schizophrenia will soon be resolved by the discovery of 'some primary but unknown abnormality' (1988: 176) in the neurochemistry of schizophrenic brains. Wyatt et al.'s review of the treatment of schizophrenia is equally unenthusiastic about the current state of play (treatments are 'at best palliative'; genetic findings are 'tentative' and 'nonspecific'), but hopeful for the future: 'Our knowledge continues to grow.... Improved care is on the horizon' (1996: 366–7).

One final example: when Harrow et al. (1990) found that one of the most taken-for-granted 'facts' in psychiatry, the supposed prophylactic efficacy of lithium carbonate in mania, could not be demonstrated in clinical practice, they did not consider it necessary to question the idea of mania as a condition amenable to biological management, or to suggest that the neurochemical theory of mania (such as it is) needs to be revised. Instead, their proposals were limited to practicalities: the use of alternate drugs such as carbamazepine should be explored and blood lithium levels should be monitored more assiduously.

In a closely argued and carefully documented study suggestively titled 'The structure of psychopharmacological revolutions', Healy demonstrated that 'the catecholaminergic hypotheses of depression and dopaminergic hypotheses of schizophrenia (the latter is referred to by Wallace (1997) as "the hallowed dopamine hypothesis") appear irrefutable. While apparently testable, negative evidence to date has had little effect and there is almost infinite scope to resist refutation' (1987: 367). Much research in the field appears to operate on 'the assumption that amines *will* be found to be deranged in the affective disorders despite the evidence ... that the original pharmacological basis for the expectation no longer warrants an exclusive focus on amines' (Healy, 1987: 359). He concludes that, like the Oedipal hypothesis in psychodynamic psychiatry, these hypotheses will never be refuted, no matter how overwhelming the weight of contradictory evidence, but will at best fade away, just as psychodynamic psychiatry faded away when research interest moved on to other fields.

## 'A strange antirational period': discounting the recent past

A catalogue of how biological psychiatry has remained unmoved by 'specific questions of fact', such as those presented above, prompts a sceptical response to claims by Guze

(1989) and others that psychiatry has loosened itself from the fetters of philosophy and will henceforth operate along strictly scientific lines. However, a tendency to oversell the internal coherence of research work is not by any means unique to biological psychiatry, and equally damaging accounts have been given, for instance, of biology (Meyers, 1990) and physics (Gross, 1991).

Like other scientific historiographies, the one constructed to explain and justify biopsychiatry also locates speculative, philosophical and superstitious behaviour in the discipline's past, with rational and scientific approaches supposedly becoming more prominent as one approaches the present. Critical historians of science have argued that 'preconceptions of science as necessarily antagonistic to superstition [have] resulted in a misperception of historical data' (Kirsch, 1980: 359), and that the passage of time has rendered practices such as a belief in demonology and witchcraft sufficiently exotic so that it is easy to forget that they were once considered established fact by such scientific luminaries as Copernicus, Kepler, Napier, Boyle and Newton.

What is rather special about the New Biological Psychiatry, however, is that it places the era of superstition not in the sixteenth or seventeenth centuries, but only two or three decades away from the present. The culmination of these superstitious tendencies was, so the story goes, the deinstitutionalisation debacle of the 1960s and 1970s. Cancro speaks of 'this strange antirational period of massive denial and grandiose expectations' (1989: vii) and of the 'near delusional beliefs' of those psychiatrists who participated in it. Deinstitutionalisation's failure appears to represent a powerful warning that to trivialise mental illness as anything other than a serious biological disease is to advocate the gross neglect of psychiatric patients. Thus Trimble feels compelled to explicitly warn fellow biopsychiatrists against again becoming 'submerged and lost in a quagmire of new, old or revived psychological theorising' (1988: xii).

To make things worse, psychiatry is presented as having lost its head not only for a decade or so after the 1960s, but for the better part of a century. The trouble started, as Trimble explains, with 'psychological theorising, which arose on the neoromantic tide of the turn of the century. This culminated in the psychoanalytic movement, which for a considerable time became synonymous with psychiatry' (1988: xi). This 'considerable time' lasted from the 1920s until well into the 1970s, a fact which historians of the New Biological Psychiatry believe should be seen in the context of a much longer period of relative sanity: 'this era has provided psychiatry with a legacy that it does not deserve, the main trend of the tradition for over 2000 years being medical and neuropathologically based' (Trimble, 1988: xi–xii). It is doubtful if any other scientific discipline, medical or otherwise, has had to admit to such a sizeable recent dip in what is usually presented as the steadily rising line of scientific conquest, and in this respect the New Biological Psychiatry clearly differs from psychiatry in general.

Another curiosity is that the main physical treatments in psychiatry, the treatments that have given biopsychiatry such a central place in everyday psychiatric practice, were instituted not before or after the 'strange antirational period', but while it was still in full swing: electroshock in 1938, lithium in 1949, chlorpromazine in 1952 and imipramine in 1958. Cancro explains this anomaly by presenting biopsychiatric research as an ongoing enterprise that, although periodically repressed, continued over the years with the painstaking task of scientific-knowledge accumulation:

The period was primarily dominated in America by psychoanalytic thinking. Biological studies were going on, but they were not in the mainstream. It was not until the mid-1950s, with the introduction of pharmacologically effective compounds, that American psychiatry began to move into the pantheon of medicine. Despite this scientific movement of the 1950s, the exuberance of the 1960s swept much of the previous rational enquiry and evolutionary growth aside (1989: vii).

Is it true that psychiatry has just returned from a half-a-century-long psychoanalytic detour, in the course of which it lost contact with the grand old traditions of its biomedical past, or are both the detour and the grand old traditions New Biopsychiatric inventions?

That psychoanalysis had a certain prestige in psychiatry in the period from the 1920s to the 1970s, and that it in turn conferred a degree of prestige on the psychiatric profession, cannot be denied. However, it is clear that somatic views of mental illness were by no means discounted. Among the more horrific treatments advocated and administered by biopsychiatrists during the 'neoromantic' period are pre-frontal lobotomy, of which over 50 000 had been performed by the mid-1950s and hydrotherapy, which (in one of its variations) required that patients be kept tightly cocooned for up to four hours in sheets that were regularly drenched, first with cold and then with hot water. Then as now, it was only a small minority of hospitalised patients who were ever psychoanalysed. For the vast majority of hospitalised patients, the facts of psychiatric life revolved around closed wards, restraint and somatic treatment.

Two textbooks for lower-level psychiatric personnel published on the eve of deinstitutionalisation are suggestive of the sorts of things left out of biopsychiatric accounts of what we are asked to believe was a neoromantic/psychoanalytic interregnum. Rodeman starts her guide for American psychiatric aides with the following confident assertion, so very reminiscent of latter-day biopsychiatric statements: 'The history of the care and treatment of psychiatric patients reveals that this care has progressed from abuse and punishment in the early days to the present-day care and treatment based on scientific knowledge and understanding of human behaviour' (1956: 1). She goes on to advise aides to bear in mind that psychiatric patients perspire more than ordinary people, to never show either approval or disapproval of patients' behaviour ('remember always that he is ill and that his behaviour is a symptom of his illness' (1956: 13)), and so on. Much attention is given to the mechanics of preparing patients for insulin-coma therapy and hydrotherapy, and aides are repeatedly urged to 'reassure the patient and emphasize that this is a treatment' (1956: 44), and to 'avoid any details of the treatment which might frighten the patient' (1956: 98). In case there are some aides who harbour doubts of their own, Rodeman is quick to reassure them: 'It is not yet known how the insulin coma produces improvement in the patient, but improvement occurs in all aspects of his personality' (1956: 97).

The second textbook, by Houliston (1955), matron at Crichton Royal Mental Hospital at Dumfries, was written for British psychiatric nurses, but the picture she paints is very similar. Confinement, seclusion, supervision of patients with 'tendencies to wander or escape' – these are presented as the stock-in-trade of a nurse's life in a mental hospital. Psychotherapy gets just more than a page, in which the reader is informed that it has two varieties: suggestion and persuasion. All in all, Houliston is as confident as Rodeman that science is still carrying us all upwards and forwards and that things are much better now than they were in the bad old days: 'The modern treatments available to mental patients include such things as electro-shock, insulin therapy, prolonged narcosis, hydro-therapy, occupational and recreational therapy, the various forms of psychotherapy, and prefrontal leucotomy, the brain operation recently introduced in psychiatry with success' (1955: 7).

Rodeman's and Houliston's textbooks were chosen for purposes of illustration, but are not unique. For instance, a similar ethos pervades Ingram's (1949) *Principles of Psychiatric Nursing* and Altschul's (1957) *Aids to Psychiatric Nursing*, although Trick and Obcarskas' (1968) more recent *Understanding Mental Illness and its Nursing* is perhaps not quite in the same category. A somatic orientation towards mental illness during the 'neoromantic' period is not confined to nursing texts either, as is demonstrated by the preface to the sixth edition of Henderson and Gillespie's *Text-book of Psychiatry*, in which they state that 'The dramatic successes attained by methods of physical treatment, such as those conducted by chemically or electrically induced convulsions and by surgical division of the white matter of the frontal lobes, have prompted us to add a special chapter on these triumphs of empiricism' (1944: vii).

Interestingly, both Rodeman and Houliston have historical introductions in which psychiatry's imagined progression from superstition to science is mapped out. Houliston's historiography is particularly interesting in that she divides psychiatric history into various eras ('demonological', 'political' and so on), locating the then present firmly in the scientific era. Ironically, this era is said to have started with the dawn of the 20th century, just at the precise moment that Trimble (1988) sees the 'neoromantic tide' coming in.

If the story about psychiatry's neoromantic aberration is illusory, then what about the grand-old-tradition story? The short answer to this question is that, with the exception of clearly organic brain syndromes such as Alzheimer's disease and general paralysis of the insane (cerebral syphilis), which as early as 1822 was understood to be a physical disease and by 1909 'had moved from the stormy waters of psychiatry into the safe harbor of neurology' (Gilman, 1988: 211), the neurological basis of mental illnesses remains unexplicated. Similar views have been expressed by Kleinman (1988) and Kleinman and Cohen (1997). Kleinman states the case quite bluntly: 'There is still, after more than 30 years of intensive biological investigation, no clear-cut understanding of the biology of schizophrenia .... This does not deter psychiatrists and those who write the advertisements for drug companies from asserting without any hesitation that schizophrenia is a biologically based disorder. This belief is a central tenet of professional orthodoxy' (1988: 188).

Trimble (1988) is probably correct in stating that the main trend in psychiatry over the past 2000 years has been neuropathological, but unfortunately there is little in this tradition, except for its general sentiment, that is of much use to modern biopsychiatry. Hippocrates and Galen may have set an example in their insistence that mental illness has a somatic origin, but their aetiological ideas concerning the correct mixture of phlegm, bile and so on now seem fanciful. The same goes for the 17th-century British biopsychiatrist Thomas Willis, the details of whose theory relating to animal spirits circulating through the cortex are of course no longer accepted. The list goes on: Griesinger (insanity is caused by changes in circulation, nervous irritation or disturbed nutrition); Morel (insanity is a hereditary form of 'degeneration'); Foville (neuroses are localised nervous-system diseases) and so on.

It is instructive to look at the original texts of some of these great figures from the prehistory of biopsychiatry, for instance that of James Prichard (1837/1973). Prichard is mainly famous for creating the now-defunct disease of moral insanity, 'consisting in a morbid perversion of the natural feelings, affections, inclinations, temper, habits, moral dispositions, and natural impulses, without any remarkable disorder or defect of the intellect or knowing and reasoning faculties, and particularly without any insane illusion or hallucination' (1837/1973: 16). The great danger in moral insanity is that 'persons labouring under this disorder are capable of reasoning or supporting an argument upon any subject within their sphere of knowledge that may be presented to them; and they often display great ingenuity in giving reasons for the eccentricities of their conduct, and in accounting for and justifying the state of moral feeling under which they appear to exist' (1837/1973: 21). A typical example of moral insanity would be a previously submissive adolescent girl who runs away from home or a housewife who questions her husband's authority; and for many decades after the publication of Prichard's book, the concept of moral insanity was referred to by psychiatrists making commitment decisions in such cases.

Although it was accepted that social and psychological factors could play a role in moral insanity, at root it always had a physiological cause: the person's inherent 'temperament', a 'natural predisposition', or perhaps 'some disorder affecting the head, a slight attack of paralysis, a fit of epilepsy, or some febrile or inflammatory disorder' (Prichard, 1837/1973: 21). And what is to be done about insanity, moral or otherwise? Prichard endorses the whole plethora of what now appear to be wilfully cruel and senseless treatments: bleeding, cold showers, purgatives ('no fact in medical practice has been longer established than the utility of purgatives in madness' (1837/1973: 195)), emetics, digitalis, opium, mercury and the rotating chair.

## ■ 'A thing of the past': millenarian qualities of the New Biological Psychiatry

In his foreword to the fifth edition of Kaplan and Sadock's *Comprehensive Textbook of Psychiatry* (1989), Robert Cancro refers to 'this brief historical summary' (vii). However, the preceding two paragraphs are historical only in the sense that they rehearse the by-now familiar idea of an irreconcilable difference between 'theological' intuition and rational science. Instead, pride of place goes to Neural Science (Chapter 1) and Neurology (Chapter 2), with history relegated to the last 21 pages of the two-volume work.

This was not always the case. Stepping back a mere decade, one finds that the third edition, published in 1980, opened with a lavishly illustrated historical chapter by George Mora, spread over 94 pages. By the fourth edition, five years later, this had been cut to 20 pages and moved to the end of the book, although the opening chapter still tackled 'theoretical trends' in psychiatry. The fifth edition, as has been mentioned, gets straight to business with Neural Science and Neurology, and the history chapter at the end, no longer by Mora, has degenerated into a lack-lustre catalogue of great men and their achievements. The seventh edition of Kaplan and Sadock (Kaplan *et al.*, 1994) has no separate history chapter and opens with a full-colour guide to commonly prescribed drugs.

Why have history's shares, as reflected in the 'bible' of American psychiatry, dropped so precipitously over the past two decades? At one level it is no doubt simply a matter of space. To accommodate the mass of new material being produced in fields such as brain imaging and neurochemistry, it is only natural that 'old-news' items such as history and philosophy should be jettisoned. At another level, it is an ideological shift that requires that psychiatry distance itself from aspects of its own history in order to 'make itself anew'. This is essentially the same conclusion as that arrived at by Foucault, who asks: 'Why should an archaeology of psychiatry function as an "anti-psychiatry", when an archaeology of biology does not function as an anti-biology? Is it because of the partial nature of the analysis? Or is it not rather that psychiatry is not on good terms with its own history, the result of a certain inability on the part of psychiatry, given what it is, to accept its own history?' (1980: 192).

The gradual silencing of history's voice in the halls of biopsychiatry is not due to a loss of faith in the essentials of psychiatric historiography (i.e. progress through rational scientific discovery), but to a certain discomfort with regard to that history. There is little that the NBP can do with psychiatric history before 1955, except to warn against the dangers of unscientific theorising, or to show that for a very long time psychiatrists have believed in organic aetiologies and treatments of one sort or another despite the lack of empirical warrant.

For biopsychiatry, the past is shrinking, while the future is looming ever larger. The little history chapter at the end of the fifth edition of Kaplan and Sadock is called 'Psychiatry: past and future', and from the 'future' section we learn: 'The good news is that, because of progress both in scientific understanding and in clinical practice (all of which is likely to continue at the present brisk pace), the public will increasingly see mental illness as illness and psychiatrists as physicians who treat mental illness – more and more effectively. The stigma that was once attached to the psychiatric profession is likely to become, fairly soon, a thing of the past' (Pardes, 1989: 2157).

Pardes may well be right. Popular magazines such as *Time* and *Scientific American* and television programs such as *Beyond 2000* increasingly reproduce biopsychiatric orthodoxies regarding the aetiology and treatment of syndromes like schizophrenia and the major affective disorders. They also reproduce the promissory notes that biopsychiatrists almost routinely append to the end of their research reports. This is how, for example, Gershon and Rieder conclude their *Scientific American* article: 'We expect our understanding of the biology of schizophrenia and mood disorders to expand dramatically, fuelled by the impressive advances in neurobiology, cognitive neuroscience and genetics' (1992: 95).

Similar expressions of hope and expectation are very common in the professional literature. Some examples from genetic studies: 'There is good evidence, especially from studies of twins and adopted children, that genetic factors are important in minor psychiatric disorders … the recent tentative location of genetic sites associated with manic-depressive psychoses gives hope that such sites may also exist, and be found, for the cyclothymic and dysthymic traits' (Hare, 1991: 44); 'Once a gene is identified a whole new era will begin' (Mellon, 1989: 155); 'It seems likely that if major genes operate on schizophrenia, these will be identified in the next few years' (Murray et al., 1988: 176); 'We can be confident that, if genes of major effect are involved reasonably commonly in the aetiology of schizophrenia, they will be detected and localised during the next few years' (McGuffin et al., 1995: 681).

Despite the passing of each successive 'next few years', the putative genetic mechanisms behind schizophrenia and other psychiatric disorders continue to remain elusive, and much the same is true concerning a viable theory of the neurochemical mechanisms involved and of the effects of psychotropic medications (Wyatt et al., 1996). Ingleby speaks of 'the myth which helps to keep orthodox psychiatry on the move: the belief that what we need are simply more "findings" – that round the corner lies some vital new fact which will settle the arguments once and for all' (1981: 23). While persuasive evidence may yet become available in the 'next few years' (for instance, from the human genome project), the New Biological Psychiatry has manoeuvred itself into a position where a post-millenarian scenario, in which it becomes evident that the arguments will not or cannot be settled, is at least conceivable.

## ■ 'More than a science': the new anti-biopsychiatry

At the start of the chapter, it was mentioned that not all psychiatrists and other mental-health workers are equally comfortable with biopsychiatry's rampant successes. In an article in the *British Journal of Psychiatry*, Robert Cawley (1993), emeritus professor of Psychological Medicine at the University of London, argues that psychiatry is more than a science – more even than an applied science – and that certain aspects of the assessment, management and prognosis of mental illness can therefore not be reduced to (or deduced from) scientific findings. Like other practitioners of a possibly embryonic new anti-biopsychiatry, Cawley is circumspect in his criticism. A formula commonly used in this emerging literature is to start by acknowledging the achievements of biopsychiatry up front. So already in the second paragraph, Cawley talks of 'the neurosciences, in which we have seen staggering advances in the last couple of decades' (1993: 154). Similarly, Gabbard, in his rearguard defence of psychodynamic psychiatry, refers in the first sentence of his article to the 'remarkable discoveries from the neurosciences [that] fill the pages of our journals' (1992: 991); Person starts his argument against mindlessness in psychiatry by admitting that 'psychoanalysts cannot ignore the biological revolution that has occurred in academic psychiatry' (1989: 182); Hartmann refers to 'continuing excellent but unbalancing advances in brain biology' (1992: 1137); while Wallace speaks of the 'gargantuan literature' in the field of biopsychiatry and the 'tremendous scientific and clinical fruit' (1997: 92) borne by this branch of the discipline.

Such attempts to downplay differences occur throughout nominally critical texts now found in psychiatric journals. Cawley (1993) readily admits that psychiatry is a science, asking only that we don't forget that it is also *more* than a science, while Gabbard, who argues not against biopsychiatry, but against the '"either-or" polarization of the psychodynamic and the biological' (1992: 991), strenuously attempts to blend the discourses of neuroscience, psychodynamics and behaviourism, as exemplified by the following: 'Painful events, such as separations and losses, early in life may sensitize receptor sites, leading to vulnerability to recurrent depression in adulthood ... ideas and images associated with depressive states could ultimately act as conditioned stimuli capable of eliciting a major depressive episode without a concrete loss or external stressor in the environment' (1992: 992).

While speaking of subjective early childhood experiences and receptor sites in one breath may at first seem strange, it is a distinct possibility that an amalgamation of bio- and psychojargon may become common in psychiatric circles, with the language of neurology gradually taking on metaphorical meanings, particularly if a hard scientific understanding of mental disturbance continues to elude researchers.

Sensitive to the requirements of the times, Shevrin (1988) attempts to imbue psychoanalysis with neuroscientific respectability, and neuroscience with psychoanalytic meaning, using what might previously have been seen as absurd methods such as event-related potentials to prove the existence of the unconscious. Another example in this genre is Post's work, which attempts to straddle the gap between the literatures on psychosocial stress and neurological deficits in affective disorders, with formulations such as the following being common: '[Social] stressors and the biochemical concomitants of the episodes themselves can induce the proto-oncogene c-fos and related transcription factors, which then affect the expression of transmitters, receptors, and neuropeptides that alter responsivity in a long-lasting fashion' (1992: 999).

Abroms describes at length how he reconciles psychodynamic and biological approaches in his psychiatric practice, devoting entire chapters to topics such as 'staging the treatment' and the 'dynamics of drug therapy', pointing out, in terms reminiscent of moral treatment, that 'therapists may have to work hard to become better attuned to the patient's special needs, to provide the support and tenderness that enlists cooperation, and the caring firmness that curbs rebellion' (1993: 160). According to him, without such precautions, drug treatment may fail due to psychodynamic factors such as 'performance anxiety', 'castration anxiety', 'oral rage', the 'incest taboo' and 'fear of penetration'. A case study of 'Carla, the lonely, divorced patient' ends as follows: 'Her psychotic mother was so poisonous that Carla regarded all gifts of food or medicine emanating from a parental figure as bad milk. After much reassurance and insight, she was finally able to swallow her antidepressant and let it work' (1993: 169).

While most biologically oriented psychiatrists would perhaps balk at using this kind of formulation, they are happy to concede that the giving of medication has to be seen in a psychological and social context: 'We are fully aware that current biological treatments work best when they are combined with psychosocial intervention, and expect that future biological treatments will also involve appropriate non-biological considerations' (Wyatt et al., 1996). In addition to suggesting that therapy might help pills to work, it is equally commonly suggested that the relationship between the two modes of treatment runs the other way around. Cooper, for example, says that 'in instances in which an underlying biologic malfunction is suspected, there is powerful warrant to attempt a biologic intervention that may then facilitate psychological interventions' (1989: 209). Alternately, a peaceful coexistence may be achieved by carefully demarcating separate professional and philosophical territories for mind and brain: 'Psychoanalysis is a powerful instrument for research and treatment, but not if it is applied to the wrong patient population' (Cooper, 1989: 216).

Where the new anti-biopsychiatry offers alternatives to hard-core biopsychiatry, these tend to be quite low-key and bland, a far cry from the strong medicine once prescribed by anti-psychiatrists. Cawley's (1993) list of those aspects of psychiatry that are beyond science include, for example, individuality, subjectivity, self-awareness, interpersonal processes, empathy and communication. Since, according to Cawley, these are the 'six, and only six, crucial aspects of our discipline which are in principle unrelated to the basic sciences and yet are central to what we are doing' (1993: 155), one must assume that such stocks-in-trade of anti-psychiatry as free will, morality and creative deviance are amenable to scientific treatment, are not crucial aspects of psychiatry, or are not central to what psychiatry is doing.

It may, in fact, be overstating the case to claim that such a thing as the new anti-biopsychiatry exists, even in embryonic form. The impression of important scientific advances having been made in the last three decades, and of even more important advances being imminent and inevitable, is so strong that all concerned can now afford to be magnanimous in allowing diverse views a place in the psychiatric sun.

APA president Hartmann's (1992) appeal for a return to Engel's (1979) bio-psychosocial model is perhaps more typical of the discourse one can continue to expect from psychiatry than Guze's (1989) polemical biologism. Joseph English, then APA president-elect, called for balance and tolerance in the mind-brain debate and praised the average psychiatrist as 'the most tolerant of medical specialists' (1992: 1142). This is the kind of middle-ground discourse where psychiatrists and psychiatric commentators have long been accustomed to meet. Both Arthur Kleinman (1988) and Sander Gilman (1988), neither of whom are anywhere near the psychiatric mainstream, can for instance be seen to be calling for much the same thing as the APA president: 'The extreme relativism of some antipsychiatry anthropologists is as outrageously ideological as is the universalistic fundamentalism of some card-carrying biological psychiatrists' (Kleinman, 1988: 33); 'I find the middle ground – where culture and biology reciprocally interact – the best vantage point from which to make sense of the cross-cultural data base and to avoid the excesses of its extremist neighbors' (Kleinman, 1988: 187); or 'Such writers as Thomas Szasz and R. D. Laing began to see mental illness as an artifact of society. Then the resurgence of a biologically oriented psychiatry in the past decade has led to the illusion that mental illness is simply an artifact of biology. Both views ignore the fact that the *idea* of mental illness structures both the perception of disease and its form' (Gillman, 1988: 18–19).

To the extent that a new anti-biopsychiatry might therefore exist, it is at most an attempt to tone down the shrillness of extreme biological positions, and to ensure that the baby is not thrown out with the bath water. At the same time, it provides a back door for psychiatry, should the strong biological programme not deliver on its promises. Rather than a millennial religion, prone to falling apart when its prophecies are not fulfilled, the New Biological Psychiatry may have the capacity to expand back into psychosocial territory should this prove necessary. Wallace explains how such a feat could be justified: 'A species-specific physiology, ethology, and ecology of *Homo sapiens* must encompass the image- and symbol-laden dimensions of both personal experience/behavior and its sociocultural surround. In short, the naive and energy-wasting warfare between "biological" and "psychosocial" psychiatrists is founded on a breathtakingly constricted construct of human biology and on an unacknowledged "mind-body" split' (1997: 90).

Drob identified six possible ways for psychiatry to deal with theoretical diversity, of which three seem to describe the positions reviewed in this chapter: relativism ('The emergence of a single dominant paradigm for psychiatry, if it occurs at all, will be determined by historical, economic, sociological, and other nonscientific factors' (1989: 63) – i.e. the traditional outsider historiographical position), commensurability (the best theory will win – i.e. the 'hard' biopsychiatric position) and reductionism (different modes of understanding can ultimately be translated into each other – i.e. the new anti-biopsychiatry or the 'soft' pro-biopsychiatric position).

A new scientific language for psychiatry, which may create the conditions for using apparently hard-edged neuroscience terms as metaphorical codes for mental concepts, is being forged not only as a by-product of projects such as Post's (1992) stress-deficit work, but also quite consciously in the *Diagnostic and Statistical Manual of Mental Disorders* (4th ed.) (DSM-IV). Spitzer *et al.* (1992) describe their proposal for doing away with the term 'organic mental disorders' in DSM-IV, arguing that psychiatry has now superseded the Cartesian mind-body duality, formerly reflected in 'the two great divergent trends in psychiatry during the later part of the nineteenth century' (1992: 240), namely 'brain psychiatry' and psychodynamics. While the inclusion of 'organic mental disorders' in DSM-III and DSM-III-R (the revised edition) may not be meant to imply that the other disorders are non-organic, Spitzer *et al.* are seriously concerned that such connotations may nevertheless exist:

> The connotative meaning of the word 'organic' always returns to its historical roots, which imply a functional/structural, psychological/biological, and mind/body dualism .... These original dichotomies may have been valuable when we had little understanding of how the CNS functions, but they are at variance with the growing body of evidence of the importance of biological factors in the etiology of the major 'non-organic' mental disorders (1992: 241).

Spitzer *et al.*'s proposed solution is a trichotomy, classifying all disorders as either primary (e.g. schizophrenia proper), secondary (i.e. secondary to some non-psychiatric medical disorder, e.g. dissociative disorder due to epilepsy) or drug-induced (e.g. cocaine-induced erectile dysfunction). The beauty of this system, now by and large implemented in DSM-IV (which no longer uses the term 'organic mental disorders' (Kaplan *et al.*, 1994)), is that it eliminates any remaining suggestion that the major psychiatric disorders are non-organic, without on the other hand explicitly identifying them as *necessarily* organic. DSM-IV, as the official style manual of psychiatric discourse, has yet again moved along with the new biopsychiatric fashion, without having committed itself to an extreme biological view that may eventually prove untenable.

Throughout its history, psychiatry, more so than the rest of medicine, appears to have been unable to operate without an attendant anti-psychiatry. As Dain (1989) points out, hostility to psychiatry even predates the establishment of psychiatry as a profession in 1844, and has often come from psychiatrists themselves – sometimes taking on a relatively benign (although influential) form, as was the case for the group of psychiatrists around Clifford Beers at the turn of the 20th century, and sometimes involving a thorough-going rejection of most of psychiatry's scientific and institutional basis, as was the case more recently with Szasz, Laing and company. As Rose (1986b) has argued, opposition to psychiatry has in fact been central to its modernisation.

From the current evidence, it seems likely that the future new anti-biopsychiatry, if it is to be led by psychiatrists, will be of the Beers rather than the Szasz variety. However, it remains possible that the more radical challenge from outside psychiatry, particularly from ex-patient groups and their allies, may gain in power. According to Parker and Burman, who have worked extensively with groups critical of psychiatry, such groups are currently defining community-based treatment of mental illness as a thinly disguised device for regulation and control, and the concerned academic's job should therefore be 'to publicize the analyses presented by these groups rather than expropriate them, rather than presenting them as if they were *ours*' (1993: 165).

Unfortunately, some patient and family lobby groups, such as SANE (Schizophrenia – A National Emergency), seem at present as likely to adopt conservative positions. Dain's gloomy prognosis perhaps best summarises the state of play: 'What form both psychiatry and anti-psychiatry will take in the future is unclear. It is probably safe to say that short of achieving definitive knowledge about mental disorder and how to treat and prevent it and without the public will to care adequately for mentally disabled persons, both psychiatry and anti-psychiatry do have a future' (1989: 19).

## References

Abroms, E. M. (1993). *The Freedom of the Self: The Bio-existential Treatment of Character Problems.* New York: Plenum.

Alexander, F. G. and Sheldon, S. T. (1966). *The History of Psychiatry: An Evaluation of Psychiatric Thought and Practice from Prehistoric Times to the Present.* New York: Mentor.

Allderidge, P. (1990). Hospitals, madhouses and asylums: Cycles in the care of the insane. In R. M. Murray and T. H. Turner (eds), *Lectures on the History of Psychiatry*, pp. 28–46. London: Gaskell.

Altschul, A. (1957). *Aids to Psychiatric Nursing.* London: Bailliere, Tindall and Cox.

American Psychiatric Association (1980). *Diagnostic and Statistical Manual of Mental Disorders* (3rd edn). Washington, DC: American Psychiatric Association.

American Psychiatric Association (1987). *Diagnostic and Statistical Manual of Mental Disorders* (3rd edn, rev.). Washington, DC: American Psychiatric Association.

American Psychiatric Association (1994). *Diagnostic and Statistical Manual of Mental Disorders* (4th edn). Washington, DC: American Psychiatric Association.

Barham, P. (1992). *Closing the Asylum.* Harmondsworth: Penguin.

Brush, S. G. (1974). Should the history of science be rated X? *Science*, 183, 1164–72.

Cade, J. F. J. (1949). Lithium salts in the treatment of psychotic excitement. *Medical Journal of Australia*, 36, 349–52.

Cancro, R. (1989). Foreword. In H. I. Kaplan and B. J. Sadock (eds), *Comprehensive Textbook of Psychiatry* (5th edn), Vol. 1, pp. vii–viii. Baltimore: Williams and Wilkins.

Cawley, R. H. (1993). Psychiatry is more than a science. *British Journal of Psychiatry*, 162, 154–60.

Charlton, B. G. (1990). A critique of biological psychiatry. *Psychological Medicine*, 20 (1), 3–6.
Cockerham, W. C. (1981). *Sociology of Mental Disorder*. Englewood Cliffs: Prentice-Hall.
Colp, R. (1989). History of psychiatry. In H. I. Kaplan and B. J. Sadock (eds), *Comprehensive Textbook of Psychiatry* (5th edn), Vol. 2, pp. 2132–53. Baltimore: Williams and Wilkins.
Cooper, A. M. (1989). Will neurobiology influence psychoanalysis? In A. M. Cooper, O. F. Kernberg and E. S. Person (eds), *Psychoanalysis: Toward the Second Century*, pp. 202–18. New Haven: Yale University Press.
Dain, N. (1989). Critics and dissenters: Reflections on 'anti-psychiatry' in the United States. *Journal of the History of the Behavioral Sciences*, 25, 3–25.
Drob, S. L. (1989). The dilemma of contemporary psychiatry. *American Journal of Psychotherapy*, XLIII (1), 54–67.
Engel, G. L. (1979). The biopsychosocial model and the education of health professionals. *General Hospital Psychiatry*, 1, 156–65.
English, J. T. (1992). Response to the presidential address: Patient care for the twenty-first century. *American Journal of Psychiatry*, 149 (9), 1142–4.
Foucault, M. (1980). *Power/Knowledge: Selected Interviews and Other Writings by Michel Foucault, 1972–1977*. Worcester: Harvester Press.
Gabbard, G. O. (1992). Psychodynamic psychiatry in the 'decade of the brain'. *American Journal of Psychiatry*, 149 (8), 991–8.
Gershon, E. S. and Rieder, R. O. (1992). Major disorders of mind and brain. *Scientific American*, 267 (3), 89–95.
Gilbert, G. N. and Mulkay, M. (1984). *Opening Pandora's Box: A Sociological Analysis of Scientists' Discourse*. Cambridge: Cambridge University Press.
Gilman, S. L. (1988). *Disease and Representation: Images of Illness from Madness to Aids*. Ithaca and London: Cornell University Press.
Gross, A. G. (1991). Rhetoric of science without constraints. *Rhetorica*, 9 (4), 283–300.
Guze, S. B. (1989). Biological psychiatry: Is there any other kind? *Psychological Medicine*, 19 (2), 315–23.
Hare, E. (1991). The history of 'nervous disorders' from 1600 to 1840, and a comparison with modern views. *British Journal of Psychiatry*, 159, 37–45.
Harrow, M., Goldberg, J. F., Grossman, L. S. and Meltzer, H. Y. (1990). Outcome in manic disorders. *Archives of General Psychiatry*, 47, 665–71.
Hartmann, L. (1992). Presidential address: Reflections on humane values and biopsychosocial integration. *American Journal of Psychiatry*, 149 (9), 1135–41.
Healy, D. (1987). The structure of psychopharmacological revolutions. *Psychiatric Developments*, 4, 349–76.
Henderson, D. K. and Gillespie, R. D. (1944). *A Text-book of Psychiatry for Students and Practitioners* (6th edn). Oxford: Oxford University Press.
Houliston, M. (1955). *The Practice of Mental Nursing*. Edinburgh: E. and S. Livingstone.
Ingleby, D. (1981). Understanding 'mental illness'. In D. Ingleby (ed.), *Critical Psychiatry*, pp. 23–71. Harmondsworth: Penguin.
Ingram, A. (1991). *The Madhouse of Language: Writing and Reading Madness in the Eighteenth Century*. London: Routledge.
Ingram, M. A. (1949). *Principles of Psychiatric Nursing*. Philadelphia and London: W. B. Saunders.
Johnson, A. B. (1990). *Out of Bedlam: The Truth about Deinstitutionalization*. London: Basic Books.
Kaplan, H. I., Freedman, A. M. and Sadock, B. J. (1980). *Comprehensive Textbook of Psychiatry* (3rd edn). Baltimore: Williams and Wilkins.
Kaplan, H. I. and Sadock, B. J. (1981). *Modern Synopsis of Comprehensive Textbook of Psychiatry* (3rd edn). Baltimore: Williams and Wilkins.
Kaplan, H. I. and Sadock, B. J. (1985). *Comprehensive Textbook of Psychiatry* (4th edn). Baltimore: Williams and Wilkins.

Kaplan, H. I. and Sadock, B. J. (1989). *Comprehensive Textbook of Psychiatry* (5th edn). Baltimore: Williams and Wilkins.

Kaplan, H. I., Sadock, B. J. and Grebb, J. A. (1994). *Synopsis of Psychiatry: Behavioral Sciences and Clinical Psychiatry* (7th edn). Baltimore: Williams and Wilkins.

Kiloh, L. G., Smith, J. J. and Johnson, G. F. (1988). *Physical Treatments in Psychiatry*. Melbourne: Blackwell.

Kirsch, I. (1980). Demonology and science during the scientific revolution. *Journal of the History of the Behavioral Sciences*, 16, 359–68.

Kleinman, A. (1988). *Rethinking Psychiatry: From Cultural Category to Personal Experience*. New York: Free Press.

Kleinman, A. and Cohen, A. (1997). Psychiatry's global challenge. *Scientific American*, March, 86–9.

Kuhn, T. S. (1962). *The Structure of Scientific Revolutions*. Chicago: University of Chicago Press.

Light, D. W. (1982). Learning to label: The social construction of psychiatrists. In W. R. Gove (ed.), *Deviance and Mental Illness*, pp. 33–48. Beverly Hills: Sage.

MacDonald, M. (1990). Insanity and the realities of history in early modern England. In R. M. Murray and T. H. Turner (eds), *Lectures on the History of Psychiatry*, pp. 60–81. London: Gaskell.

Martin, R. (1988). Truth, power, self: An interview with Michel Foucault. In L. H. Martin, H. Gutman and P. H. Hutton (eds), *Technologies of the Self: A Seminar with Michel Foucault*, pp. 9–15. Amherst: University of Massachusetts Press.

McGuffin, P., Owen, M. J. and Farmer, A. E. (1995). Genetic basis of schizophrenia. *Lancet*, 346, 678–82.

Meador-Woodruff, J. H. and Watson, S. J. (1997). Editorial. *Journal of Psychiatric Research*, 31 (2), 157–8.

Mellon, C. D. (1989). Genetic linkage studies in bipolar disorder: A review. *Psychiatric Developments*, 7 (2), 143–58.

Meyers, G. (1990). *Writing Biology: Texts in the Social Construction of Scientific Knowledge*. Madison: University of Wisconsin Press.

Miller, P. (1986) Critiques of psychiatry and critical sociologies of madness. In P. Miller and N. Rose (eds), *The Power of Psychiatry*, pp. 5–17. Cambridge: Polity Press.

Mishler, E. G., Amarasingham, L. R., Osherson, S. D., Hauser, S. T., Waxler, N. E. and Liem, R. (eds) (1981). *Social Contexts of Health, Illness, and Patient Care*. Cambridge: Cambridge University Press.

Murray, R. M., Kerwin, R. W. and Nimgaonkar, V. L. (1988). What have we learned about the biology of schizophrenia? In K. Granville-Grossman (ed.), *Recent Advances in Clinical Psychiatry*, pp. 161–84. London: Churchill Livingstone.

Pardes, H. (1989). Future of psychiatry. In H. I. Kaplan and B. J. Sadock (eds), *Comprehensive Textbook of Psychiatry*, pp. 2154–7. Baltimore: Williams and Wilkins.

Parker, I. and Burman, E. (1993). Against discursive imperialism, empiricism and constructionism: Thirty-two problems with discourse analysis. In E. Burman and I. Parker (eds), *Discourse Analytic Research*, pp. 155–72. London: Routledge.

Person, E. S. (1989). The crucial role of mentalism in an era of neurobiology. In A. M. Cooper, O. F. Kernberg and E. S. Person (eds), *Psychoanalysis: Toward the Second Century*, pp. 181–202. New Haven: Yale University Press.

Pincus, H. A., Henderson, B., Blackwood, D. and Dial, T. (1993). Trends in research in two general psychiatric journals in 1969–1990: Research on research. *American Journal of Psychiatry*, 150 (1), 135–42.

Post, R. M. (1992). Transduction of psychosocial stress into the neurobiology of recurrent affective disorder. *American Journal of Psychiatry*, 149 (8), 999–1010.

Prichard, J. C. (1837/1973). *A Treatise on Insanity and Other Disorders Affecting the Mind*. New York: Arno Press.

Rodeman, C. R. (1956). *A Guide for Psychiatric Aides*. New York: Macmillan.

Rose, N. (1986a). Psychiatry: The discipline of mental health. In P. Miller and N. Rose (eds), *The Power of Psychiatry*, pp. 43–84. Cambridge: Polity Press.

Rose, N. (1986b). Law, rights and psychiatry. In P. Miller and N. Rose (eds), *The Power of Psychiatry*, pp. 177–213. Cambridge: Polity Press.

Scull, A. (1991). Psychiatry and its historians. *History of Psychiatry*, II, 239–50.

Shevrin, H. (1988). Unconscious conflict: A convergent psychodynamic and electrophysiological approach. In M. J. Horowitz (ed.), *Psychodynamics and Cognition*, pp. 117–67. Chicago: University of Chicago Press.

Spitzer, R. L., First, M. B., Williams, J. B. W., Kendler, K., Pincus, H. A. and Tucker, G. (1992). Now is the time to retire the term 'organic mental disorders'. *American Journal of Psychiatry*, 149 (2), 240–3.

Trick, K. L. L. and Obcarskas, S. (1968). *Understanding Mental Illness and its Nursing*. London: Pitman Medical.

Trimble, M. R. (1988). *Biological Psychiatry*. Chichester: John Wiley.

Vandermeersch, P. (1991). The victory of psychiatry over demonology: The origin of the nineteenth-century myth. *History of Psychiatry*, II, 351–63.

Wallace, E. R. (1997). Psychiatry's sickness and its biological cure. *Psychiatry*, 60, 89–99.

Woodward, W. R. (1986). Disciplinary history. *Journal of the History of the Behavioural Sciences*, 22, 212–14.

Wyatt, R. J., Apud, J. A. and Potkin, S. (1996). New directions in the prevention and treatment of schizophrenia: A biological perspective. *Psychiatry: Interpersonal and Biological Processes*, 59 (4), 357–70.

Zilboorg, G. and Henry, G. W. (1941). *A History of Medical Psychology*. New York: Norton.

# CHAPTER 3

# The political conundrums of post-traumatic stress disorder

*Gillian Eagle*

## ■ Introduction

The diagnostic category of 'post-traumatic stress disorder' (PTSD) finally appears to be here to stay after its incorporation and moderation in three successive versions of the American Psychiatric Association's *Diagnostic and Statistical Manual of Mental Disorders* (DSM). Several authors have pointed to an historical cyclical rise and decline in the recognition of the disorder, which seems to gain prominence in the aftermath of major wars or globally publicised catastrophes (Herman, 1992a; Wilson, 1994). Over time, there has been considerable refinement of what has come to be recognised as the syndrome, with the latest version of DSM, DSM-IV (i.e. the 4th edition), including the two categories of 'acute stress disorder' and 'post-traumatic stress disorder', the latter further divided into 'acute', 'chronic' and 'delayed onset' types, depending on time-frame issues (American Psychiatric Association, 1994). The inclusion of the category 'disorders of extreme stress not otherwise specified' (DESNOS) (Herman, 1992b) was also considered in order to do justice to the recognition of more complex forms of traumatic stress not easily encompassed within present parameters, although due to lack of agreement and clarity, no formal classification was entered. However, the conceptualisation and description of post-traumatic stress as a disorder characterised by intense anxiety in the aftermath of a serious life stressor has become part of popular consciousness, to the extent that it has been described in popular magazine articles and even attributed to characters in American and local South African television dramas such as *Egoli*.

The impetus for this paper arises out of a personal response to working within the field of violence intervention in South Africa over a period of almost 20 years and the influence of the introduction of post-traumatic stress conceptualisations into this area of intervention. The arguments presented reflect some of my own and other clinicians' struggles to engage with what sometimes feels like a form of co-option into mainstream psychiatric discourse and the implications for intervention following the adoption of this perspective. Many of the issues raised for discussion have been brought to the fore by other writers within the field (Kleber *et al.*, 1995) and raised in conference debates, however this chapter aims to draw together and extend disparate arguments and to examine their application to the South African context in particular. Given the historical climate of violence impact and intervention in South Africa, some of the political debates arising from work within this country appear to have particular salience for maintaining a critical perspective on post-traumatic stress work.

## Brief contextualisation

Prior to the period of the unbanning of the African National Congress (ANC) and the demise of the formal apartheid system, a large proportion of therapeutic work in the area of violence intervention overlapped with progressive political agendas. Thus problems that later fell under the rubric of post-traumatic stress were initially conceptualised as event-specific areas of intervention deserving particular explanation and understanding. My experience, which is not uncharacteristic of other counsellors who became involved in violence intervention in the 1980s, was that my first exposure to such work was through involvement in a range of rape-crisis organisations across the country. Such organisations were explicitly feminist in ideology, and a large proportion of their training involved understanding the social location of violence against women from the perspective of gender socialisation and oppression. Counselling methods, although broadly framed within a crisis-intervention understanding, were informed by a politicised perspective on rape and involved a degree of what could be called 'consciousness raising', in that clients' feelings of self-blame and guilt were reframed in terms of problems in gender politics and attributions of blame. Given organisational feminist agendas, individual intervention was also complemented by educational work designed to bring about attitude change and a range of media campaigns, and there was a commitment to democratic and progressive practices in the operation of the organisation/s. While organisational membership was almost exclusively restricted to women, and tended to be largely middle-class and predominantly white, there was a flattening of hierarchy in the use of non-professional counsellors and the recognition of all members as bringing value on the basis of their life experiences. Overall, within rape-crisis organisations, therapeutic intervention was underpinned by an explicitly feminist ideology and was complemented by further activist strategies.

The 1980s in South Africa saw the rise of a different form of organisational structure designed specifically to address the casualties of forms of state repression and violence. The Organisation for Appropriate Social Services in South Africa (OASSSA) and Psychologists Against Apartheid (with some additional alternative aims) drew in a range of mental-health professionals who were explicitly committed to serving the oppressed in South Africa and overtly critical of aspects of the apartheid-state policy. In addition, there were also detainee support groups established in several large centres. Within OASSSA (with whose organisational work and structure I am most familiar), two major foci of intervention were the counselling of ex-political detainees and the training of township groups (particularly youth activists) in crisis-counselling skills as part of emergency service interventions that also included training in first aid and the taking of legal statements. Many of the trainee counsellors had been directly traumatised themselves, and training workshops were designed to allow time for personal and group counselling as well as skills training. Many of the detainees had been tortured during their periods of incarceration and most had been kept in solitary confinement, exposed to sensory and interpersonal deprivation designed to break down psychological defences. Intervention for both trainees and ex-detainees was broadly located within a crisis-intervention framework, although at this time there tended to be a growing awareness of post-traumatic stress conceptualisations. However, the work with detainees in particular was generally understood within the framework of physical and psychological torture, and this was the area of theory most influential in informing intervention. Similarly to rape crisis, the work of OASSSA was underpinned by a specific ideological stance, in this case what could be termed a broadly 'progressive' ideology incorporating commitment to a non-racial democracy, the reduction of wealth disparity and the institution of a human-rights culture. Also in keeping with rape-crisis practices, OASSSA complemented direct service work with advocacy work involving media presentations, research, conferences and court appearances, among other interventions. Organisational structures were also designed to function democratically, accountably and, as far as possible, non-hierarchically. So the parallels in both organisational forms are clearly apparent.

For a range of reasons too complex to address within this chapter, but including, significantly, the political transition of the 1990s, OASSSA and Psychologists Against Apartheid dissolved in the early 1990s. One or two rape-crisis organisations are still functioning in an altered, generally more professionalised form, but the national feminist culture surrounding the work of early rape-crisis structures no longer exists. Seemingly in the place of such almost entirely volunteer-based organisational forms, more formal non-governmental organisations (NGOs) have arisen, such as the Trauma Clinic attached to the Centre for the Study of Violence and Reconciliation in Johannesburg, the Cape Town-based Centre for Survivors of Torture and Political Violence and the KwaZulu-Natal-based Survivors of Violence project, among others. Many of these NGOs were initiated by some of the same people who had been involved in OASSSA and related organisations, but their orientation has clearly changed with their establishment as professionally based, fully funded organisations. A further change, the one most central to the debate in this chapter, has been a shift towards understanding the impact of violence in terms of acute and post-traumatic stress disorders as evidenced in the language of training and increasing attendance at traumatic-stress conferences, both international and local, although the latter are a very recent introduction.

The implications of subscription to the conceptualisation of violent victimisation under the rubric of traumatic stress are complex, and I believe warrant some scrutiny if interventionists are not to run the risk of divorcing their practice from contextual and activist concerns. The rest of this chapter is devoted to exploring potential political problems stemming from uncritical adoption of what has become the dominant discourse in the area of the psychological impact of violence: 'The concept post-traumatic stress disorder has become so fashionable that it is dominating the debate worldwide about human responses to catastrophic events' (Kleber *et al.*, 1995: 4). However, as will also become clear in the course of the discussion, there are also clinical/therapeutic and even political imperatives that provide some support for the instantiation of the dominant discourse of post-traumatic stress. The interrogation of these issues is divided into two major sections, the first of which is devoted to the limitations of the diagnostic formulation and encompasses what could be called the '-isations' involved, and the second of which addresses the more *overtly* political role implied in utilisation of the diagnosis.

## The descriptive limitations of the diagnosis of traumatic stress: the '-isation' problems

Many of the issues addressed in this section have been cogently raised by Summerfield (1995) in a chapter entitled 'Addressing human response to war and atrocity: Major challenges in research and practices and the limitations of Western psychiatric models'. In his chapter he points out that irrespective of whether trauma is human induced or stems from natural disaster, the bulk of people affected by traumatic events tend to be impoverished or oppressed in other ways in their pre-existing life circumstances. He also notes that in contemporary armed conflicts 'over 90% of all casualties are civilians, typically from the poorest sectors of society' (Summerfield, 1995:17). In this respect, he argues that the majority of traumatic-stress-inducing events have a political location in the sense that victimisation is reflective of more general power imbalances in societies. The casualties of ongoing conflicts in many countries on the African continent (largely ignored in terms of global politics), the alarmingly high incidences of rape and violence against women in South African society and statistics indicating that crime levels are still highest in impoverished, under-resourced communities in South Africa would seem to bear out this premise at a number of levels. Within this broad framework, Summerfield argues for a recognition that post-traumatic stress diagnosis is culture-bound, drawing from what could be referred to as a Westernised, individualised and medicalised paradigm typical of mainstream American and Eurocentric psychiatry. Such concerns are certainly not unique to Summerfield, and have been raised by numerous trauma workers, usually from so-called underdeveloped countries, but remain marginalised within dominant traumatic-stress forums such as the conferences of the International Society of Traumatic Stress Studies (ISTSS) and their *Journal of Traumatic Stress*. While such critiques are aired, they tend to be understood as addenda to mainstream conceptualisations, qualifying rather than challenging fundamental premises. It is useful, then, to examine the validity of these points of criticism.

### The medicalisation of trauma

While there is clearly a whole field of medicine devoted to the treatment of physical trauma to be distinguished from the kind of trauma related to psychological disturbance, the establishment of the psychiatric classification of post-traumatic stress has arguably located a psychosocial phenomenon within the domain of biological psychiatry. Debates about whether to locate traumatic stress within a dissociative- or anxiety-related taxonomic categorisation reinforce the perception that trauma has been firmly incorporated within the psychiatric domain. When reading the literature in the field of traumatic stress, it is often strikingly apparent that one is working within a domain of multiple conceptualisations, perhaps more diverse than most other areas of psychiatric diagnosis, largely because of the somewhat unique inclusion of the precipitating factor/s as part of the diagnostic criteria. Therefore, in some instances trauma is described in terms of neurological functioning, and in others in terms of presenting assimilative difficulties in cognitive schemata. Perhaps the greatest tension is between the dominant diagnostic description of symptoms involving manifestations of intrusion, avoidance and hyper-arousal, and the more humanising conceptualisations of trauma as involving an extreme experience of loss of control and ruptures to meaning. Although DSM-IV does allow for the characterisation of feeling responses as involving 'intense fear, helplessness or horror' (American Psychiatric Association, 1994: 428), the dominant language is that of symptoms involving demonstration of behavioural and physiological indicators.

The medicalisation of trauma requires the categorisation of experience into classifiable indicators, rendering certain presentations legitimate and others outside of the norm. While the alterations to the diagnostic descriptions of traumatic stress across DSM-III, DSM-III-R (the revised 3rd edition) and DSM-IV demonstrate that diagnostic categorisation is contestable at any point in time, the veracity of a person's experience of traumatic stress is to some extent measured by the degree to which their 'symptoms' conform to the pre-eminent diagnostic entity. The medical categorisation therefore becomes a benchmark against which to measure experience as well as a framework within which to locate distress. As Levett (1987) has pointed out in relation to engagement with incest and arguably through the lens of the work of Foucault – particularly the text *Madness and Civilization* (1973) – the apparent humanising of medical constructions of these phenomena renders them apolitical and decontextual. By extension, this robs 'damaged' or 'sick' individuals of justifications of their condition as a response to oppression and exploitation. The medicalisation of traumatic stress appears to carry similar contradictions, offering legitimisation of the experience of victims in a constrained form, in many instances at the expense of the identification of the exploitative power enactments that their positions represent.

To date, the trauma field has at least remained open to favouring psychotherapeutic rather than pharmacological methods of intervention, so avoiding the most narrow of biological frameworks. However, increasingly popular studies using neuroimaging and exploring neurophysiological processes suggest that there may be a return to more biomedical interventions in the treatment of trauma, alienating the field further from socio-political concerns. The turn to detailed examination of brain functioning may provide a useful piece of knowledge in the puzzle, but should not be allowed to subsume other valid conceptualisations or to support the acceptance of individual medicalised interventions as sufficient in addressing trauma. While this concern may be viewed as parodying psychiatric perspectives, consistent debates about the apolitical stance of the dominant research and intervention bodies in the area suggest that splits between medical and political perspectives remain. In sum, then, the already well-articulated critiques of medical models of mental illness pertain to the diagnosis of post-traumatic stress disorder, with perhaps additional relevance in that the origins of disturbances in trauma are so clearly to be found in power abuses, as outlined in the introduction to this section.

### Individualisation
Related to the medicalisation of trauma, but somewhat differently focused, are concerns around the individualised orientation of post-traumatic stress disorder. The categorisation of the disorder makes provision for the diagnosis of a specific individual, which may be viewed as problematic at two different levels. Firstly, those theorists concerned with systemic understandings of normality and abnormality

would assert that traumatised individuals are traumatised units of a system, which is in turn affected by the impact on the individual. So family, colleagues, friends and community members are indirectly or vicariously affected by traumatised members of the group, and need to be taken into account in more meaningful ways than the diagnosis allows (despite references to 'witnessing' or being 'confronted with' trauma-inducing events in the diagnostic criteria). The traumatisation of families or significant others tends to be studied as secondary rather than primary in research into trauma, reinforcing notions of the individual as the site of experience and distress and, in a sense, establishing hierarchies in entitlement to concern and reparation. So, for example, direct victims usually present at clinics for psychotherapy, and it is often only incidentally that interventionists discover that other family members are suffering from related symptoms. Clearly, such individuals have not viewed themselves as entitled to their distress or to help-seeking in the same way as the directly affected person.

The second basis for critique is a more radical one, linked in some respects to appreciation of cross-cultural dimensions of understanding post-traumatic stress. Increasingly, theorists are beginning to write about and are attempting to formulate responses to mass-scale trauma such as the genocide in Rwanda and the devastation in Kosovo. In such contexts, the whole social fabric of a society may be ruptured, with dramatic changes to population demographics, mass displacement of people and ongoing disruption to basic conditions of social, political and economic life. Attempts to encompass the experience of individuals and communities in these circumstances under the rubric of post-traumatic stress seem grossly inadequate. Individuals may demonstrate characteristic post-traumatic stress symptoms, but is this understanding particularly helpful to those people undergoing such social rupture or to those attempting to intervene? While it is difficult to assert what alternative framework is ideal, aid and healthworkers may sometimes hold doggedly to post-traumatic stress conceptualisations in response to feeling powerless or overwhelmed, perhaps increasing their separation from communities rather than allowing for flexibility in engagement (Weine, 2000). Under these circumstances, the individualisation of the descriptive framework may be an inhibiting and limiting factor. Similarly, attempts to understand the impact of forced removals and political conflicts affecting whole communities, such as those between Inkatha- and ANC-aligned groupings in South Africa, also highlighted the inability of the diagnosis to capture the impact of such mass-scale phenomena. Interestingly, however, there were some studies that attempted to draw attention to the ravages of such conflicts by means of demographic surveys of symptom reporting, such as Dawes and Tredoux's (1989) study that examined the impact of attacks on Crossroads squatter camp on resident children and mothers. Such studies appeared to have political aims beyond clinical concerns, in that they were designed to create a climate of public outrage and draw attention to state-supported abuses. I will return to such strategic uses of post-traumatic stress diagnoses and their implications later in the discussion.

## Westernisation

As Summerfeld points out, as with other diagnostic categories formulated within Western or Eurocentric assumptive systems (Kleinman, 1987), the symptoms categorised as meeting the diagnosis of post-traumatic stress are to some extent culture-bound. Although the reference to 'instinctive fight-flight responses' to extreme threat as characterising part of the basis for traumatic-stress symptoms, for example hyper-arousal, has contributed to assumptions about the universality of such responses, it is clear that the presentation of symptoms is culturally mediated. Even at the level of gender differences between people of the same class and ethnic origin, it has been observed that men tend to present with more anger following trauma exposure and women with more fear (Janoff-Bulman and Frieze, 1987).

Among non-Western societies, such as those researched in South and Central American, Asian and African contexts, it is apparent that there are both subtle and dramatic differences in expressions of distress and also in understandings as to why traumatic events occur, which in turn have implications for presentation. Among more traditional African people at a broad level of generalisation, it can be argued that the two primary differences in symptom presentation lie in the area of the soma and in the social-network implications of trauma. Given the integrative world view or cosmology of African society, in which psyche-soma or body-mind splits are absent, it is not surprising that many traumatised African people present with somatic symptoms, such as chest and back pains or feelings of faintness or dizziness, as integral to their distress. Such presentations are not encompassed within the frame of PTSD, although, as with all categorisations, there is reference to the fact that diagnosticians need to be open to culturally specific forms of presentation. In addition, since African cosmology holds that all people operate as integrally related forces, with animistic links to the natural and spiritual world (Ngubane, 1977; Shutte, 1994), the experience of harm or misfortune is understood as a rupture within this whole field of forces, representing an imbalance that needs to be rectified. At a concrete level, this may manifest as deep concern about having alienated one's ancestral community or as suspicion of others within one's immediate social network, resulting in a form of social alienation that goes beyond the notion of social withdrawal identified as a symptom within the PTSD cluster C (American Psychiatric Association, 1994: 428). These examples point yet again to inadequacies in a diagnostic formulation that by virtue of its origins could be seen as colonising the domain of responses to extreme stress.

Once again, it must be acknowledged that this level of critique tends to parody psychiatric practice, in which there are clearly practitioners who are sensitive to cultural biases. However, the fact remains that this Westernised conceptualisation of response tends to dominate assessment, intervention and research in the area, marginalising other understandings, which remain qualifiers or aberrations rather than mainstream formulations. The culturally specific nature of the dominant system of explanation is unacknowledged, except when explicitly challenged from outside the framework. This, in turn, does have political implications for the diagnosis of people from 'other' cultures, for example, refugees requiring psychiatric evaluation to confirm their legitimacy in a host country, or people outside the Western mainstream seeking to claim damages for misfortunes inflicted upon them. In such instances, the links between psychiatric discourse and legal rights may become powerful determinants of the claimants' legitimacy. In these and other respects, the Westernisation of the diagnosis has both ideological and material import.

## Literalisation

In addition to the concerns raised so far, which pertain predominantly to the symptom criteria of PTSD, it is also worth noting the implications of criterion A, i.e. the nature of the stressor conditions that comply with a positive diagnosis. From the more generalised description of stressor events of DSM-III-R: 'an event outside the range of normal human experience' (American Psychiatric Association, 1987: 238), to that of DSM-IV: 'an event or events that involved actual or threatened death or serious injury, or a threat to the physical integrity of self or others' (American Psychiatric Association, 1994: 427), there has been a shift in the specificity of the kind of event that warrants the diagnosis. While this narrowing of the definition represents progress in the refinement of the diagnostic entity, it also highlights the emphasis placed on the presence of an objective, consensual and, to some extent, measurable origin for the condition. In keeping with past attempts to measure stressor severity by means of ranked events (Ghaziuddin et al., 1990), there have been attempts to assess the relative severity of impact of different types of trauma (Green, 1994), with some evidence that threat to life and physical injury are predictive of greater vulnerability to PTSD (Kilpatrick and Resnick, 1993).

Theorists writing from more psychodynamic and cognitive perspectives have challenged this somewhat mechanistic interpretation of traumatic events, arguing that the subjective meaning of exposure is crucial to comprehending the impact of trauma, be this in terms of pre-existing cognitive schemata (Horowitz, 1992; McCann and Pearlman, 1990) or in terms of prior psychic history and intrapsychic functioning (Garland, 1998). These kinds of debates appear to replicate contestation within psychological theory between positivist and subjectivist/hermeneutic perspectives, and highlight the location of traumatic-stress studies within yet another set of value-bound debates. More recently, social-constructionist perspectives have extended these controversies (Burr, 1995; Gergen, 1985), deconstructing the role of language and discursive frameworks in formulations of experience and challenging claims to versions of reality and truth. Within the trauma field, such debates have surfaced primarily with regard to the historical retrieval of memories of abuse and the recognition of what has been termed 'false-memory syndrome'.

In an article examining the history of PTSD, Wilson (1994) follows the trajectory of the role of the recognition of objectively established abusive events, beginning with the debated reality of allegations of sexual abuse in Freud's writings: 'Between 1895 and 1897 Freud shifted emphasis in his thinking away from a PTSD paradigm of neurosis to one that centred around intrapsychic fantasy' (Wilson, 1994: 683). This shift influenced diagnostic opinion away from acceptance of the normality of the traumatic response in the face of overwhelming stress, towards a more pathogenic conceptualisation of the individual, whose predisposition to the development of disorder was understood to predate exposure to trauma. This view was epitomised in DSM-II, and the contestation between models of traumatic stress that emphasised the stressor impact as opposed to pre-existing personality deficiencies is evident in traumatic-stress writings from the early 1900s up until the present (Kinzie and Goetz, 1996). To some extent, DSM-III's and DSM-IV's recognition and articulation of the role of the stressor event and its impact on 'almost anyone' has destigmatised traumatised individuals, who are no longer viewed as personally weak or psychically flawed. However, this emphasis on the objective external origin of the condition has also had its drawbacks, as I argued earlier.

Simpson writes: 'The DSM has been (and remains) consistently ambivalent in both recognising and denying the essential component of subjective perception within the construct, and about how to allow for the obviously relevant issue of the individual's specific and general vulnerabilities, while wishing to exclude patently trivial stresses from recognition as traumatic' (1995: 196). In attempting to exclude such trivial stressors, the definition of the scope of events pertinent to diagnosis has become further narrowed with DSM-IV, and implies that individuals presenting with clear evidence of symptoms who do not meet the stressor criterion have to be excluded from diagnosis. This tension is somewhat reminiscent of criticisms aimed at the South African Truth and Reconciliation Commission concerning the range of events that were considered to fall within the scope of 'gross human rights violations'. So forced removals and pass-law arrests were not considered sufficiently gross to warrant inclusion, and some have argued that the pervasive abusiveness of the apartheid system was almost condoned by the exclusive focus on *extreme* abuses. Similarly, with traumatic stress, it may be that less-dramatic causes of traumatic stress disqualify sufferers from social sanction.

Focusing on engagement with post-traumatic stress in cases of torture and repression under the apartheid regime, Simpson highlights the degree to which the stressor criterion has been open to misinterpretation. In certain instances, the lack of evidence of an exceptional stressor or stressors was used as a justification for the inability to diagnose: 'A psychiatrist working for the South African government insisted that it was impossible to make the diagnosis because, he argued, one cannot ever diagnose PTSD unless there is "objective, collateral proof" of the existence of the stressor (a requirement invented by him and highly convenient in hiding the effects of torture)' (Simpson, 1995: 198). In other instances, the stressor criterion was open to alternative abusive interpretation: 'A state psychiatrist in South Africa has testified that, because political detentions without trial, solitary confinement, and police assaults have been common in the black community, these experiences are therefore not exceptional and thus cannot meet criterion A' (Simpson, 1995: 197). While such distortions of diagnostic formulations cannot be laid at the door of the originators of the diagnosis, Simpson argues that the 'producers of the DSM industry' have failed to take account of these ethical considerations. Similarly, feminist critiques of the conservatism inherent in 'false-memory syndrome' propositions and their role in detracting from the publicisation of the prevalence of incestuous abuse and related gender politics also point to the moral implications of taking up certain scientific positions.

The literalisation of trauma as epitomised in the insistence upon, and definition of, accepted stressor-event criteria instantiates contradictory costs and benefits, and lays the diagnostic category open to potential abuses when the neutrality of diagnostic formulations is assumed rather than problematised. Much of the basis for diagnostic specificity pertains beyond the need for agreed-upon research and treatment parameters to the demands made by the legal system on diagnostic formulations.

## Legalisation

Parallel with the formalisation of the diagnosis of post-traumatic stress has been the incorporation of the category into the legal domain, initially in response to compensation claims, and more recently in the service of both the defence and the prosecution in criminal cases: 'The damage claim laws, first in Europe and then in the United States, that allowed compensation for damages from accidents coincided with the medical professions' increasing awareness of traumatic neurosis' (Kinzie and Goetz, 1996: 173). So, throughout its development as a diagnosis, traumatic stress has been subject to the scrutiny of legal experts, and many of the debates within the medical field have been initiated by contestation within the legal domain. The need for a clearly categorised descriptive entity as discussed in terms of medicalisation, individualisation and Westernisation, as well as the insistence on rigorously defined stressor criteria, all to some extent stem from conformity to the legal requirements of the diagnostic entity. Therefore, the legalisation of post-traumatic stress disorder is inextricably bound up with many of the critical issues raised so far. However, as in many of the other categories discussed, there are both emancipatory as well as limiting aspects to litigious conceptualisations: 'PTSD has also proved an effective tool in attacking traditional legal restrictions on liability for intentional and negligent infliction of psychic harm. More broadly, the PTSD diagnostic conception offers the law a scientific rationale to support the sociopolitical ideology of victimization and to justify the growing recognition of victims' rights' (Stone, 1993: 24). Although writing about the American context, much of what Stone argues has general applicability, and in post-apartheid South Africa, one of the new agendas is what is known as 'victim empowerment'.

The use of PTSD diagnoses in legal settings has continued to highlight some of the contradictions inherent in the category (which I have alluded to already under the literalisation debate), particularly when PTSD has been invoked as a criminal defence. In some instances, lawyers have argued that PTSD was a normative response to an abnormal stimulus, for example, for an abused woman, 'the characteristic response of the "reasonable" woman' (Stone, 1993: 26), and that consequent aggression directed towards the batterer was not an aberrant feature. However, in other instances, battered women and Vietnam veterans who have committed violent acts have pleaded insanity (as a consequence of their exposure to trauma) as a defence. Stone argues that the 'two faces of PTSD evidence: syndrome as "sickness" and syndrome as "normal" response under the circumstances' (1993: 26), carry not only legal, but also political weight, as evidenced in feminist engagement with battery debates. In yet other instances, the presence of PTSD may be used to establish the veracity of victimisation, as in a court case where the presence of rape-trauma syndrome was used to refute the possibility of consensual sex: 'As PTSD in the defendant can exculpate or mitigate, so PTSD in the victim can lead the government to prosecute, the jury to sentence, and the judge to punish' (Stone, 1993: 28). In South African history, as will be elaborated in the next section, evidence around the presence of psychiatric disturbance of the nature of PTSD was sometimes invoked in order to establish the likelihood that the accused had been tortured, and in some cases to question the validity of confessions and evidence garnered by the police. While such evidence usually required physical or alternative substantiation, one can apprehend the parallels in these instances with the rape survivor or abductee who reinforces his/her evidence by means of demonstration of such 'psychological scars'. In this respect, it is clear that the invocation of PTSD can act to protect victims' rights and to lend greater weight to human- and victim-rights agendas. At the same time as recognising the usefulness of this legitimisation, it is important to bear in mind metacritiques concerning the hegemony of legal discourse and the degree to which this discourse delegitimates alternative presentations.

Having examined a range of problematic themes in relation to the politics of the diagnosis of PTSD, it is important to acknowledge that there are both merits and demerits to the categorisation, and that the contestation around the definition of the disorder lends itself to supporting points of political resistance rather than purely to co-option. It is to some of the more overtly political uses of the diagnosis that the discussion now turns, extending some of the debates alluded to in the legalisation section of the chapter with specific reference to South African examples.

## ■ Overtly political ramifications of the employment of PTSD categorisation

In some instances, usually in the context of making legal arguments for asserting the human rights of victims, overtly political and clinical/psychological goals coalesce. In a somewhat different domain from PTSD, during the 1970s and 1980s, psychological theory was drawn upon to mitigate culpability of people who were charged with crimes as part of mass action. In some instances, psychological testimony about crowd behaviour and theories of disinhibition and loss of personal will were cited to argue that individuals could not be held solely accountable for actions such as necklacings and stonings. The critical social psychologist, Steve Reicher (1987), has pointed out how such theoretical constructions of the 'crowd' as a primitive, impulsive and wayward entity tend to rob the activity of the group of its meaning, for example, political protest, and to downplay the interactional role of forces in opposition, for example, the role of the police. Therefore, the alignment of psychologists with anti-apartheid activists who required defending against charges of 'common purpose' brought by the state may have simultaneously detracted from the meaning of their actions, while acting in their interests with regard to the severity of the sentences they were handed down. This tension reflects that raised by Stone in his discussion around the use of PTSD to explain a 'normal', purposeful response to a context, as opposed to invoking the diagnosis to explain actions as 'insane' or out of character and irrational.

Similar tensions emerge when one looks at the role of diagnosticians relative to the status of refugees in countries such as Australia and Canada, and may come to apply to South Africa, given the influx of refugees from other African conflicts. One of the grounds for acquiring refugee status in Australia is evidence of victimisation and ongoing risk to the individual. In some instances, brutalisation or oppression is inferred not only from personal accounts, but also from the evidence of traumatic-stress symptoms. Not only is diagnosis in this instance fraught with the problems of cultural difference alluded to earlier, but the clinician is in the invidious position of wanting to heal the patient, but also wanting to prove that the patient is sufficiently disturbed to provide the basis for his/her material protection from return to the stressor condition. This tension was also evidenced in clinicians' responses to political detainees under apartheid who became sufficiently mentally ill to warrant hospitalisation. The hospitalisation allowed them to escape the persecutory and abusive environment of solitary confinement and interrogation (often accompanied by torture), but the diagnosis was often experienced as shameful, as a sign of weakness. In addition, the clinician's role in restoring the patient to health, with the associated return to the stressor environment, was an ambiguous one. In such instances, the political alignment of the diagnostician becomes significant in a way that challenges injunctions to neutrality and objectivity in clinical diagnosis and practice.

In yet further instances, also alluded to in the section dealing with legal evidence above, the presence of PTSD may be employed to retrospectively establish that abuse or criminal activity took place. Under apartheid, it was common for the police to collect evidence for prosecution by means of confessions extracted under interrogation, in many instances involving torture (Simpson, 1995). In most instances, any witnesses to such abuses were implicated in their practice, leaving the victim the sole source of evidence of allegations of abuse. In such circumstances, the evidence of clinicians was crucial in establishing the likelihood of the veracity of such confessions, and occasionally in bringing civil charges against state interrogators. However, as I mentioned earlier, the degree of malleability in the diagnosis of PTSD lent itself to uses and abuses by professionals on both sides of the political divide:

> There was no lack, in South Africa, of white Afrikaans doctors and psychiatrists who were happy to assist by skilfully and emphatically finding nothing wrong with political detainees, no matter how severe their symptoms, and by testifying that they were perfectly fit, no matter how damaged they might be. There was also an almost total lack of doctors willing to take the risk of working with human rights lawyers to testify as to the facts of such trauma (Simpson, 1995: 208).

Such observations further strengthen challenges to the neutrality or apolitical nature of clinical practices. It is also worth noting, in common with Simpson, that there is ongoing evidence of abusive interrogation by the police in South Africa, documented by human-rights organisations, although currently criminal suspects and 'aliens' appear to bear the brunt of these abuses.

In a further examination of the politico-legal employment of PTSD diagnosis in South Africa, issues to do with mitigation and exculpation also deserve mention, in keeping with some of the legal dilemmas posed by Stone (1993) and mentioned earlier. PTSD employed as a defence can again act in the interests of both victims and victimisers, and herein lies the rub. In certain instances, violence committed in the service of anti-apartheid ends was accounted for by expert psychological witnesses in terms of past brutalisation and oppression. So acts of violence were justified as defensive, in response to the damage inflicted by the apartheid system, either in relation to specific acts of brutalisation or more general oppression (in keeping with the defensive arguments put forward on behalf of battered women who inflict harm upon their partners). Such testimony often served to mitigate the severity of sentences imposed on anti-apartheid activists, and in this context could be viewed as serving progressive political ends. However, more recently, as underscored by evidence led by amnesty applicants to the Truth and Reconciliation Commission, similar arguments have been invoked by agents of the apartheid state. For example, Eugene de Kok, a senior Vlakplaas commander, self-admittedly responsible for numerous deaths and acts of brutality, claims to be suffering from PTSD with associated intrusive symptoms such as nightmares and vivid memories of events. It could be argued that there is a significant difference in enacting violence from a structural and perceived position of powerlessness as opposed to a position of power. Lack of control and helplessness are generally accepted as cornerstones of the psychological experience of traumatisation. Therefore, it is difficult to comprehend how De Kok can lay claim to the crucial feeling dimension of intense 'fear and helplessness', although horror may have conceivably been present in some of the incidents in which he participated. In recognition of the expectation that victims are required to demonstrate a lack of choice in their exposure to events, De Kok, and others like him, have claimed that they were afraid to the extent that they were lackeys in a chain, who faced inordinate pressures if they contested their role in the exercise of violence. Such arguments are difficult to entertain in the face of the evidence of the extremity of violence employed by agents in carrying out their so-called 'duties'. In such instances, turning to another psychiatric label, it seems that the rhetoric of PTSD may be serving anti-social ends and may be employed with calculated or unconscious cynicism. Opening the door to the employment of PTSD as a diagnostic justification for the enactment of violence conceivably provides the basis for a blurring of boundaries between victims and victimisers. While such a perspective may be more realistic, it tends to obscure the moral codes employed to judge the justifiability of different acts of violence. It is clear that whether the litigious employment of the diagnosis of PTSD is considered a use or abuse of the category is determined by political and moral criteria, rather than scientific parameters. This highlights the need for those employing the diagnosis to be self-conscious of their own assumptions and political and moral convictions.

In the context of anti-apartheid politics, those who did champion victims of state repression had recourse to some organisational base such as the National Medical and Dental Association (NAMDA) (for medical professionals) and organisations like OASSSA and Psychologists Against Apartheid referred to in the introductory section of this chapter. In addition to its employment in individually focused advocacy work, PTSD was also invoked at a broader social level to highlight the plight of victims by drawing attention to the psychological damage they suffered. Mass studies of the presence of traumatic-stress symptoms among ex-detainees (Foster et al., 1987), children living in townships affected by political conflict (Dawes and Tredoux, 1989; Gibson, 1987; Rock, 1997) and internally displaced people (Michelson, 1994), all served both academic and intentionally political aims. Researchers in these instances were guided by an activist agenda that aimed at embarrassing the government by drawing national and international sympathy and attention to such victims of human-rights abuses. However, again there was a tension in the apparent scientific neutrality of such studies, which required of researchers not to assert overtly political agendas, lest they be accused of bias and their research denied credibility. Such activism had to be taken up at other levels, such as through the popular media, if academic integrity was to be maintained. This tension continues to beset traumatic-stress researchers and practitioners, as evidenced in a debate at the recent Third World Congress of the Society for Traumatic Stress Studies (Melbourne, March 2000) about whether it was the role of the organisation to protest against the imposition of laws arguably antithetical to human rights (in Australia in this instance, but more generally in a world context). The status quo, as outlined by Simpson, appeared to hold sway in this international gathering of experts: 'The literature on torture and state terrorism is very limited and is excessively concentrated on the atypical experiences of distant centres profitably treating refugees and largely rather obsessively engaged in cataloguing the categories of cruelty and the associated symptoms, while avoiding serious study of or engagement with the universal political element of such trauma, or in work realistically likely to help prevent such events' (Simpson, 1995: 200). However, the fact that the issue was given plenary attention at the Australian conference and that the central theme of the last European conference held in Instanbul, Turkey (June 1999) was 'Human Rights', indicates that increasing pressure is being brought to bear on the traumatic-stress industry to take a more proactive political position. In this respect, the conferences of OASSSA and Psychologists Against Apartheid that took place in the 1980s in South Africa prefigured such developments some 15 years ago. While certainly not unique in world terms, the South African political context propelled mental-health practitioners into engagement with the politics of their practices in ways that stimulated a more critical engagement with issues of normality and abnormality generally, and the impact of trauma in particular. Returning to the introduction, it is clear that traumatic stress highlights such political tensions in clinical diagnosis and intervention precisely because victims are not indiscriminately chosen and abuses of power are so evident in the causal chain of the disorder.

# Conclusion

Simply stated, the conclusions of this chapter are twofold. Firstly, the chapter has argued that the scientific status of PTSD as a diagnostic entity is questionable, as emphasised by the cultural bias of the symptoms described and problems in refining the stressor criterion. This is not a new argument, and is a central feature of the book *Beyond Trauma: Cultural and Societal Dynamics* (Kleber *et al.*, 1995). However, given the paucity of such writings and the ongoing marginalisation of such critiques, they are worth reiterating. In addition, I have attempted to point out that the alleged lack of rigour in the diagnosis may also allow for more space for resistance and subversion. In its inception, traumatic-stress diagnosis was essentially liberatory, in that it rendered the experiences of hundreds of victims normative and acceptable, rather than continuing to place responsibility for distress at the door of the deficient individual. In recognising such a category, psychiatry and medicine made admissible the fact that governments were directly or indirectly responsible for inflicting psychological damage on individuals in the service of their own ends, for example, in waging wars. Despite its co-option into more conservative discourses, this potentially challenging role should not be overlooked and may be rediscovered.

The second broad aim of the chapter has been to make visible the moral and political choices and actions inherent in the employment of the diagnosis of PTSD, in some instances more glaringly evident than others. While such considerations have been acknowledged in the literature, as in a debate in the *Journal of Traumatic Stress* concerning the *Intifadah* and issues to do with Holocaust survivors, led by a piece entitled 'Ideological bias in the *Journal of Traumatic Stress*' (Milgram, 1994), they still tend to be marginalised by scientific and professional agendas. The introduction of politics into academe is understood to be antithetical to sound scholarship, and there appears to be considerable anxiety about the possible organisational conflicts that may ensue should international traumatic-stress societies adopt overtly political standpoints. While it is clear that dodging such positioning is difficult in the international arena, I would argue that it is well nigh impossible in South Africa, largely because of the political history of trauma work outlined at the outset of the chapter.

In the absence of a clear ideological imperative, as exemplified in the feminist politics of rape-trauma organisations and the anti-apartheid stance of other groupings prevalent in the 1980s, it would seem that a revised contextual and moral base needs to inform current practices in South Africa. Despite its liberal associations and the somewhat tempered nature of its imperatives for action, the discourse of human rights appears to embody the most viable set of moral principles to inform trauma intervention in South Africa in the 21st century. Human-rights agendas have served the needs of anti-racist activists in the 1960s in America, campaigners for laws against the exploitation of women and proponents of anti-atrocity agreements in the United Nations, among others. In keeping company with such activists against oppression, it would seem that trauma workers would be well served to make such a stance, along with all its complications, part of their overt commitment in their engagement with victims and survivors. Simpson's quote from Montaigne is an apt assertion with which to conclude this chapter, which hopefully has illustrated the political complexity of normative diagnoses with specific reference to PTSD: 'Science without conscience is but the death of the soul' (1995: 209). How that conscience is determined will of course be influenced by the material and ideological imperatives of a particular social system at a particular point in history. Without constant attention to and articulation of one's motives in PTSD practice, interventionists remain vulnerable to co-option. Such a stance may in part be achieved by remaining responsive to political agendas and by keeping company with others who seek to subvert psychological assumptions. To practise psychology politically is to be willing to be called out by comrades, colleagues, survivors and one's own sense of conscience.

# References

American Psychiatric Association (1968). *Diagnostic and Statistical Manual of Mental Disorders* (2nd edn). Washington, DC: American Psychiatric Association.
American Psychiatric Association (1980). *Diagnostic and Statistical Manual of Mental Disorders* (3rd edn). Washington, DC: American Psychiatric Association.
American Psychiatric Association (1987). *Diagnostic and Statistical Manual of Mental Disorders* (3rd edn, rev.). Washington, DC: American Psychiatric Association.
American Psychiatric Association (1994). *Diagnostic and Statistical Manual of Mental Disorders* (4th edn). Washington, DC: American Psychiatric Association.
Becker, D. (1995). The deficiency of the concept of post-traumatic stress disorder when dealing with victims of human rights violations. In R. J. Kleber, C. R. Figley and B. P. Gersons (eds), *Beyond Trauma: Cultural and Societal Dynamics,* pp. 99–110. New York: Plenum.

Brom, D. and Witztum, E. (1995). When political reality enters therapy: Ethical considerations in the treatment of post-traumatic stress disorder. In R. J. Kleber, C. R. Figley and B. P. Gersons (eds), *Beyond Trauma: Cultural and Societal Dynamics*, pp. 237–48. New York: Plenum.

Burr, V. (1995). *An Introduction to Social Constructionism*. London: Routledge.

Dawes, A. and Tredoux, C. (1989). Emotional status of children exposed to political violence in the Crossroads squatter area during 1986/1987. *Psychology in Society*, 12, 33–47.

Foster, D., Davis, D. and Sandler, D. (1987). *Detention and Torture in South Africa: Psychological, Legal and Historical Studies*. Cape Town: David Philip.

Foucault, M. (1973). *Madness and Civilization*. New York: Random House.

Garland, C. (1998). *Understanding Trauma: A Psychoanalytic Approach*. London: Gerald Duckworth.

Gergen, K. J. (1985). The social constructionist movement in modern psychology. *American Psychologist*, 40, 266–75.

Ghaziuddin, M., Ghaziuddin, N. and Stein, G. S. (1990). Life events and the occurrence of depression. *Canadian Journal of Psychiatry*, 35, 239–42.

Gibson, K. (1987). Civil conflict, stress and children. *Psychology in Society*, 8, 4–26.

Green, B. L. (1994). Psychosocial research in traumatic stress: An update. *Journal of Traumatic Stress*, 7 (3), 341–62.

Herman, J. (1992a). *Trauma and Recovery: The Aftermath of Violence from Domestic Abuse to Political Terror*. London: Basic Books.

Herman, J. (1992b). Complex PTSD: A syndrome in survivors of prolonged and repeated trauma. *Journal of Traumatic Stress*, 5 (3), 377–420.

Horowitz, M. (1992). *Stress Response Syndromes* (2nd edn). New York: Aronson.

Janoff-Bulman, R. and Frieze, I. H. (1987). The role of gender in reactions to criminal victimization. In R. C. Barnett and G. K. Baruch (eds), *Gender and Stress*, pp. 159–84. New York: Free Press.

Kilpatrick, D. G. and Resnick, H. S. (1993). Clinical phenomenology: Clinical manifestations in different patients. In J. R. Davidson and E. D. Foa (eds), *Post-traumatic Stress Disorder: DSM-IV and Beyond*, pp. 57–146. Washington, DC: American Psychiatric Press.

Kinzie, J. D. and Goetz, R. R. (1996). A century of controversy surrounding post-traumatic stress-spectrum syndromes: The impact of DSM-III and DSM-IV. *Journal of Traumatic Stress*, 9 (2), 159–79.

Kleber, R. J., Figley, C. R. and Gersons, B. P. (1995). *Beyond Trauma: Cultural and Societal Dynamics*. New York: Plenum.

Kleinman, A. (1987). Anthropology and psychiatry: The role of culture in cross-cultural research on illness. *British Journal of Psychiatry*, 151, 447–54.

Levett, A. (1987). Childhood sexual abuse: Event, fact or structure? *Psychology in Society*, 8, 80–102.

McCann, L. and Pearlman, L. (1990). *Psychological Trauma and the Adult Survivor: Theory, Therapy and Transformation*. New York: Brunner/Mazel.

Mendelson, G. (1987). The concept of post-traumatic stress disorder: A review. *International Journal of Law and Psychiatry*, 10, 45–62.

Michelson, C. (1994). Township violence, levels of distress and post-traumatic stress disorder amongst displacees from Natal. *Psychology in Society*, 18, 47–55.

Milgram, N. A. (1994). Ideological bias in the *Journal of Traumatic Stress*. *Journal of Traumatic Stress*, 7 (3), 467–72.

Ngubane, H. (1977). *Body and Mind in Zulu Medicine*. London: Academic Press.

Reicher, S. (1987). Contact, action and racialization: Some British evidence. In M. Hewstone and R. Brown (eds), *Contact and Conflict in Intergroup Encounters*, pp. 64–87. Oxford: Blackwell.

Rock, B. (1997). *Spirals of Suffering*. Pretoria: Human Sciences Research Council.

Shutte, A. (1994). *Philosophy for Africa*. Cape Town: University of Cape Town Press.

Simpson, M. A. (1995). What went wrong? Diagnostic and ethical problems in dealing with the effects of torture and repression in South Africa. In R. J. Kleber, C. R. Figley and B. P. Gersons (eds), *Beyond Trauma: Cultural and Societal Dynamics,* pp. 187–212. New York: Plenum.

Stone, A. A. (1993). Post-traumatic stress disorder and the law: Critical review of the new frontier. *Bulletin of the American Academy of Psychiatry and the Law*, 21 (1), 23–36.

Summerfield, D. (1995). Addressing human response to war and atrocity: Major challenges in research and practices and the limitations of Western psychiatric models. In R. J. Kleber, C. R. Figley and B. P. Gersons (eds), *Beyond Trauma: Cultural and Societal Dynamics*, pp. 17–30. New York: Plenum.

Weine, S. (2000). *When History is a Nightmare.* New York: John Wiley.

Wilson, J. P. (1994). The historical evolution of PTSD diagnostic criteria: From Freud to DSM-IV. *Journal of Traumatic Stress*, 7 (3), 681–98.

Yehuda, R. and McFarlane, A. C. (1995). Conflict between current knowledge about post-traumatic stress disorder and its original conceptual basis. *American Journal of Psychiatry*, 152 (12), 1705–13.

# A critical re-reading of post-traumatic stress disorder from a cross-cultural/community perspective

*M. Brinton Lykes*

## ■ Introduction

In 1983, the International Symposium of Children and War reported that 5% of all casualties in the First World War were civilians, whereas such casualties reached 50% in the Second World War and over 80% in the Vietnam War (UNICEF, 1986, in Summerfield, 1995). The United Nations Children's Fund (UNICEF) has documented the shifts in victims characteristic of modern warfare, arguing that today over 90% of all casualties are civilians (UNICEF, 1996). Those marginalised from power and resources in a society are disproportionately affected by wars. The metanarrative of the Cold War and the Doctrine of National Security that legitimised horrific violations of human rights, including torture, massacres, disappearances, etc. of those aligned with 'communism' or opposed to a state's 'national project' have ceded ground to multiple narratives emergent from contemporary conflicts waged at the intersices of economic, political and ethnic or racial conflicts. One of these multiple narratives that dominate 'post-war' discourse within the West is that of the 'victim/survivor' who suffers from 'post-traumatic stress disorder' (PTSD) (American Psychiatric Association, 1994). So, within the arena of modern warfare, mental-health workers (including psychiatrists, psychologists and social workers) can be found in zones of armed conflict and, more specifically, as protagonists in the multiple arenas of recovery, reparations and reconciliation that characterise the wake of such terror.

Contemporary psychologists and mental-health workers offer one set of responses to survivors of the type of horror experienced in modern warfare. Typically they focus on the *effects* of war on civilian populations, describing psychological symptoms and behaviours observed. This set of responses first emerged in the study of soldiers' responses to warfare and has a long tradition within psychiatry and psychology. Some, including Starcevic and Durdic (1993), trace its origins to soldiers' 'irritable heart[s]' in the wake of the US Civil War. There is consensus (see, for example, Kleinman, 1995; Bracken *et al.*, 1995, among others) that characterisations of the psychological effects of the First World War for soldiers described as 'shell shock' or 'war neurosis' and of fighters in the Second World War as 'survivor syndrome', 'combat exhaustion' or 'battle fatigue' are clinical antecedents of the symptoms and syndromes reflected by the diagnosis known as PTSD. Other antecedents have been traced to, for example, Lindemann's discussion of the psychological sequelae of surviving the nightclub fire in Boston in the 1940s (Lindemann, 1979).

When the creators of the third edition of the *Diagnostic and Statistical Manual of Mental Disorders* (DSM-III) (American Psychiatric Association, 1980) introduced the term in 1980 in association with major stressors, including concentration-camp experiences, torture, bombings and natural disaster, they subsumed previous diagnostic categories including post-torture syndrome and rape-trauma syndrome under PTSD. Therefore, this apparently contemporary illness discourse for survivors of political violence is neither altogether new, nor recent. What is perhaps 'new' is the extent to which it has been popularised within Western culture, and the extent to which psychologists, psychiatrists and other mental-health workers have convinced international agencies, including the United Nations, of the importance of incorporating mental-health work within the rapid and long-term responses to war, natural disasters and other 'exceptionally difficult circumstances'.

This strategy for dealing with the effects of trauma, applied in many parts of the world to children and adults in situations of organised violence, is embedded in traditional Anglo-Saxon medical conceptions of illness, where selected symptoms and behavioural indices provide evidence of PTSD or other 'diseases'. Although this is not, on the surface, a 'bad' or problematic thing, many have suggested that the tendency to understand the effects of war, state-sponsored violence and structural oppression within the biomedical framework of PTSD deeply constrains the understandings available to those who seek to accompany survivors, medicalising and pathologising what are fundamentally political, economic, cultural and psychological phenomena.

Bracken *et al.* (1995), among others, have critiqued the assumptions underlying the PTSD model in biomedicine and psychiatry. Briefly, this critique demonstrates that the model's ontology reveals an individual at the centre of morality and cosmology, as well as a presumed universalism of forms and content of mental disorder. However, as Kleinman (1987) observed, simply because we can identify a similar phenomenon in different situations does not mean that it is universal. Despite this, therapeutic modalities developed to respond to these syndromes, drawing primarily on 'talking cures' or 'biomedical interventions', are presumed to be relevant across cultures. Marsella and White (1982/1989), Bracken (1993) and Kleinman (1995), among many others, have argued to the contrary (see also Eagle's essay in this volume). This chapter contributes to the current debate surrounding PTSD by focusing on selected resources within psychology and the social sciences more broadly that break epistemological and ontological set with current normative uses of PTSD. It argues that we can better understand and more effectively respond to war and state-sponsored violence and their psychosocial sequelae through a critical reading of the socio-political, historical and cultural contexts that are defining of and defined by these experiences of violence. Specifically, the chapter suggests ways in which symbolic representations, constructivist theories, human-rights discourse and liberation psychology constitute resources for a resituating of 'trauma'. Through a specific example of intercultural community-based participatory research among rural Mayan Ixil women in Guatemala, the chapter demonstrates how the critical perspective it describes informed an intervention with local survivors, and how that intervention contributes to rethreading life in a local community and to retheorising trauma. Finally, it explores parallel possibilities for meaning-making and praxis within South Africa.

## Breaking epistemological set?

Despite the contributions made through the recognition of the psychological needs of survivors of war and state-sponsored violence, multiple researchers and field workers have argued that current constructions of war's sequelae are inadequate or misrepresentative of the complex realities attendant to such experiences. I begin my discussion by clarifying some of the limits of PTSD suggested by those who study war's effects from within this limited discursive environment.

### Contextualising the subject

Jensen and Shaw's (1993) review of research on the effects of war on children and youth concluded that advances have been made in correcting earlier methodological flaws in this research, e.g. lack of adequate controls and problems with self-report and retrospective data, so facilitating greater understanding of the complex range of responses of children and youth in situations of war. They recommended extending the individual focus on children and youth to include family and community, and, further, that we shift from a predominant interest in psychopathological consequences of war (dominant in much of the literature) to studying war's effects on children's attitudes, values and development. Cairns makes similar suggestions in his multiple studies of 'children of the troubles' in Northern Ireland (Cairns, 1996). This recommended shift to a contextualised model (following Bronfenbrenner, 1979) and to more positive variables, including values and beliefs, is a step away from the pathologising of the victim described above and in early research assessing PTSD in children, but nonetheless tends to perpetuate a focus on an individual who is affected by exogenous variables from a social context and either possesses or does not possess a resulting trait or characteristic. So, despite some advances, the discourse remains constrained by the individualism of a Western ideology critiqued above.

### Historicising PTSD

Herman analysed the emergence of PTSD as a model of meaning-making about the effects of political and domestic violence within the context of two United States social movements: popular resistance to the Vietnam War and the contemporary women's movements, particularly the violence against women movements. She argues that:

> The systematic study of psychological trauma therefore depends on the support of a political movement. Indeed, whether such study can be pursued or discussed in public is itself a political question. The study of war trauma becomes legitimate only in a context that challenges the sacrifice of young men in war. The study of trauma in sexual and domestic life becomes legitimate only in a context that challenged the subordination of women and children (Herman, 1992: 9).

Her historical contextualisation of this theory's origins clarifies one important contribution to the reconstruction of PTSD, in response to traditional psychiatric theories that failed to acknowledge environmental sources of extreme trauma. Her analysis was one of the first to clarify the social and historical embeddedness of this 'scientific construct', in contrast to those who attribute the development of the classification system exclusively to objective, professional, scientific reflection. Through her own research and clinical practice, Herman also extended existing understandings of trauma by emphasising its continuing and chronic character, particularly in contexts of, for example, ongoing war or family abuse. Yet, despite these contributions, she supports a medicalised model for making meaning of trauma and its effects and fails to capture trauma's community and social dimensions, characteristics that remain exogenous variables within her model.

### Approximating a new framework: historicising the subject

Research on the Holocaust (Fine, 1998) and the US internment of those with Japanese ancestry during the Second World War (Nagata, 1993) provides critical insight into how political trauma in the past lives on in the present, in the psyche and life course of those who experienced the trauma directly, as well as their offspring. The past is brought into the present through the intergenerational dynamics of families. In both instances, silence has been found, perhaps paradoxically, to be a source of transmission of the unspeakable. Silence protects the survivor, and yet silence 'gives voice' in the imaginations of the children of survivors, and even their offspring, in which fantasies and speculations sometimes approximate or surpass historical horrors and lived experiences.

The private lives of individuals and significant periods of political conflict and social trauma are brought together in this research. In Erikson's terms, according to Hareven (1992: 271), they draw attention to 'the meeting between individual life history and the historical movement'. Viewed from the perspective of critical psychology, they rejoin the decontextualised individual of modern psychological inquiry (Gergen and Davis, 1985) and the historical, collective experience of identity-giving groups (see Liem, 1999 for elaboration of these ideas and another example).

### Trauma as collective experience

Punamaki's introduction to a three-volume special issue of the *International Journal of Mental Health* identified several severe limitations of traditional psychological and psychiatric theories of stress and trauma. She suggested that traditional (i.e. Anglo-Saxon) theories 'portray the *essence* of being a *victim* of politically induced violence and repression' (1989: 4; my emphasis). The theories' 'implicit concept of the human being, the assumption of the universality of psychological responses, and the inability to describe accurately the interaction between social-political and psychological developments and to catch both the collective and the individualistic dimensions of the human psyche' (Punamaki, 1989: 5) limit their usefulness in understanding war and its effects. The inability to describe what Punamaki calls the 'collective ... dimensions of the human psyche' is echoed in recent work by Summerfield (1995), who draws on his experiences in Nicaragua as well as his reading of the survivors of Vietnam, the Falklands/Malvinas war of 1982, the Palestinian *Intifadah* in Gaza and on the West Bank and apartheid-state violence against the inhabitants of Soweto. In each context, he argues that it is not only the individual that is traumatised, but the social setting, in which social and cultural institutions are ruptured. Therefore, any understanding of trauma must be read within its social, cultural and political contexts over time, not as a relatively static entity located and to be addressed within affected individuals. In the rest of the chapter, I will argue that in order to develop such a re-reading of trauma, one must reposition oneself as a knower within the historical, cultural and political contexts of that which one seeks to know, situating one's work within an interdisciplinary framework, and drawing on alternative psychological epistemologies and practices with survivors.

## Deconstructing and reconstructing: positionalities of knowers and known

As a white, female, educated UnitedStatesian[1] whose government sponsored the overthrow of the democratically elected government of Guatemala in 1954, I am aware of my situated 'otherness' in my field work in rural Guatemala. This position of difference within a praxis of solidarity and collective struggle informed the development of a participatory action research methodology in the field that has enabled me to re-read trauma in rural Guatemala, exploring some of the symbolic or non-functional aspects of terror and multiple meanings of trauma co-constructed with Mayan women and children whom I have accompanied from my position as social scientist and solidarity activist.[2]

Research grounded in positivist assumptions and a medical model hypothesises a separate subject (e.g. a child) who experiences an object (e.g. terror) in timeless space, and creates meaning from the atrocities and terror through descriptions of their effects at the level of the individual, relying on delimited instruments to inform understanding. In contrast, relationships constructed between researcher and subject in time constitute sources of data that approximate more adequate bases for knowing than data gathered with more traditional research instruments. As importantly, the relationship between the researcher and the survivor creates a context in which some of the latter's multiple versions of survival are constructed and/or enacted. In the ensuing discussion, I briefly summarise contributions to repositioning myself within an interdisciplinary framework and describe how my relationship as researcher-activist in community with survivors has contributed to facilitating a re-reading of the meanings of trauma within one rural Mayan context. Finally, I explore implications or possible applications of such work within a South African context.

### Understanding terror: inscriptions on the body

As I indicated earlier, civilians constitute the majority of those affected by contemporary warfare and the unequal social relations of power and resources that have given rise to many of today's civil wars. The annual reports of UNICEF (see http://www.unicef.org/sow00/), as well as a wide range of people's atlases (see, for example, Kidron and Segal, 1995; Seager, 1997; Smith, 1997), document high infant-mortality rates, dramatic levels of absolute and extreme poverty, foreshortened life expectancies, poor health care and high levels of illiteracy, particularly in rural areas and among women in the majority world, sites where many of the armed struggles of the concluding decades of the 20th century have occurred. The engendered nature of violence in these wars has also recently been highlighted (see Agger, 1994; Aron *et al.*, 1991; Lykes *et al.*, 1993), and the case of Guatemala is no exception. Women's extreme poverty as well as serious violations of women's human rights have been amply documented by both the Commission for Historical Clarification (CEH, 1999) and the report of the Archdiocese of Guatemala, *Never Again* (ODHAG, 1998). Given their embeddedness within local communities and historic marginalisation, many women similar to those in Guatemala are less likely to testify about violence committed against themselves, focusing rather on their families and communities as the sites of violation. Despite this, we know from key informants that girls and women were repeatedly raped, fetuses torn from pregnant women's stomachs and beaten against trees to kill them and women tortured in front of their children, and children in front of their parents (ODHAG, 1998, 1: 91–2, among others). Moreover, women were more likely than men to survive these terrors, facing the added burdens of the psychosocial and material consequences of violence.

### Understanding terror: symbolic readings

Such economic and human-rights indicators situate the material costs of war. Some anthropologists have sought to read the symbolic meanings of such inscriptions within their historical contexts, offering important images that have informed the thinking and practice of a small but growing number of psychologists who seek alternative models for conceptualising trauma. For example, in his analysis of the Guatemalan counterinsurgency, Davis describes terror's 'objectives' as being 'to generate an attitude of terror and fear – a "culture of fear" – in the Indian population, ensuring that never again would it support or ally itself with a Marxist guerrilla movement' (1988: 24). Adams (1988, 1989) described the functioning of the 'culture of fear' that permeated life in Guatemala for nearly half a century as a part of the dynamics of ladino-Mayan relations[3] that have been intentionally manipulated by the army. Its genesis lies, according to Adams, in the conquest that sought not only to conquer but to ensure the survival of native labour.

Falla (1984) referred to similar experiences of terror as a 'partial genocide'. This term suggests both the military's intention to destroy and sow fear, thereby controlling an entire population, *and* to maintain a cheap labour force to support a repressive, inegalitarian economic system in the country. The army's 'Guns and Beans Program' of the 1980s – intense repression accompanied by benevolent assistance – exemplifies these dual objectives (see, for example, America's Watch Committee, 1982), and for many contemporary Maya not only signifies contemporary counterinsurgent strategies but resymbolises earlier repressive relations between the Spaniards and their ancestors. Further, 'A conquest that fails to exterminate or assimilate the conquered inevitably leaves a population of divided identities' (Adams, 1988: 284).

One cannot understand war in Guatemala without approximating an understanding of its symbolic meanings as they resonate through time at the point where past and future converge, i.e. in the seemingly never-ending present. Terror, thus, creates a situation of 'normal abnormality' (Martín-Baró, 1989; Taussig, 1986/1987) or 'terror as usual'. The state silenced the population through terror, exploiting fear in a particular way.

In his exploration of terror and its functions within the years of the most recent Argentinian dictatorship (1976–1983), Suárez-Orozco (1990, 1991) considers terror's symbolic ability to threaten culture and social subjectivity. His work extends both the spatial and the temporal dimensions within which terror is traditionally conceptualised. Terror's destructive forces affect the community and the culture across generations, not only the individual within his or her lifetime (Danieli, 1998). As I have argued previously (Lykes, 1996), terror not only destroys the present, but forces a rethinking of the past and deeply threatens the future through its destructive effects on the next generation's capacity to culturally affirm itself.

## Re-reading trauma from a liberatory perspective

Within such contexts, liberation psychology and community-based participatory research strategies, grounded in the protagonism of local actors, challenge a medical model and positivist, universalist, objective and laboratory-based research strategies and their applications. Martín-Baró (1990), a Salvadoran social psychologist, argued that the after-effects of political repression carried out by governments was one of the thorniest problems confronting Latin American states hoping to establish democratic governments. He emphasised that in addition to damage to personal lives, harm had been done to the social structures themselves, i.e. to the norms, values and principles by which people are educated, and to the institutions that govern the lives of citizens: 'Social trauma affects individuals precisely in their social character; that is, as a totality, as a system' (Martín-Baró, 1994: 124).

Parallels between Martín-Baró's work and earlier writing by Fanon (1967) in Algeria and more recent liberatory psychology in the anti-apartheid movements of South Africa have been identified (see Dawes, 2001; Lykes *et al.*, in press). These works situate the struggles of oppressed people within systemic and structural relations, depart from individualised constructions of problems characteristic of dominant psychological paradigms and focus on collaborative relations between local communities and psychologists. The latter are urged to develop new competencies and roles, including, but not limited to, those of advocates and watchdogs.

Within this alternative framework, trauma is not primarily or exclusively an intrapsychic phenomenon, but rather is conceived of as psychosocial. Psychosocial trauma reflects a dialectic process, i.e. it 'resides in the social relations of which the individual is only a part' (Martín-Baró, 1994: 124). Martín-Baró suggests further that 'psychosocial trauma can be a normal consequence of a social system based on social relations of exploitation and dehumanising oppression' such as those in wartime El Salvador (1994: 125). Trauma becomes a usual event, not an aberration. Under normal circumstances, the slaughter of individuals, the disappearance of loved ones, the inability to distinguish what one's experience is from what others say it is (and, when one does, the fear of speaking one's point of view), the militarisation of institutions and the extreme polarisation of social life are seen as abnormal. One of the effects of war in El Salvador, according to Martín-Baró (1994), is that the typical person comes to accept these experiences as normal.

Drawing on Latin American liberation theology and pedagogy (e.g. Freire, 1970, 1973; Gutiérrez, 1973/1988), Martín-Baró posited that a psychology that could explain and respond to these realities should include: 1) a focus on the liberation of a whole people (i.e. the collectivity) as well as personal liberation; 2) a new epistemology in which the truth of the popular majority is not to be found, but created, i.e. wherein truth is constructed 'from below'; and 3) a new praxis, in which we place ourselves within the research-action process alongside the dominated or oppressed rather than alongside the dominator or oppressor (Martín-Baró, 1994).

## Reflexivity and contemporary constructions of trauma

Within a liberatory psychology, we are challenged to clarify the meanings we make from below. Social constructivists argue that these meanings are not adequately represented by labelling symptoms or syndromes (Aron et al., 1991). Rather, they are co-constructed by those who experience them in relationships (e.g. the therapist with her client) in a particular socio-historical time, culture and place (Agger, 1994; Gergen, 1994, 1997). Dialogue and engagement are critical strategies for constructing knowledge and understanding that are inherently value-laden, not value-neutral. This meaning-making process can, therefore, best be understood within the historical and cultural contexts of the actors, i.e. through the thick descriptions of events or re-enactments of experiences as they are constructed or reconstructed by the survivors in dialogue and/or interaction with those who accompany them, in our case, psychologists (Lykes, 1996).

Feminist psychologists and critical theorists argue that, as psychologists, we are challenged to analyse the effects we have within the knowledge-generating contexts in which we work, as we engage with clients in therapeutic activities or with participants in our research (see Fine, 1992; Lather, 1991; Maguire, 1987, among others). The practice of reflexivity within local communities in contexts of war and peacemaking has contributed in particular ways towards understanding psychosocial trauma (see, for example, Lykes, 1996; Zur, 1998). An example from Perú illustrates this point within therapeutic discourse.

Kreimer (1994), a Peruvian anthropologist and therapist, argues that, as 'other', she frequently represents and resignifies the oppressor for her clients, i.e. the source of the marginalisation, oppression or violence that created the situation of the survivor. From her position of 'outsider' she had to learn to stand within the multiple meaning-systems of the marginalised, i.e. to recognise the meaning of reparation or recovery within their cultural experiences. To accompany a healing or reparatory process with *Quechua* communities affected by state violence in Perú, for example, required her to understand that, for these communities, healing can entail reconsideration of all aspects of life and effectively beginning everything anew. This understanding is embedded in their language and is central to their social experiences. Failure to understand the internal logic and vision of life of the people with whom we work risks misinterpreting the 'problems' or doing the opposite of what we seek to do.

Kreimer found that thinking culturally and reflexively about work among indigenous communities also implicitly affirms the rights of these indigenous peoples to their collective beliefs, i.e. their vision of life. Yet, as Long and Zietkiewicz (2002) caution, we should not replace reductionist biomedical thinking with a similarly reductionist reading from indigenous or traditionalist meaning systems. As 'outsiders', we Westerners need to be attentive to the multiple readings present within the context of psychosocial trauma, readings that include how we are being read as 'other' and how we re-read our colleagues, our collaborators and ourselves in this co-constructed space.

## Constructing alternative meanings of trauma with local communities

My access to Mayan meaning-making is both constrained and facilitated by many years of knowing survivors and their caretakers in rural Guatemala. Those relationships have deeply shaped my experiences of Guatemala, both contributing to my understanding about life within a context of war and reminding me of the limits of my knowledge.

Previous researchers had found that the psychological effects identified in Guatemalan child survivors, for example, do not differ significantly from those identified in survivors from other countries (see Lykes, 1994, for a summary of these findings). Yet, as I have argued above, listing symptoms or diagnosing syndromes barely scratches the surface of this reality. What does it mean for a Mayan child to lose her land, to watch her home and crops and traditional dress burn, and see her animals killed? This is not simply the cumulative effect of traumatic experience. The Mayan collective body has been deeply wounded, i.e. a body that is constituted in its deepest particularity in the individual lives of survivors, a body that is profoundly communal. It is that collective body – made up of the ants, the trees, the corn, the domestic animals and the human beings gathered across generations – that has been ripped from its roots and wanders the earth. And this earth has been burned and scarred, both reflecting and constructing the communities' scars. The burning of crops reflects not only the destruction of subsistence or physical survival, but also an attack on a symbol that most fully represents the people, i.e. that reflects Mayan social subjectivity. Therefore, what has been destroyed is broader in scope than the notion of individual, internal trauma, i.e. it is collective and cultural. Just as importantly, psychosocial trauma is extended in time. The destruction of cultural archetypes and metaphors annihilates or deeply limits the next generation's possibility of affirming aspects of their cultural lives. Only a deeper reading of Mayan life and traditions can yield more adequate theories for work with these child survivors.

Traditional social-science methodologists recommend longitudinal, controlled studies with representative samples for testing hypotheses derived from theory and/or field experiences. Given the political, economic and ethical realities of war and the criticisms described above of the medical model and positivist social-science methods, I have, in contrast, proposed 'activist participatory research' or 'passionate scholarship' (see DuBois, 1983; Lykes, 1989). Most simply, this is a process through which the researcher accompanies the participant or subject over time, participating and observing while providing resources to the participant and his or her community. It reflects a willingness to risk entering another's life-space and allowing him or her to enter one's own. Understanding, and one's possibilities for continuing engagement, are co-constructed in experiences of conflict and contradiction as well as shared subjectivity.

## A brief description of the context: situating collaborative work

The town of Chajul, where I worked with Mayan women and children between 1992 and 2000, lies deep in the Guatemalan Highlands. It is one of three towns comprising an area that the Guatemalan military designated as the 'Ixil Triangle' in the 1970s and 1980s, referring to the Ixil language and culture of the area's three largest towns, Nebaj, Cotzal and Chajul. The population of Chajul is predominantly Ixil Maya, comprising local survivors, refugees returning from Mexico, people descending from the Communities of Populations in Resistance,[4] and others who had been displaced both within the country and beyond its borders. At a local level, community members are working through many of the regional and national dynamics that have deeply marked their lives and have surfaced in new ways after the ending of a protracted war.

Space does not permit an extensive discussion of these eight years of collaboration, which began with workshops using drama, art and movement with a small group of Mayan women, survivors of the violence described above. They sought to respond to their own and other women and children's economic needs, yet realised that the multiple wounds inscribed on their bodies and in their communities limited them. They hoped to develop a corn mill, enabling women to grind corn by machine, for a lower fee, rather than by hand, thereby freeing them for other income-generating activities. In a recent co-authored paper, I and my fellow authors describe this early work, the other two economic development projects we began as well as two psychosocial and educational projects, one for children and the other with and for the women of the Association of Maya Ixil Women – New Dawn (ADMI) (Lykes et al., 1999). This latter project the women called 'PhotoVoice'.

## Shifting historical realities create new opportunities

The Peace Accords signed by the Guatemalan government and the guerilla forces (URNG) in December of 1996 included the establishment of a Commission for Historical Clarification (CEH, 1999), which complemented the Archdiocesan Committee on the Recuperation of Historical Memory (ODHAG, 1998) and created more spaces for breaking silence about the war and the multiple human-rights violations and trauma suffered in many areas of the country. Trained interviewers fanned out into the Guatemalan countryside to take testimonies from survivors, hoping to create contexts where those silenced by war could speak their truths and begin complex processes of recovery, reintegration and reconciliation. Many women in Chajul declined to participate – some out of continuing fear, others because those taking testimonies represented religious groups or political tendencies that they did not accept or share. Some of this latter group, including some women of ADMI, indicated that the interviewers were interested in the violence of decades ago, not the everyday violence of hunger that they and their children suffered continuously in the here and now. They expressed a desire to document the experiences of 'la violencia' (the violence) and its effects within Chajul, to share their stories with each other in a way that would enable them to better understand the causes of such horror, and to develop responses towards rebuilding local communities. They also sought to communicate the stories of horror and survival to future generations who had not experienced it first hand and to those beyond Chajul not privy to this history. They sought, in this way, to 'give witness', offering spaces for sharing and healing to women who had not yet told their stories, as well as remembering (or re-membering) their own pasts as resources towards preventing the repetition of such violence in the future.

Existing language differences and limited literacy, as well as local traditions of storytelling and dramatisations, had contributed to the women's embrace of creative resources within previous workshops. I introduced them to a method of community photography, called 'Talking pictures' or 'PhotoVoice' (Wang and Burris, 1994; Wang et al., 1996), which had been developed in China with non-formally educated women, where photographs were used to influence local health and education policies. The visual image is unlike other forms of communication, as cameras are increasingly accessible and photographs are universally comprehensible and can be used to facilitate discussion, document experience and facilitate critical analysis of social reality and problem solving.

We decided to use a variation of the PhotoVoice technique to tell the story of Ixil women, and to document and communicate the Ixil realities through the images and text that women of ADMI would create. We wanted to document the experiences of violence, displacement and loss described above, and its effects among women and children who are now living in Chajul and its neighboring villages. We adapted participatory research strategies and PhotoVoice to local realities, envisioning pictures as vehicles for self- and communal reflection, initially among the group of participants, and then among ever-widening circles of women within and beyond Chajul.

Through the experiences of 'telling stories' about their pictures, participants have learned how to put visual images into words, and, just as importantly, how to move from an internalised, private image often developed within a system of state-imposed silence to a shared understanding of their social reality developed with others. The particular content of many of the photographs has facilitated the sharing of deeply held feelings about the violence and its effects, some of which had not been previously socialised within the community. Participation has therefore been an opportunity for individual participants' growth and development through sharing stories, comparing differing versions of survival and rethreading and reintegrating community through the development of a shared vision towards collective action for change. Ana Caba Mateo, one of the participants, described the project in the following way:

> The project PhotoVoice is very important for us because, as the name explains, PhotoVoice is both photographs and voice. The voice explains what a photo is and what it means. It's a road, a guide that is giving us direction in the search for a solution to our needs as women. Because through the photographs that can be read in a book, one can see what women do, how they customarily do their work, what their needs are, and what their problems are. Through the photographs with which they have been working, the women themselves speak of their reality ... .
>
> We women or other people who have endured *la violencia* [the violence] are remembering, through means of the PhotoVoice project, what we have seen or experienced and we are establishing a memory of it. This is very important because there are many young people who are growing up now who did not see this suffering and, because they didn't live through it, they doubt that it happened. In contrast, people like us, who lived and suffered in our own flesh, remember it very well. And so, interviewing the people who suffered through it and who saw their family members die offers a

sort of relief for them, because they recount what happened to another person. You think or feel that in sharing that person is asking, hoping, that this violence, this war, never again return … . This PhotoVoice project is our search for a way for the people from around the world to lend their support so that this violence and the massacres that took place never happen again. That is why this project is so very important for us (Women of PhotoVoice/ADMI and Lykes, 2000: 103).

## ■ Comparisons beyond Guatemala: questions for future work

This chapter outlines initial steps in a process of re-reading trauma from a concrete praxis within and among Mayan survivors of war and state-sponsored terror. This reading draws heavily on theories and constructs unknown to the Maya with whom I have been working. Rather than imposing these frameworks on our praxis, I have sought to use them to deconstruct dominant psychological discourses about trauma into which I as a UnitedStatesian, upper-class, white, academic psychologist have been socialised. I have sought to create a strategy that enables us as cross-border collaborators to retell stories wherein we develop a textured and complex discourse that can be read by others (see Women of PhotoVoice/ADMI and Lykes, 2000, for a concrete example of this). Our collaborative praxis has generated spaces within which the survivors have privileged their language and their systems of knowing through accessing resources that have emerged within the professional world of post-modern capitalism, i.e. the camera and the photograph. Through this work, we have begun to interrogate dominant discourses within the Ixil Triangle today, e.g. discourses of war, military repression, guerrilla warfare, Mayan nationalisms, economic repression, women's traditional roles and repressed discourses, gendered violence, racial conflict between ethnic groups and religious differences.

This is not a simple or linear process of 'giving voice', but rather a collaborative exploration informed by multiple discourses within psychology, human-rights work, development theory and the practices and indigenous knowledge systems of rural Mayan communities. Women from diverse life experiences have worked together and generated concrete practices that are informed by and inform ways of thinking about trauma and its particular, collective effects in Chajul. We are thereby developing and documenting some women's ways of responding to these particular forms of psychosocial trauma. Just as importantly, we are changing the material conditions for some women and children of these communities.

Similar examples can be drawn from South Africa. As I suggested above, theoretical contributions from North Africa inform a liberatory psychology and informed psychologists engaged in the South African anti-apartheid movement. Just as significantly, a local network of community-based survivor self-help groups, Khulumani, has contributed to lifting up survivors' voices within nation-wide processes seeking truth and reconciliation within post-1994 South Africa. The work of Khulumani (see Hahn and Segal, 1995; Segal *et al.*, 1997; Hamber *et al.*, 2000) further exemplifies the social construction of survival and the mediated nature of all language (see Lykes *et al.*, in press, for additional comparisons and discussion of this point). Just as significantly, despite dramatic political and cultural differences between

Guatemala and South Africa, the majority populations in each country have given voice to their experiences of oppression and resistance, speaking out against repression and marginalisation.

My work in Guatemala and more recently in South Africa has helped me to 'think culturally' about experiences of terror and survival and to identify three distinct theoretical contributions towards reconceptualising trauma and recovery. Firstly, by challenging the traditional Western psychological focus on individual identity, 'selfhood' is voiced and enacted through story and in relationship as inherently social. To speak of 'who I am' invokes family, community, the animal kingdom, one's traditions and language, and the earth. Subjectivity is collectively constituted and the experiences summarised here suggest that the 'self' of the Mayan or the rural, black South African is characterised as 'social subjectivity'. There is, of course, a growing critique of traditional Western theories of self which, although extensive (e.g. Gergen, 1991; Hermans and Kempen, 1993; Markus and Kitayama, 1991; Sampson, 1993), has not significantly influenced psychological theories of trauma and its effects. The work with Maya in Guatemala and among blacks in South Africa suggests a connection that could be productively developed to extend such a critique.

Secondly, in addition to the common functions of terror identified by human-rights activists and scholars, consideration of terror's symbolic dimensions clarifies terror's threat to culture and to social subjectivity. This work extends both the spatial and the temporal dimensions along which we conceptualise terror. Terror's destructive forces affect community and culture, not only internal, individual well-being. Further, terror not only destroys the present and forces a rethinking of the past, it deeply threatens the future through its destructive effects on the next generation's capacity to affirm aspects of their cultural lives. Attention to the symbolic dimensions of terror are therefore critical for approximating knowledge of Mayan stories of victimisation and survival, and contribute to our broader theorising about trauma, its consequences and the healing process.

Thirdly, work among the women and children of Chajul as well as the work of others with families of political prisoners and blacks tortured and murdered in South Africa critically challenges those who would pathologise and medicalise survivors of state-sponsored violence and war. Although some of the women participants in the project described here or others in survivor groups in South Africa might evidence symptom constellations that fit the criteria of PTSD, this constellation of physical and psychological responses captures only one small dimension of who they are, and of what and who they are becoming. Just as importantly, as Summerfield has argued, 'post-traumatic symptoms are not just a private and individual problem but also an indictment of the social contexts which produced them' (1995: 26).

Psychologists seeking to work within a context of psychosocial trauma and its wake must see beyond discourses of victimology that dominate our field and our society, and should engage with survivors in work that enables them to reconstruct social and economic networks and their cultural identities. Psychological recovery is threaded within a woof of societal reparation and social justice, and the resultant cloth is woven from the lives of survivors and those in the mental-health field who seek to accompany them. Just as importantly, these efforts change over time. None of the constitutive social and cultural structures or systems is static. Post-war environments both limit and facilitate co-constructions of new social structures and social identities. Our collaborative work as UnitedStatesian and Maya Ixil and Ki'che' women and children in Chajul and its surrounding villages provides one small example of these ongoing processes of recuperation, reintegration and social reparation.

# Endnotes

1. The term is a translation of the Spanish term *est a dounidense*. It is used here rather than the more common 'American' since this latter term includes reference to all citizens of the Americas – Canada, México, Central and South America, and the United States of America. (See Gugelberger, G. M. (ed.) (1996). *The Real Thing: Testimonial Discourses and Latin America*. Durham, NC: Duke University Press.)
2. Several cautionary words: I have spoken and written of many examples of Guatemalans engaged in activist-based resistance – organised in labour unions, Mayan and peasant organisations, church groups and in the Communities of Populations in Resistance in the Guatemalan Highlands, etc. The ideas presented here in no way negate my deep respect and admiration for the witness of these courageous people who break silence through overt resistance and/or rebellion or for those Mayan communities, e.g. some Ki'che' towns, including Nahualá, that were not as directly impacted by war and that responded through greater unity. In this chapter I seek, rather, to explore a more silent underside of terror and *other* versions of survival, silence and voice.
3. A full discussion of ethnic and interethnic relations within Guatemala is beyond the scope of this chapter. See CEH (1999); Bastos, S. & Camus, M. (1996). *Quebrando el silencio: Organizaciones del pueblo Maya y sus demandas (1986–1992)*. (Breaking the silence: Maya organizations and their demands) Guatemala: FLACSO; Fischer, E. F. & Brown, R. Mck. (1996). *Maya Cultural Activism in Guatemala*. Austin, Texas: University of Texas Press; Warren, K. (1999). *Indigenous Movements and their Critics: Pan-Mayanism and Ethnic Resurgence in Guatemala*. Austin, Texas: University of Texas.
4. The Communities of Population in Resistance refers to the more than 30 000 civilians who fled to the mountains and the jungle within Guatemala in the early 1980s, seeking to escape the army's persecution while remaining within their country of origin. They organised communities based on principles of a just society and have survived despite the ongoing civil war and repeated direct attacks by the Guatemalan military who accused them of collaborating with the guerillas. In the 1990s, they descended from the mountains as organised groups and demanded protection from the government, initiating a slow process of re-initiation into Guatemalan civil society.

# References

Adams, R. N. (1988). Conclusions: What can we know about the harvest of violence? In R. M. Carmack (ed.), *Harvest of Violence: The Maya Indians and the Guatemalan Crisis*, pp. 274–91. Oklahoma City: University of Oklahoma Press.

Adams, R. N. (1989). The reproduction of state terrorism in Central America. Paper no. 89-01, University of Texas at Austin, Texas.

Agger, I. (1994). *The Blue Room: Trauma and Testimony Among Refugee Women: A Psycho-social Exploration*. London: Zed Books.

American Psychiatric Association (1980). *Diagnostic and Statistical Manual of Mental Disorders* (3rd edn). Washington, DC: American Psychiatric Association.

American Psychiatric Association (1994). *Diagnostic and Statistical Manual of Mental Disorders* (4th edn). Washington, DC: American Psychiatric Association.

Americas Watch Committee (1982). *Human Rights in Guatemala: No Neutrals Allowed*. New York: Americas Watch Committee.

Aron, A., Corne, S., Fursland, A. and Zewler, B. (1991). The gender-specific terror of El Salvador and Guatemala: Post-traumatic stress disorder in Central American refugee women. *Women's Studies International Forum,* 17, 37–47.

Bracken, P. J. (1993). Post-empiricism and psychiatry: Meaning and methodology in cross-cultural research. *Social Science and Medicine,* 36 (3), 265–72.

Bracken, P. J., Giller, J. E. and Summerfield, D. (1995). Psychological responses to war and atrocity: The limitations of current concepts. *Social Science and Medicine,* 40 (8), 1073–82.

Bronfenbrenner, U. (1979). *The Ecology of Human Development: Experiments by Nature and Design.* Cambridge, Mass.: Harvard University Press.

Cairns, E. (1996). *Children and Political Violence.* Oxford: Basil Blackwell.

CEH (Comisión para el Esclarecimiento Histórico (Commission for Historical Clarification)) (1999). *Guatemala, Memory of Silence, tz´inil na ´tab´ al: Report of the Commission for Historical Clarification: Conclusions and Recommendations.* Guatemala City: CEH (The entire report is available in Spanish on the Internet at http://hrdata.aaas.org/ceh. All citations in this paper are from the English version of the report released by the CEH, 25 February 1999, in Guatemala City.)

Danieli, Y. (ed.) (1998). *International Handbook of Multigenerational Legacies of Trauma.* New York: Plenum.

Davis, S. H. (1988). Introduction: Sowing the seeds of violence. In R. M. Carmack (ed.), *Harvest of Violence: The Maya Indians and the Guatemalan Crisis,* pp. 3–36. Oklahoma City, Oklahoma: University of Oklahoma Press.

Dawes, A. (2001). Psychologies for liberation: Views from elsewhere. In D. J. Christie, R. V. Wagner and D. DuN. Winter (eds), *Peace, Conflict, and Violence: Peace Psychology for the 21st Century,* pp. 295–306. Upper Saddle River, NJ: Prentice-Hall.

DuBois, B. (1983). Passionate scholarship: Notes on values, knowing and method in feminist social science. In G. Bowles and R. Klein (eds), *Theories of Women's Studies,* pp. 105–16. Boston: Routledge.

Eagle, G. (2002). The political conundrums of post-traumatic stress disorder. In this volume.

Falla, R. (1984). Vision of an indigenous people who suffer genocide. In S. Jonas, E. McCaughan and E. S. Martinez (trans. and eds), *Guatemala: Tyranny on Trial: Testimony of the Permanent People's Tribunal.* (condensed English version) pp. 112–19. San Francisco: Publicaciones Sinthesis.

Fanon, F. (1967). *Black Skin, White Masks.* New York: Grove Press.

Fine, E. (1998). Transmission of memory: The post-Holocaust generation in the Diaspora. In E. Sicher (ed.), *Breaking Crystal: Writing and Memory after Auschwitz,* pp. 185–200. Chicago: University of Illinois Press.

Fine, M. (1992). *Disruptive Voices: The Possibilities of Feminist Research.* Ann Arbor: University of Michigan Press.

Freire, P. (1970). *Pedagogy of the Oppressed.* New York: Seabury Press.

Freire, P. (1973). *Education for Critical Consciousness.* New York: Seabury Press.

Gergen, K. J. (1991). *The Saturated Self: Dilemmas of Identity in Contemporary Life.* New York: Basic Books.

Gergen, K. J. (1994). *Toward Transformation in Social Knowledge* (2nd edn). Thousand Oaks, CA: Sage.

Gergen, K. J. (1997). *Realities and Relationships: Soundings in Social Construction.* Cambridge, MA: Harvard University Press.

Gergen, K. J. and Davis, K. (1985). *The Social Construction of the Person.* New York: Springer-Verlag.

Gutiérrez, G. (1973/1988). *A Theology of Liberation: History, Politics and Salvation.* Maryknoll, NY: Orbis Books.

Hahn, H. and Segal, L. (1995). *Khulumani – Speak Out* (video). Johannesburg: Centre for the Study of Violence and Reconciliation.

Hamber, B., Nageng, D. and O'Malley, G. (2000). 'Telling it like it is ...': Understanding the Truth and Reconciliation Commission from the perspective of survivors. *Psychology in Society,* 26, 18–42.

Hareven, T. (1992). The search for generational memory. In P. Leffler and J. Brent (eds), *Public History Readings*, pp. 270–283. Malabar: Kreiger.

Herman, J. (1992). *Trauma and Recovery*. New York: Basic Books.

Hermans, H. and Kempen, J. G. (1993). *The Dialogical Self: Meaning as Movement*. San Diego, CA: Academic Press.

Jensen, P. S. and Shaw, J. (1993). Children as victims of war: Current knowledge and future research needs. *Journal of the American Academy of Child Adolescent Psychiatry*, 32 (4), 697–708.

Kidron, M. and Segal, R. (1995). *The State of the World Atlas* (5th edn). London and New York: Penguin Group.

Kleinman, A. (1987). Anthropology and psychiatry: The role of culture in cross-cultural research on illness. *British Journal of Psychiatry*, 151, 447–54.

Kleinman, A. (1995). *Writing at the Margin: Discourse between Anthropology and Medicine*. Berkeley: University of California Press.

Kreimer. E. (1994). Proceso social y reparacion (Social processes and reparation). In C. Aldana, M. J. Oyague and C. Torres Llosa (eds), *Infancia y Violencia 2: Experiencias y Reflexiones Sobre los Niños y la Violencia Política en el Perú* (*Childhood and Violence, Part 2: Experiences and Reflections on Children and Political Violence in Perú*), pp. 105–12. Lima: Cedapp-Centro de Dessarrollo y Asesoría Psicosocial (Center for Development and Psychosocial Assistance).

Lather, P. (1991). *Getting Smart: Feminist Research and Pedagogy with/in the Postmodern*. New York: Routledge.

Liem, R. (1999). *History, Trauma, and Identity: The Legacy of the Korean War for Korean Americans*. Unpublished manuscript.

Lindemann, E. (1979). *Beyond Grief: Studies in Crisis Intervention*. New York: Aronson.

Lock, M. (1982). Models and Practice in Medicine: Menopause as syndrome or life transition? *Culture, Medicine and Psychiatry*, 6 (3), 261–280.

Long, C. and Zietkiewicz, E. (2002). Unsettling meanings of madness: Competing constructions of South African insanity. In this volume.

Lykes, M. B. (1989). Dialogue with Guatemalan Indian women: Critical perspectives on constructing collaborative research. In R. Unger (ed.), *Representations: Social Constructions of Gender*, pp. 167–85. Amityville, NY: Baywood.

Lykes, M. B. (1994). Terror, silencing and children: International multidisciplinary collaboration with Guatemalan Maya communities. *Social Science and Medicine*, 38 (4), 543–52.

Lykes, M. B. (1996). Meaning making in a context of genocide and silencing. In M. B. Lykes, A. Banuazizi, R. Liem and M. Morris (eds), *Myths about the Powerless: Contesting Social Inequalities*, pp. 159–78. Philadelphia: Temple University Press.

Lykes, M. B., Brabeck, M. M., Ferns, T. and Radan, A. (1993). Human rights and mental health among Latin American women in situations of state-sponsored violence: Bibliographic resources. *Psychology of Women Quarterly*, 17, 525–44.

Lykes, M. B., Caba Mateo, A., Chavez Anay, J., Laynez Caba, A., Ruiz, U. and Williams, J. (1999). Telling stories – rethreading lives: Community education, women's development and social change among the Maya Ixil. *International Journal of Leadership in Education*, 2 (3), 207–27.

Lykes, M. B., Terre Blanche, M. and Hamber, B. (in press). Narrating survival and change in Guatemala and South Africa: The politics of representation and a liberatory community psychology. *American Journal of Community Psychology*.

Maguire, P. (1987). *Doing Participatory Research: A Feminist Approach*. Amherst, MA: Center for International Education.

Markus, H. and Kitayama, S. (1991). Culture and the self: Implications for cognition, emotion, and motivation. *Psychological Review*, 98 (2), 224–53.

Marsella, A. J. and White, G. M. (eds) (1982/1989). *Cultural Conceptions of Mental Health and Therapy*. Dordrecht: D. Reidel.

Martín-Baró, I. (1989). La institucionalización de la guerra (The institutionalisation of war). Paper presented at the annual meeting of the InterAmerican Psychological Association, Buenos Aires, June/July.

Martín-Baró, I. (1990). Reparations: Attention must be paid: Healing the body politic in Latin America. *Commonweal*, 117 (6), 184, 186.

Martín-Baró, I. (1994). *Writings for a Liberation Psychology*. Cambridge, MA: Harvard University Press.

Nagata, D. K. (1993). *Legacy of Injustice: Exploring the Cross-generational Impact of the Japanese-American Internment*. New York: Plenum.

ODHAG (Oficina de Derechos Humanos del Arzobispado de Guatemala (Office of Human Rights of the Archdiocese of Guatemala)) (1998). *Nunca Más: Informe Proyecto Interdiocesano de Recuperación de la Memoria Histórica* (*Never Again: Report of the Interdiocesan Project on the Recovery of Historic Memory*), Vols. 1–5. Guatemala City: ODHAG.

Punamaki, R-L. (1989). Special Issues: *International Journal of Mental Health*, 17 (4) and 18 (1–2).

Sampson, E. E. (1993). *Celebrating the Other: A Dialogic Account of Human Nature*. Boulder, CA: Westview Press.

Seager, J. (1997). *The State of Women in the World Atlas* (2nd edn). London and New York: Penguin Group.

Segal, L., Hamber, B. and Hahn, H. (1997). *SisaKhuluma: We are still Speaking* (video). Johannesburg: Centre for the Study of Violence and Reconciliation.

Smith, D. (1997). *The State of War and Peace Atlas* (3rd edn). London and New York: Penguin Group.

Starcevic, V. and Durdic, S. (1993). Post-traumatic stress disorder: Current conceptualization, an overview of research and treatment. *Psihijatrija Danas*, 25 (1–2), 9–32.

Suárez-Orozco, M. M. (1990). Speaking of the unspeakable: Toward a psychosocial understanding of responses to terror. *Ethos*, 18 (3), 353–83.

Suárez-Orozco, M. M. (1991). The heritage of enduring a 'dirty war': Psychosocial aspects of terror in Argentina, 1976–1988. *Journal of Psychohistory*, 18 (4), 469–505.

Summerfield, D. (1995). Addressing human response to war and atrocity: Major challenges in research and practices and the limitations of Western psychiatric models. In R. J. Kleber, C. R. Figley and B. P. R. Gersons (eds), *Beyond Trauma: Cultural and Societal Dynamics*, pp. 17–29. New York and London: Plenum.

Taussig, M. (1986/1987). *Shamanism, Colonialism, and the Wild Man: A Study in Terror and Healing*. Chicago and London: University of Chicago Press.

UNICEF (1996). *Impact of Armed Conflict on Children: Report of Graça Machel*. Available online at: http://www.unicef.org/graca/.

Wang, C. and Burris, M. (1994). Empowerment through photo novella: Portraits of participation. *Health Education Quarterly*, 21 (2), 171–86.

Wang, C., Burris, M. and Ping, X. Y. (1996). Chinese village women as visual anthropologists: A participatory approach to reaching policymakers. *Social Science and Medicine*, 42 (10), 1391–400.

Women of PhotoVoice/ADMI and Lykes, M. B. (2000). *Voces e Imágenes: Mujeres Mayas Ixiles de Chajul/Voices and Images: Mayan Ixil Women of Chajul*. Guatemala City: Magna Terra.

Zur, J. (1998). *Violent Memories: Mayan War Widows in Guatemala*. Boulder, CA: Westview Press.

# SECTION 2

# PATHOLOGY AS POLITICS

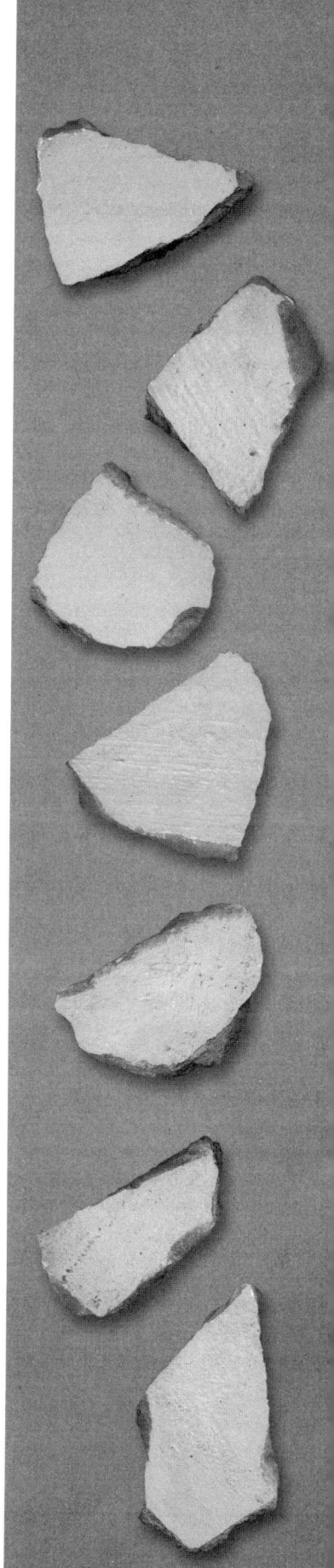

# CHAPTER 5
# Rewriting the body, reauthoring the expert: Reading the anorexic body

*S. Fuller & Derek Hook*

> The anorexic, starving in the midst of plenty, has become the enigmatic icon of our times, half heroine, half horror (Ellman, 1993: 2).

## ■ Introduction

The confounding image of a skeletal, anorexic figure, coming to know herself as 'sharp enough to look after herself' (*Discorder*, 1995: 28) as her ever-bonier frame reveals the potentials of her body as weapon[1] is a suggestive one for the position taken in this chapter. We consider anorexia in terms contrary to those that dominate the field, where, for the most part, the anorexic is seen as a victim, and passively so, of a consumer culture in which male preferences heavily influence expectations of women. We do not seek to deny that women in contemporary culture, and beyond, are subject to dominating discourses and negative events and representations, but we argue with interpretations that see women as passively accepting situations of inequality, and unresistingly taking on roles assigned them. We argue that anorexia is a strategy – although defying easy universal narration – that challenges, subverts and transgresses, spurning patriarchal structures and the feminine slimness ideal even as it hints at collaboration with these privileged forms. Recognising the anorexic as also a resisting and transgressing subject who contests her more general lack of control, and who seeks a strategy that opposes a situation in which she is left no position from which to speak – here drawing on the arguments of Gayatri Spivak in her work done in the field of Subaltern Studies – we consider anorexia to be a miming-turned-mockery of the upheld ideal.

Many women diagnosed as anorexic feel they have been made invisible through the relations of power in which they are located. By adopting the strategy they do, their seeming act of disappearance ironically comes back writ large to haunt those implicated in the discourses of domination. So, re-reading anorexia in terms of a post-colonial and post-structural feminist approach, it can be examined as a mocking of the 'masters' discourse' of the female body, and can be viewed as a particular form of mimesis that confronts the social disorder of the particular power/knowledge relations between the coloniser and the colonised.

As is the case with any risky strategy or action, the anorexic subject may not fully internalise her (possible deadly) outcomes, and her motivations, like those of most subjects, may be ambivalent in their configurations and complex in their origins. To make this argument, we draw on the work of Bhabha (1994), recognising that in this context it could be that, like other colonial subjects mouthing the discourse of post-Enlightenment English colonialism, it is the anorexic who is speaking with a tongue that is forked (Bhabha, 1994: 85). We take his analysis not merely to reproduce this argument in a different discourse or context, but rather to take the spirit of his argument and think it elsewhere. With anorexia, it is the colonised rather than colonising subjects who produce irony, mimicry and repetition with their iteration of a centred discourse of authority, turning from the ideal in the process.

Bhabha argues that mimicry mocks the power of the monument as model, with profound and disturbing effect on the authority of colonial discourse. This mode of colonial discourse – which Bhabha calls mimicry, and in which colonialism repeatedly exercises its authority through figures of farce, producing in the process texts rich in irony – is an ironic compromise. It represents a double articulation and a complex strategy that appropriates the 'other' as it visualises power. It is also a mark of the inappropriate. It is this difference, almost the same but not quite, that poses a threat to normalised knowledges, disciplinary powers and the continually reiterated norm (Bhabha, 1994).

The discourse of mimicry, then, which Bhabha sees as 'at once resemblance and menace', is constructed around an ambivalence, so that in order to be effective it 'must continually produce its slippage, its excess, its difference' (1994: 86). Using this approach, which is based on an ambivalence of what is always in place and already known – but which must nevertheless be anxiously repeated – the anorexic subject can be seen as not merely engaged in an attempt to copy the dominant culture's ideal through the reiteration of the slim norm, but as engaged in an act that transforms what it resembles. This is a transformation that is both similar *and* dissimilar. It destabilises that which it mimes, calling into question the systemic closure and the self-grounding pretensions of a particular system of meaning (cf. Butler, 1993). So, in Bhabha's (1994) conception, what we are talking of here is a difference that is almost the same, but not quite; indeed not the slim ideal, not quite. Bhabha's analysis teaches that the colonial discourse's rendition of stereotypes is also its moment of fear and anxiety, i.e. that moment when the mimicry of the colonised image turns to mockery and where the authority of the coloniser suddenly comes under severe stress.

The same ridiculing by supposed imitation is in evidence in what is continually demanded of the anorexic by the discourses of health that measure, monitor and discipline. This is a ridiculing that appears to challenge the adequacy of these discourses and these (health) professionals in dealing with the disorder of anorexia nervosa. Anorexics in treatment, for example, seem to repeat the inner disciplining, measuring and surveying generally associated with modernity and, more specifically, with psychiatry, but often do so with scornful deliberation, as when they painstakingly measure themselves or count their calories. This 'female obedience', these imitations 'of the letter' but not 'of the spirit', appear to be a further reiteration that leads further away from, rather than closer to, the goals of the 'ideal' and of normalisation. Ironically, these actions then continue to call for normalising interventions by health professionals, and as such these desperate reiterations (or re-iterations) may be read as a form of mockery.

As Prakash (1995) argues, power exists in a form of relationality in which the dominance of one is never complete. Adopting such a post-colonial and post-structural approach has advantages and consequences. Firstly, by incorporating the ambivalence and indeterminacy associated with these positions – i.e. with a disavowal of dualistic and essentialist thinking – this approach allows for a fluidity between and deconstruction of categories, which counters absolutism. In this way, the anorexic may no longer be seen as merely a victim, but as a transgressor and a resister as well.

This theoretical attitude provides a complex reformulation of anorexia: in particular, it enables one to escape the stark alternatives generally offered in the literature in the field. It is an irony, given that the dangers of dualistic thinking are so frequently recognised in feminist theory, that women with anorexia are still so often portrayed as positioned within a world of bald oppositions. This dualistic conceptualisation leads to forms of theory and therapeutic practice that do little more than straitjacket anorexics.

A second advantage of this approach is that it works against the contemporary Western bias evident in dominant accounts of the phenomenon, where a 'fat phobia' and a concerted focus on consumer society lead to the failure to recognise that anorexia is differently configured according to changes in history and geography. Not surprisingly, this bias, which occurs in much of the theory and cultural criticism on anorexia – in which the focus is on 'fat phobia' as a central feature of anorexia – is in evidence within the discipline of psychiatry. In the manual central to both its status and its practices, the *Diagnostic and Statistical Manual of Mental Disorders* in its various editions, the discipline defines the condition of anorexia nervosa as having the essential features of:

- A distorted body image and disturbance in the way in which one's body weight, size or shape is experienced. For example, the person claims to 'feel fat' even when emaciated and believes that one area of the body is 'too fat' even when obviously underweight.
- Refusal to maintain body weight over a minimal normal weight for age and height.
- Intense fear of gaining weight or becoming fat, even though underweight.
- In females, absence of at least three consecutive menstrual cycles when otherwise expected to occur (American Psychiatric Association, 1987: 65).

These essentialist emphases dominate the fields of social theory, cultural criticism and the psychotherapeutic profession. They exacerbate the neglect of the phenomenon's contradictory and multifarious aspects, pushing practitioners to a less, rather than more, complex position. In so doing, they produce interpretations that ironically may result in the further disempowerment of girls and women. These conceptualisations can be contested if anorexia is thought of in *contradictory terms*. That is, we may avoid these pitfalls if we think of anorexia beyond the dualist and essentialist categorisations by which the anorexic either rejects her body with its appetites by attempting to transcend it, or rejects *herself* when falling prey to its desires.

Interpreting anorexia through the act of mime turned to mockery allows one to do this. Here there is the appearance of a reiteration of the gestures of the dominant, which, at the same time is 'its slippage, its excess, its difference' (Bhabha, 1994: 86). In this way, one might facilitate an argument of agency and resistance, while at the same time calling into question the system in which the anorexic, the theorist and the therapist are located. In other words, an offshoot of this form of conceptualisation is that it might enable the destabilising of patriarchal culture, of the categorisations and norms of the medical profession, and of orthodox philosophy's essentialist and dualistic social theory. It is this releasing of the category of the anorexic from fixity that may, paradoxically, allow the rethinking of an 'anorexic agency'.[2]

The re-reading presented here is underpinned by a number of assumptions. The first, following Touraine's (1977) position as laid out in his *Return of the Actor: Social Theory in Postindustrial Society*, is the idea that acts in contemporary society are not confined to the reproduction of social structures, but are characterised also by social action and resistance, transformation and indeterminancy. The second such assumption is the idea that the body is constructed by the moral, medical and scientific knowledges of the time, and that it is coded such that even medical perceptions of the body are based upon readings of its signs rather than a knowledge of its essence.[3] Therefore, the re-reading is informed by Foucault's (1979) critique of the rule of modernity, and the vital and necessary role that the body plays in its various disciplinary practices. Here the body is seen as a changing product of culture with cultural practices inscribed upon it. Furthermore, its sexuality in this conceptualisation (Foucault, 1979) is a construction rather than an essence, based on an active agency that follows from the position that while subjects may be constituted, they are not wholeheartedly determined. Extending this view, Butler (1993) claims that the constituted nature of the subject is the very precondition for its agency. Furthermore, following Mouffe (1995), social agents are constituted by an ensemble of subject positions that can never be completely fixed in a closed system of differences, and are constructed by a diversity of discourses among which there is no necessary relation, but a constant movement of overdetermination and displacement. All of these positions work against an essentialising, colonising discourse that desires the reformation of the 'other', and provide a strong underpinning of the argument that places the focus on anorexia as an *act* rather than a *condition*. These positions therefore provide a hopeful potential basis for viewing the anorexic as exhibiting a critical agency against an oppressive power and knowledge. They enable us to view the anorexic not merely as a passive subject simply reiterating the norm, but as an agent making a choice to use her body as a site of resistance.

## ■ A critique and reformulation; and an argument for active agency

To consider the implications of this alternative reading for theory and therapeutic practice, it is useful first to survey the dominant narratives about anorexia in these fields. In the accounts that portray anorexics as having little agency and as drawing passively into themselves the messages and negative representations that surround them – in both the language used to talk about self-starvation and the assumptions that underpin these narratives – anorexics are seen as facing contradictory but polarised options. On the one hand, they are conceived of as dissociated from their alien bodies, yet, on the other, they are thought of as haunted by their appetites. What research has been done on what the health profession sees as a 'difficult' research community indicates that women diagnosed with eating disorders have often been sexually abused and are thus the victims of the appetites of others, rather than of their own. Like hysteria, which has also been seen as an option women have taken to voice opposition to their situations, only one in 10 of those diagnosed with anorexia are male, which brings the gendered nature of the phenomenon and its analysis sharply into focus, and strengthens the appropriateness of the use of a post-colonial approach to it. The youth of anorexics in particular indicates a further disadvantage in regard to power. The onset of anorexia occurs often at about the age of 15, and it is most commonly developed by the age of 25 (Turner, 1984).

Anorexics are often described as passively internalising the taunting missives of lack, as they construct taut and sparse bodies either to approximate the male form that, through history, has been put forward as that of the perfected sex, or to conform to that which is put forward by patriarchal consumer culture as the feminine ideal. This is so much the case that anorexics are typically seen to exhibit a fear of going out of control by becoming fat, and hence ruining their chances for love and career, because being thin in contemporary society is equated with being successful, competent and loveable. Food is seen as a source of anxiety for millions of women, simultaneously an object of dread and intense desire, and women as engaged in an ongoing battle with it: craving it, fearing it and letting it control their lives. The battle between abstinence and indulgence is waged on a daily basis, and this interpretation is contrasted with former fears around the erstwhile 'forbidden fruit' – sex. Therapists such as Meadow and Weiss (1992) argue that this battle is similar to the time when sexual fantasies fuelled the imagination and women became obsessed with having sexual intercourse. The agony and the ecstasy of succumbing to the passions of the flesh were, seemingly, ever-present in women's imaginations. Sex was at once the ultimate danger and the ultimate delight for women, creating a continuous struggle between experiencing sexual pleasure and risking their futures. The paradox for women was that, to be loved by a man, they had to deny themselves the most basic way of experiencing love – they had to deprive themselves of their sexual appetites. Meadow and Weiss (1992) argue that this constant repression of normal bodily drives resulted in a variety of sexual disorders in women, including the inability to achieve orgasm and a complete lack of sexual desire. Ironically, Meadow and Weiss, like the medical professions more generally, focus on the role of food, arguing for a similarity between contemporary eating problems and the sexual conflicts of past decades, with women still repressing their basic needs – whether oral or sexual – in order to be loved. Recounting a narrative that appears to be extremely disempowering for women, they claim that in their therapy practices they are witnessing the new 'Good Girls Don't' phenomenon revolving around eating and dieting – a shift in women's central preoccupation from sex to food.

Bordo, whose work (1993a, 1993b) in the discipline of philosophy is well established in the field of anorexia, also ascribes a significant role to food. She argues (1993a) that anorexia, which often manifests itself after an episode of sexual abuse or humiliation, can be seen at least in part as a defence against the 'femaleness' of the body and a punishment of its desires, which have, in her view, frequently been culturally represented through the metaphor of female appetite. The extremes to which the anorexic takes the denial of appetite (i.e. to the point of self-starvation) suggest to theorists such as Bordo the dualistic nature of the anorexic's construction of reality:

either she transcends body totally, becoming pure 'male' will, or she capitulates utterly to the degraded female body and its disgusting hungers. If fat in contemporary society is the sign of failure to control the bodily appetites that are so important for the privileging of reason over emotion and mind over body, then it is a burden that weighs more heavily on women than did the previous burden of repressing sexual appetites in Victorian times (Bordo, 1993a).

Cultural critics outside of the academy generally tell a similar story. Graydon, the former national president of Media Watch, the Canadian organisation that polices demeaning images of women in the media, robs anorexics of agency when she describes anorexia as a 'monster' out to 'destroy' teenage girls, 'to kill them before they reach adulthood' (1995: 12). Located as a cultural critic of the media – a task generally associated with empowering women by countering the dominant discourse around them – Graydon argues that this monster is insidious and operates 'with the tacit support of corporate America and the girls' family and friends' (1995: 13). For her, young women are without agency, as the 'monster' of anorexia, 'speaking in a million voices', 'worms its way into their heads' (1995: 13), infecting their minds and turning them against their bodies. Meadow and Weiss similarly attribute enormous power to the media, and little to anorexics. They present food advertisements as tantalising women, as fuelling their consuming passions for forbidden foods, just as romance magazines, novels and films previously served to keep the obsession with sex alive in women's imaginations (1992).

Many women diagnosed as anorexic, however, give a very different view. One such woman, in response to an open letter by a therapist in which he constructed a woman he was working with as being 'within the deadly hold of anorexia', argued in a letter to the therapist: 'I find this all so demeaning and patronizing. By separating anorexia and depression away from S it seems to me that you are taking away any of her own responsibility and putting her squarely into the victim role. Obviously S is not to blame for the horrible circumstances that have transpired in her life, but she has made choices – one of them being anorexia'.

Exhibiting the Western bias discussed earlier, Meadow and Weiss (1992) claim that in the 1950s, conflict over whether to eat or not was non-existent. Eating disorders at this time were rare, and bulimia was almost unheard of. Other accounts, in stark contrast, argue that self-starvation stretches back centuries, and was, for example, practised by saints (Bell, 1985). Yet other accounts take issue with studies that give primacy to 'fat phobia' as a central explanation for diminished food intake (Lee, 1995). Such studies suggest that extreme forms of self-starvation can be traced across place as well.

Even on the occasions when some form of agency is recognised within anorexia, as in portrayals of the rituals and practices of the anorexic as areas of bodily control, these actions are considered as being so compulsively driven as to severely problematise any conception of meaningful agency. Indeed, such practices and rituals are conceived of as controlling the anorexic who repeatedly performs them. For Bordo (1993a), this type of desire for control over the body demonstrated by the anorexic has strange echoes with that of female body-builders, since both place the same emphasis on will, purity and perfection, and conceptualise the body not as weapon, symbolic or otherwise, but as something alien to its owner, needing to be tamed and controlled. Bruch (1979) takes this interpretation a step further when she reports that anorexics speak of having a ghost inside or surrounding them that dictates and dominates them. Garfinkel and Kaplan (1986) depict the pursuit of a thin body as an isolated area of control in a world in which the anorexic feels ineffective. Dieting, they claim, provides the anorexic with an artificial yet dangerous sense of mastery and control. This notion of obsessive and compulsive control is one that is shared by both social theorists and therapists in their attempts to understand the anorexic: the verdict offered by the medical profession of an out-of-control attempt to control is repeated by cultural critics. In this way, the anorexic is placed in an extreme, static and polarised position in relationship to potential agency. In what appears to be a move of transference and projection, the anorexic is conceived of as unable to see a middle ground (Bordo, 1993a), and is therefore interpreted with a sense of determinancy that blinds theorists both to the transformative aspects that come with the dangers of the phenomenon and to the potential for collaboration between anorexic and clinician, or anorexic and researcher. A meaningful sense of action, resistance or agency ultimately becomes nearly impossible in such limited readings of anorexia, and the prospect of a viable and combative 'politics of anorexia' is shut down before it can even be initiated.

## Nasty girls; dirty theory

What would be the consequences of adopting an alternative interpretation of social action and active agency in which anorexics are conceived of as more 'nasty' than 'good' girls, as using their bodies in an active strategy to take control and become 'sharp enough' to look after themselves, rather than merely capitulating to myriad forms of social influence? What narratives would be needed to sustain such an argument, and in which archives would such narratives be sought? Social theory, it seems, could change in this way. Understanding the anorexic as not just the consequence of a dominating and controlling male discourse, but as also a resistant answer to it, enables the recognition of an active agency, not only in a specific and individual context, but within greater social life more generally. The anorexic then becomes not merely a victim of patriarchal culture, but instead a dissident, an antagonist, a 'resister' of this culture.

There are a number of theoretical offshoots that follow rethinking anorexia in this way. Firstly, those social theories that conceive anorexia in dualistic terms and as an *essential condition* become noticeably more limited, and are destabilised in the process. Secondly, one might broaden the range of archives from which theorists seek to explain the phenomenon of anorexia. In other words, researchers may begin to place more credence on those narratives drawn from the 'local knowledges' of those women who have experienced anorexia and its 'treatment': the type of archive referred to by a former anorexic as 'the real research of lived experience'. This is a source of 'local knowledge', to follow Foucault (1980a), that members of the psychotherapeutic community are increasingly coming to respect and value, especially as traditional means of conceiving and understanding the disorder appear ever more inadequate and ineffective. This is an approach that has been adopted both by the Eating Disorders Clinic at St. Paul's Hospital in Vancouver, Canada, and by the Vancouver

Anti-anorexia, Anti-bulimia League. Accounts from this joint archive of local knowledges – compiled by women diagnosed as anorexics – offer a narrative not of alienated or captured bodies, but of active, resistant and transgressive bodies endowed with a meaningful sense of agency.

What Hacking argues in connection with multiple personality disorder could be argued in this context as well – that the individual makes an implicit choice that fits in with his or her cultural milieu. Hacking maintains that at any time, people suffering from forms of severe psychological distress that are not organic or biological, 'choose' from socially available modes of being (1995: 73). This is an argument reinforced by the narratives of anorexics, which are, in great part, strikingly different from those of mental-health professionals who approach the disorder only from 'the outside'. Women who have experienced anorexia or bulimia suggest that they do not generally see anorexia as principally an issue of food. Lau, a former bulimic, describes eating disorders as an issue of control, not of food, and recognises the body as a site of contestation. In fact, for Lau, the body is the one site of contestation where her control cannot be taken away from her. In her account, she describes the feelings of control and pleasure that purging herself of food gave her, furthering this with a description of how purging was a displacement not only of all the food she had eaten, but her entire past (Lau, 1995).

Roberts (1995) presents similar arguments, saying that anorexia is not a slimmers' disease, but a means of gaining control in one highly visible area, when on virtually every other issue the anorexic seems powerless. MacLeod (1981) describes her body as her weapon in her bid for autonomy, and likens her actions as an anorexic to the withdrawal of labour or to strike action, the only weapon available to the labourer. In an argument that coincides with Hacking's, MacLeod describes how she chose a form of passive resistance:

> Just as the worker's ultimate weapon in his negotiation with management is his labour and the threat of its withdrawal, so my body was my ultimate and, to me, only, weapon in my bid for autonomy. It was the only thing I owned, the only thing which could not be taken away from me. My motivations were not as clear-cut as those of any contemporary workforce, but there is no doubt in my mind that I was going on strike in the only way I knew how to, and that in this sense Szasz is right to describe anorexia nervosa as a political problem (1981: 66).

At the level of 'therapy', health professionals can more easily conceive of formulating collaborative responses if those with whom they are working are seen as active agents in a common cause. Similarly, such collaborative responses are more easily facilitated if health professionals can conceive of local and universal knowledges as being mutually informed. Both of these suggestions, of course, have not been the tradition within the majority of professional approaches to anorexia. At its most basic, the practice of psychiatry, as a case in point, has traditionally involved the attempt to identify and treat a 'problem': the 'patient' has the problem and the psychiatrist the authority to give this 'problem' a name and a prospective treatment. In this way, confronted with the problem of the anorexic body, typically 'resistant' to treatment and scornful of the ability of practitioners, the therapist stares professional, intellectual and emotional lack in the face. Unable to resort to a particular or clear-cut reason, as commonly agreed upon or legitimised by their particular scientific community, health professionals have little to equip them for the challenge of 'renormalising' the anorexic body.

In sizing up traditional approaches to anorexia in this way, what we are therefore able to do is to formulate a number of basic arguments about psychopathology more generally. More specifically, we have been able to caricature the seeming futility or even 'insanity' of the modernist drive to normalisation. Additionally, we have been able to demonstrate the complicity of medical science in the production of oppressive discourse. How has this been managed? Well, in terms of exposing the futility of normalisation, the arguments above have suggested how it is not feasible to treat anorexia in the terms of the stark power differentials preferred by traditional normalising approaches. Firstly, this is because the prospects of a power struggle in trying to conceptualise the disorder seem strong; secondly, because the inability to manage a collaborative treatment/research relationship – let alone to formulate a mutually coherent understanding of the problem – seems undeniable; and thirdly, because the drive to normalisation, so seemingly mimed, mocked and taken to its extreme, starts to appear as a rather confused and redundant objective in the treatment of anorexia. Furthermore, the arguments above have shown that traditional approaches to anorexia are unable to conceptualise the disorder beyond the terms of a socially based condition that denies the 'victim' any real ability to produce meaning, struggle or agency. Such approaches to anorexia hence lock the anorexic, whether in practical or theoretical terms, into a downward spiral of radical disempowerment. From the basis of these theoretical and practical starting points, then, anorexia cannot be approached, understood, theorised or treated in any way that further dissolves the anorexic's chances at self-representation, political action or agency.

## The moments of indigestion

The failure to treat anorexics with success leads Vandereycken (1993) to speak of 'the omnipotence fantasies' of those few therapists who are successful in curing the problem. In the face of anorexia, what Malcolm (1982) calls the 'impossible profession' seems even more so. Anorexics are not only seen as clinically problematic, however. Raymond *et al.* (1994) note that women with anorexia nervosa are seen as 'difficult' for researchers as well as practitioners, a situation that points to the fact that professional and local knowledges of the clinician and the sufferer of the disorder, respectively, are still very much at opposing ends.

If anorexia is scripted around issues of control, contempt and competence, and if medical discourses, and psychiatry in particular, are those disciplinary fields *most* implicated in the naming of the 'normal' and in the control and regulation of deviant minds and bodies, then the therapeutic interchange between clinician and anorexic would appear to be always, at very least, immanently volatile. A classic structural mismatch, this encounter between political dissident and agent of social control within the bounds of an ostensibly curative relationship (which, not incidentally, would seem better suited to engendering damage) would seem always conflictual at basis, always in some ways inimical, always potentially explosive. In this sense, it seems that there is an important political history of anorexia that is yet to be written. Why?

Because, as we discussed above, anorexia seems extraordinarily capable of calling into question both the legitimacy of the order of knowledge produced by the medical profession and the accompanying role of its nominated expert, the therapist. The therapeutic profession's riposte in the face of this challenge is twofold, with practitioners typically constructing the anorexic only within the formulaic terms provided by existing diagnostic categories (as suffering victim), and by denying or minimising the severity of the challenge the disorder presents to the traditional roles they have played and the knowledges they have championed.

Of those health professionals who *do* reflect on the complexity of their interactions with anorexics, many talk of experiencing a deep sense of inadequacy and failure in such relationships. Similarly, many remark on a slippage between what is required for the 'treatment' and what is proffered by the practitioner. Both of these reflections would seem to undermine the efficacy of the practitioner and of traditional professional practice. In this way, the anorexic calls into question the profession's scientific authority and its inability to offer anything but self-contained answers. This shortfall is something recognised by both practitioner and anorexic alike, as the description of an anorexic indicates when she relates how, in sessions with her therapist, she moves at a faster pace than the therapist: 'Every time I think I'm getting a little bit ahead of you I draw back. I hesitate. I start to stutter' (Chernin, 1985: 4).

As this quotation illustrates, 'patients' may at times feel that they have a greater knowledge than the therapist, and so must themselves lead the therapist slowly to the 'problem', without losing sight of the inherent power differential that characterises the therapeutic relationship. A growing number of health professionals seem, indeed, to be attempting to cast aside the 'omnipotence fantasies' that have characterised the profession. Through the use of what has become known as narrative ideas and practices – informed by feminist post-structural theory, especially the work of Foucault, reformulated by Epston and White (1989) – therapists are attempting a transformation of their 'therapeutic' relationships. Those practitioners engaged with such a project see themselves as collaborators with their 'clients', aiming to rescript the therapeutic relationship by drawing in, and on, the knowledges of those whom they had previously acted upon in a non-consultative manner. (Such a shift is in line with the important theoretical need, as pinpointed above, to grasp a sense of agency within anorexia.)

## A therapeutic alliance?

Departing from approaches to therapy in which treatment and diagnosis flow in a one-way direction from the authoritative therapist to the subservient patient, the practitioners of narrative therapy, such as Epston and White (1989), view practitioner and patient (or rather, 'client') as equal partners in the attempt to uncover and treat the presenting problem. Indeed, in a seemingly Foucauldian fashion, narrative 'therapy' works against those therapeutic practices that tend to devalue the language, expertise and knowledge of those being treated. The collaborative work of narrative therapy begins with the joint naming and exploration of the problem: client and therapist work together in developing a mutually acceptable explanation of the problem. One of the key objectives here lies in *externalising* the problem. This is a process that sets the 'disorder' apart from the person, enabling them to reapproach, reassess and rethink their relationship to it. This method of externalising the problem, furthermore, is thought to build working alliances that will help in the combating of the problem. Together, therapist and client create a context for the client's 'reauthoring' of the problem, and they co-construct the terms and the explanatory understandings of the therapy by drawing on their respective resources. What is unusual here is not only the (relative) avoidance of the traditional therapeutic power differential, but also the extent to which therapists draw on seemingly 'non-expert' or local sources of knowledge. Therapists, for example, might collect an 'archive' of audiotapes, letters and artwork contributed by former clients. In addition, such clients are frequently used as consultants, being regarded by the therapists as experts on the 'problems' they have overcome.

These practices clearly extend beyond the clinic. An example of this is the formation of the Anti-anorexia, Anti-bulimia League in Vancouver. Stephen Madigan, a narrative 'therapy' practitioner influential in the establishment of the League, sees the project in Foucauldian terms. For Madigan, Foucault (1979, 1980a) focused on the deconstruction of dominant and culturally constructed discourses of social regulation. Foucault's critical work, more specifically, is most important to Madigan in terms of the opposition it is able to offer those forms of political and scientific discourse that act to turn people into objects of (social) scientific knowledge and practice (cf. Foucault, 1980a). In fact, it is exactly this process of psychiatric discourse 'speaking clients as objects' that, as we suggested above, characterises traditional treatment approaches to anorexia. Take for example the following comment, made by a psychiatrist (who wished to remain unnamed) visiting St. Paul's Hospital in Vancouver: 'To speak the traditional institutional discourse would be to continue to exercise control over bodies, the same control to which those who have come to them for support have been subject, indeed, an exercising of control that may well have been responsible for their condition'. Further, he claimed that he felt 'like a rapist' when confronted by the anorexic in an institutional setting. (The source of quotations and statements by Madigan and others in this paragraph and the one that immediately follows is given in the section entitled **Acknowledgements** at the end of this chapter.)

Relinquishing as far as possible an empowered or controlling position is therefore a vital commitment that must be made by the narrative therapist. This approach can frustrate therapists trained for, and by inclination predisposed to, taking the active role of the rescuer, but in the face of 'resistant' anorexics and an enterprise often destined for failure if a controlling stance is adopted, this alternative proves less frustrating and often more successful. Instead of the despair and inadequacy that traditional therapists appeared to typically experience after sessions with 'difficult' groups of anorexics, narrative therapists more frequently recounted feelings and attitudes of satisfaction after narrative group interactions. The difference here appeared to stem from narrative therapists' reliance on the 'local collaborations' of the group, rather than upon the global knowledges of psychiatry, as the basis of viable and working sources of knowledge.

The usually delegitimised knowledges of the anorexic women with whom therapists have formed a therapeutic alliance are enthusiastically embraced by them in the therapeutic relationship, with comments like, 'It was all her, I didn't do anything' and 'She was taking the role of therapist; passing on that which had been helpful to her'.

How are we best to understand these changes, given Foucault's (1980a) understanding of power and knowledge, where, for him, subjugated knowledges are distinct from any general common sense, and where the particular, local or regional aspects are stressed? How are we to understand these changes against a Foucauldian ground where discontinuous and often contradictory local knowledges are juxtaposed against a unitary body of theory that would stratify, discipline and order qualified forms of knowledges in the name of 'science'? Foucault asks: 'What types of knowledge do you want to disqualify in the very instant of your demand: "Is it a science?" Which speaking, discoursing subjects – which subjects of experience and knowledge – do you then want to "diminish" when you say: "I who conduct this discourse am conducting a scientific discourse, and I am a scientist"?' (1980a: 85).

Given the attention Foucault paid to what he terms 'subjugated knowledges' – referring to the historical contents that have been buried and the set of knowledges disqualified as inadequate or insufficiently elaborated – can these attempts at changes be seen as a consideration of local knowledges by the 'centre'? Foucault, after all, gave as an example of a disqualified local knowledge the knowledge of the psychiatric patient (Foucault, 1980a: 82). However, although he argued that these delegitimised and oppositive knowledges should be taken up, accredited and put into circulation, he also warned that they might be assimilated into the institutional discourses that they had initially challenged: 'they run the risk of re-codification, re-colonisation ... . In fact, those unitary discourses, which first disqualified and then ignored [those oppositive local knowledges] ... when they made their appearance, are, it seems, quite ready now to annex them, to take them back within the fold of their own discourse and to invest them with ... their [own] ... effects of knowledge and power' (Foucault, 1980a: 86).

With this view in mind, is it possible, then, for the 'centre' to collaborate with the 'margins'? Also, thinking with Foucault in regard to his work on the confessional (Foucault, 1980b), the agency of domination can, of course, reside in the person who listens and says nothing. Should then the work at St. Paul's be seen as a further move to control, rather than to collaborate? Indeed, how should the wider practice of narrative ideas and practices be viewed, especially given its Foucauldian inspiration?

Perhaps if one thinks with Foucault in an 'anti-science' mode, i.e. in a way that would oppose any stratifying or disciplining theory, and that would incorporate the ambiguous and seemingly incoherent, perhaps in this anti-scientific way, one might understand how anorexia can function as an effective, albeit collaborative, form of resistance that does not merely dissolve into recolonisation. Perhaps this is how the 'margins' might be brought to the 'centre' without necessarily being assimilated by it. Perhaps these different ways of knowing would successfully destabilise the disciplinary power that had previously set out to normalise knowledge – and bodies – to such an extent that effective forms of collaboration might become viable. As the argument was made for an active agency on the part of anorexics, on the basis that while subjects may be constituted, they are not determined – indeed, that the constituted nature of the subject is the very precondition for its agency – so, too, is the agency argument made for health professionals who may wish to transform the discourse within which they are located. Such a precedent has already been set, of course, in the form of the anti-psychiatry movement, in which psychiatrists themselves played key roles in resisting the formidable and institutional power of psychiatry more generally.

An attitude that sees any engagement (or collaboration) between privileged and subjugated as exclusively that of colonisation would seem to straitjacket all agents of attempted change. Foucault, for example, should surely not be seen as a mere coloniser of prisoners' knowledge, or as the single beneficiary of the other various subjugated groups with whom he worked. Nor should the move towards collaboration of narrative ideas and practices be too quickly prejudged. Indeed, to see all occurrences of engagement between powerful and disempowered as being necessarily (or merely) acts of colonisation would be at one level anti-Foucauldian, because it would simply close down the prospects for meaningful resistance, prospects that for Foucault (cf. 1980a) are always present.

## ■ Acknowledgements

This chapter drew on conversations, research and interviews since October 1994 with the health professionals working directly for, or associated with, the Eating Disorders Clinic at St. Paul's Hospital in Vancouver. Elliot Goldner gave much of his time to discussion and Stephen Madigan, too, gave of his time and allowed me to sit in on seminars conducted at Yaletown Family Therapy, as did women diagnosed with anorexia participating in group therapy and associated with the Anti-anorexia, Anti-bulimia League in Vancouver.

## ■ Endnotes

1 An illustration entitled 'What happens when an angry young woman discovers her bones' appeared in an alternative arts magazine, *Discorder*, published in Vancouver (March, 1995: 28). It portrayed a woman losing significant weight as the potentials of her bony body as weapon dawned upon her. Among the captions there appeared: 'Terms such as knee to the groin took on a whole new meaning' and 'She knew she was sharp enough to look after herself'.
2 Butler similarly, but within the field of feminism, argues that, 'Paradoxically, it may be that only through releasing the category of women from a fixed referent that something like "agency" becomes possible' (1993: 16).
3 Gayatri Spivak makes arguments of this kind in Barr (1989: 12).

## ■ References

American Psychiatric Association (1987). *Diagnostic and Statistical Manual of Mental Disorders* (3rd edn, rev.). Washington, DC: American Psychiatric Association.
Barr, L. (1989). An interview with Gayatri Chakravorty Spivak. *BLAST nuLTD*, 12, Summer.
Bell, R. M. (1985). *Holy Anorexia*. Chicago and London: University of Chicago Press.
Bhabha, H. (1994). *The Location of Culture*. London: Routledge.
Bordo, S. (1993a). *Unbearable Weight*. London: University of California Press.
Bordo, S. (1993b). Feminism, Foucault and the politics of the body. In C. Ramazanoglu (ed.), *Up against Foucault*, pp. 179–202. London: Routledge.
Bruch, H. (1979). *The Golden Cage: The Enigma of Anorexia Nervosa*. New York: Vintage.
Butler, J. (1993). Contingent foundations: Feminists and the question of postmodernism. In J. Butler and J. Scott (eds), *Feminists Theorise the Political*, pp. 3–21. New York: Routledge.

Chernin, K. (1985). *The Hungry Self: Women, Eating, and Identity*. New York: Times Books.
*Discorder* (1995). March. Vancouver.
Ellmann, M. (1993). *The Hunger Artists: Starving, Writing, and Imprisonment*. Cambridge, Mass.: Harvard University Press.
Epston, D. and White, M. (1989). *Literate Means to Therapeutic Ends*. Adelaide: Dulwich Centre Publishing.
Foucault, M. (1972). *The Archaeology of Knowledge and the Discourse on Language*. New York: Pantheon Books.
Foucault, M. (1979). *Discipline and Punish: The Birth of the Prison*. Harmondsworth: Penguin.
Foucault, M. (1980a). *Power/Knowledge: Selected Interviews and Other Writings by Michel Foucault, 1972–1977*. New York: Pantheon Books.
Foucault, M. (1980b). *The History of Sexuality: An Introduction*, Vol. 1. New York: Vintage Books.
Garfinkel, P. and Kaplan, A. (1986). Anorexia nervosa: Diagnostic conceptualizations. In K. Brownell and J. Foreyt (eds), *Handbook of Eating Disorders*, pp. 266–82. New York: Basic Books.
Graydon, S. (1995). When fashionable is a fatal attraction. *Vancouver Sun*, February 4.
Hacking, I. (1995). *Rewriting the Soul: Multiple Personality and the Science of Memory*. Princeton: Princeton University Press.
Lau, E. (1995). An insatiable emptiness. *The Georgia Straight*, Vancouver, July 21–28, 13–14.
Lee, S. (1995). Self-starvation in context: Towards a culturally sensitive understanding of anorexia nervosa. *Social Science and Medicine*, 41 (1), 25–36.
MacLeod, S. (1981). *The Art of Starvation*. London: Virago.
Malcolm, J. (1982). *Psychoanalysis: The Impossible Profession*. London: Pan.
Meadow, R. and Weiss, L. (1992). *Women's Conflicts about Eating and Sexuality: The Relationship between Food and Sex*. New York: Haworth.
Mouffe, C. (1995). Feminism, citizenship, and radical democratic politics. In L. Nicholson and S. Seidman (eds), *Social Postmodernism: Beyond Identity Politics*, pp. 315–31. Cambridge: Cambridge University Press.
Nicholson, L. (1995). Interpreting gender. In L. Nicholson and S. Seidman (eds), *Social Postmodernism: Beyond Identity Politics*, pp. 39–67. Cambridge: Cambridge University Press.
Prakash, G. (1995). Postcolonial criticism and Indian historiography. In L. Nicholson and S. Seidman (eds), *Social Postmodernism: Beyond Identity Politics*, pp. 87–100. Cambridge: Cambridge University Press.
Roberts, Y. (1995). Bad to the bone. *Guardian*, London, August 14, 4–5.
Raymond, N. C., Mitchell, J. E., Fallon, P. and Katzman, M. A. (1994). A collaborative approach to the use of medication. In P. Fallon, M. A. Katzman and S. C. Woodley (eds), *Feminist Perspectives on Eating Disorders*, pp. 231–50. New York: The Guilford Press.
Touraine, A. (1977). *Return of the Social Actor: Social Theory in Postindustrial Society*. Chicago: University of Chicago Press.
Turner, B. (1984). *The Body and Society: Explorations in Social Theory*. Oxford: Basil Blackwell.
Vandereycken, W. (1993). Naughty girls and angry doctors: Eating disorder patients and their therapists. *International Review of Psychiatry*, 5, 13–17.

# Avoiding the implicit repathologisation of male homosexuality: A politico-clinical direction for research

*Anthony Theuninck, Derek Hook & Vijé Franchi*

## ■ Introduction

Research on homosexuality is problematic on a number of counts. Indeed, in an epoch of growing tolerance for homosexuality as a variance of human sexuality, it needs to be asked anew *what the purpose is of conducting research on homosexuality*. If we are to leave behind an oppressive research industry that sought the origin and implied cure of homosexuality, then we need to readdress what it is about homosexuality (and our approach to it) that is still capable of drawing such ardent research interest. We need bear in mind, in short, that any project of knowledge production is intricately tied to, and led by, the motivating goals and objectives that have initiated the project in the first place. We might hence adopt, pragmatically, the cautioning that a politically utile knowledge cannot be obtained or informed from a position of supposedly impartial or decontextualised 'objectivity'. In a similarly pragmatic manner, we need to maintain an acute awareness and transparency regarding *the utility* of the knowledge we produce. As such, to ask what homosexuality is should ideally be informed by the provision of *what one aims to achieve* with the knowledge that will be built around this construct. (Such a provision, i.e. the implicit objectives of this project of knowledge production, will, hopefully, become increasingly overt as this chapter develops.)

Secondly, to address research on homosexuality, one needs to start by critically engaging with a definition of the phenomenon. Typically, understandings of the phenomenon vacillate between viewing homosexuality, on the one hand, as construct, and on the other, as fixed material property. The latter implies the retrograde notion that desire is prior to the social, a view thoroughly problematised by both Foucault (1976), and following from him, Butler (1990). If we are to adopt the vantage of these theorists, then what is of concern in research of this sort is the manner in which *the understandings* of homosexuality are employed. As Foucault (1976) reasoned, the power of discourse is known by its *effect* rather than its origin. Accordingly, the present chapter positions itself in respect to two important reference points: that of a Western context that is characterised by a history of medical discourse that pathologised 'homosexuality' *per se*, and that of a history of activism that has coined the term 'gay' to provide an alternative affirming construction of the phenomenon in question. It is the effect of these competing discourses upon the social and psychological experience of a person that is here framed as the necessary object of study. It is therefore not so much 'homosexuality' *per se*, as the effect of the discourses about 'homosexuality' that centres the current research interest.

In view of, and in a sense *precisely because of* these two foregoing qualifications, we will argue in this chapter that the conflict between homosexually oppressive and homosexually affirmative discourses may give rise to a vulnerability to certain forms of 'psychopathology'. For the purposes of this discussion, we will adopt a relatively conventional definition of psychopathology; the use of the notion of psychopathology here will hence refer to a 'behavioural or psychological syndrome or pattern that occurs in ... [a socio-culturally and discursively embodied person] ... and that is associated with present distress ... or disability or with a significant increased risk of suffering death, pain, disability or an important loss of freedom' (American Psychiatric Association, 1994: xxi). One will note here that a departure has been made from the standard *Diagnostic and Statistical Manual of Mental Disorders* (DSM) definition by substituting 'a socio-culturally and discursively embodied person' for the notion of the individual: this is to connote that psychopathology, or what counts as psychopathology, need not be seen as residing within the locus of a bounded, context-less individual, but might more effectively be located in a socio-cultural context.

## The 'discursive homosexual'

Present literature on homosexuality is replete with representations of homosexuals as a minority group, newly born in Western history, who almost necessarily suffer the oppressive consequences of exercising their sexual preferences in hostile socio-cultural environments (cf. Weeks, 1985). The same literature is just as typically characterised by focuses on the struggle for, and celebration of, a self-determined ownership of a homosexual identity (Weeks, 1985). The drive here is to assert that those associated with homosexual practices and/or identities should be treated equally, and should enjoy the same privileges as those who indulge in heterosexual practices and maintain heterosexual identities. Here a human-rights discourse prevails, around which homosexuality is used to create a voice, narrate a culture, establish social services and build an economic infrastructure including anything from 'gay life insurance' to alternative entertainment venues (Altman, 1982). However, whether all the people united in these representations and associated discursive practices subscribe to similar notions and identities of homosexuality is highly debatable. Not all people engaging in same-sex sexual behaviour identify themselves as being gay. Similarly, different homosexuals, despite the similarity of their sexual preferences, no doubt place differing emphases on sexuality as a prime source of identity. Further still, not all 'practitioners of homosexuality' invest so resolutely in a cultural or social matrix in which *the nature of their sexual preference* is the dominant source of commonality; indeed, a variety of other forms of social identity may take precedence. Homosexuality hence need not neatly correspond to any singular or cohesive system of meaning, just as it need not accord any basic category of popular representation or identity.

A similar situation arises within the discourse of gay rights, where claims are consistently made about the *inherent* nature of homosexuality. It would seem, however, that this supposed 'genetic inevitability' of homosexuality neither necessarily applies to all instances of homosexual behaviour, nor necessarily supersedes the discursive formation of homosexuality as a knowable object of study, practice and representation. The 'inherent homosexuality' explanation would appear to discount the prospects of homosexual experimentation on the part of those who are ostensibly heterosexual (or bisexual). Similarly, it would also seem to discount the prospects of later-life sexual-orientation change. Indeed, participation in homosexual acts need not necessarily 'a homosexual make'. Homosexual behaviour may be practised in the initiation rituals of seemingly predominantly heterosexual societies, as in Melanesia, or as in the socially sanctioned (homosexual) roles adopted by the Berdache of North America (Herdt, 1993; Whitehead, 1981). In these instances, like that of the modern gay life-style, it is highly unlikely that homosexual activities or cultures are simply genetically determined; it seems, rather (and here Butler (1990) is again useful), that sexual orientation is far more a function of discourse than we might at first have supposed, that notions, values and knowledges of homosexuality, like homosexuality itself, are already *discursive* before they attach to any necessary biological/genetic substrate.

Therefore, to investigate homosexuality as an inherent and realist concept with universal and immutable properties would be to promulgate a misguided vision of homosexuality that loses touch with the rich complexity of its practices and identities. Indeed, if we are to follow Butler (1990), to conflate the term 'homosexual' and the claims to truth that are generated around it with the real body of the individual is to miss the 'homosexual' altogether. The 'homosexual' is not the ground or basis of truth, but the effect of the enterprises of knowledge that lay claim to truth (Butler, 1990). The person who is labelled or even self-labels as homosexual is not evidence of *homosexuality*, but is merely the person who has come to be understood, or come to understand themselves, within certain systems of meaning.

This is not to say that the person has no real feelings or experiences, or that they do not feel love, desire or attraction for people of the same sex. What it does mean is that those feelings or behaviours are not in and of themselves 'homosexual'. What makes these phenomena 'homosexual' is their description within certain systems of meaning and practice. Of course, implicated within these systems are power relations that regulate and organise meaning and, as a consequence, the social and personal practices associated with them (Foucault, 1976, 1977/1991). It is in this way that descriptions of sexuality seek to regulate sexual relations between people, and do so to the benefit of certain interests (Foucault, 1976). As such, we are led back to the pragmatic suggestion made at the opening of this chapter that in researching homosexuality, the object of study is in fact *the effect of discourses of homosexuality on the person*, and not the absolute bounded truth of the person *themselves*. 'Homosexuality' and the social and psychological experiences it shapes are therefore not universal, but reliant on forms of popular and current discursive knowledge and representation.

## Gayness as discourse

In schematic terms, the West maintains two broad and counterposed discursive traditions regarding homosexuality: one that may be labelled oppressive, and one that may be labelled liberative. The oppressive discourse comprises medical, legal and religious discourses and their diverse variants that (implicitly or explicitly) argue that legitimate or warranted sexuality is limited to those practices of heterosexual copulation that may, at least potentially, yield a procreative outcome. In these terms, all non-heterosexual relations are deemed marginal, falling into categories of sickness, crime or sin. It is within the oppressive discourses that the term 'homosexual' arose. It was essentially a medical term invented by the Hungarian doctor Karoly Benkert in 1869 (Altman, 1982). The 'homosexual' was thereby rendered an individual object of study, a 'personage, a past, a case history, and a childhood' whose cause and cure were sought for most of 20th century (Foucault, 1976).

The liberative discourse has invented the term 'gay' in order to provide an alternative construction to same-sex relations and their desire. (In this sense, one might suggest that the discourse of gayness has been elaborated within the greater discourse of homosexuality.) Hence, gay discourse, in overly generalised and schematic terms, typically asserts that people given to same-sex relations and desire should have the right to such relations. This discourse has, furthermore, led to a seemingly progressive self-labelling process whereby certain proponents of same-sex desire have come to refer to themselves as 'gay'. Affirmation of this discourse allows 'free' or socially sanctioned expression of same-sex desire within systems of public and private relations that have previously been reserved for heterosexual relations. Hence, as Altman (1982) notes, identifying as 'gay' has evolved into a life-style marked by what you buy, where you shop, where you live, what you wear, who you vote for, your choice of entertainment and what you adopt as your philosophy of life. In this way, gayness might be seen as embodying a persona, a social and moral stance, promoting itself as a forceful economic and political demographic. Similarly, it has become a useful framework of meaning, practice and resistance through which to understand and validate forms of sexuality traditionally persecuted and oppressed within many Western societies. As Chauncey (1994) notes, the neophyte with homosexual desires is confronted with the need to make meaning of their feelings and direct a course of action in accordance with them; gay discourse provides a dominant positive frame of reference within which to do so.

Before we imply that gayness is in some ways an inherently more liberative form of sexuality than is, say, heterosexuality, it is important to note that being 'gay' does not necessarily signify any greater objective freedom over and above that of other forms of sexuality. Being gay is still a matter of being subject to a technology of sexuality, i.e. there are still certain agreed-upon conventions and limitations according to which sexual desire may be practised, sought out and even thought about. Gay discourse, and its accompanying ensemble of practices, like those of heterosexuality, nonetheless seeks to regulate the practice of sexuality, albeit for different sexual relations. In short, gay discourse, like discourses of heterosexuality, can be oppressive. Differences among people engaging in or drawn to same-sex relations may not all be simply assimilated within gay discourse: the axes of race, class, gender, age, etc. all differentially affect how same-sex relations are experienced.

It hence becomes important to qualify the notion of a 'gay discourse'. Gayness, no doubt, is party to numerous different and differing articulations of practice, life-style and subjectivity, and, respectful of the political stakes riding on each such articulation, we will not attempt to provide an authoritative version of what it means to be gay. Essentialising 'gayness' as a single or unitary discourse, like attempts to annex this discursive category as the epitome of any particular life-style, typically functions to obscure various complex strands of gayness and the way they intersect with other social positions. To paraphrase Butler (1990), one might suggest that it is just as impossible to separate out 'gayness' as 'gender' from the political and cultural intersections in which it is invariably produced and maintained. In this sense, the notion of 'gayness' here will remain, quite intentionally, largely unspecified and relatively underdetermined, such that the broad terms of this debate may be customised and applied to more specific terms of argument and activism. At the risk of being repetitive, it is probably worth emphasising again here that what is being engaged with in this study is the effect of discourses of homosexuality upon the person, and not the absolute, bounded truth of the person themselves, i.e. gayness as discourse rather than essential trait of identity.

Despite these qualifications of gayness, there seems little point in contesting the assertion that gay discourse *does* provide a potentially positive frame of reference from which to oppose those strands of heterosexist[1] discourse, which would attempt to marginalise and exclude same-sex relations as legitimate forms of sexuality. In this sense, gayness might be considered as the discursive experience of the self within a system of meaning dichotomised by rhetorics of oppression versus resistance, delegitimisation versus activism, marginalisation versus validation and 'the gaining of voice'. *Experiencing conflict around homosexuality is therefore a product of the opposing expectations, requirements and norms set out by opposing gay and anti-gay discourses.* Indeed, in this way, to research gayness and those strands of a heterosexist discourse that would oppose it is, largely, to engage with discursive phenomena that gain their prominence and substance largely on the bases of *personal and social struggles for meaning.* So one way of understanding psychopathology might be in terms of the 'shutting down' of discursive possibilities for self-definition and understanding; indeed, it is this form of oppression that will here be considered as particularly relevant to creating a vulnerability to psychopathology[2] in gay individuals who aspire to live out their same-sex desires and relations within a heterosexist Western context.

## Gayness as vulnerability to psychopathology

Within the broad field of psychology, this chapter therefore adopts a fairly novel approach to enquiring into the negative mental-health consequences of trying to establish a gay identity in non-conducive, heterosexist environments. The fact of such detrimental effects, and the possibility of alleviating factors in view thereof, has been taken up by a number of authors (cf. Minton and McDonald, 1984; Coleman, 1982; Cass, 1979; Troiden, 1979; Savin-Williams, 1994; D'Augelli, 1993 and 1996a; Garnets *et al.*, 1990; Radkowsky and Siegel, 1997; Martin and Hetrick, 1988). However, most of this work is marred by its failure to identify the particular stressors that gay people may be subjected to. No neat stressor typologies have been developed; similarly, the specific relations of these stressors to certain mental-health difficulties remain largely unelaborated. In fact, there has been, in general terms, a conspicuous *avoidance* regarding the linking of certain pathologies to the experience of gay labelling in Western heterosexist contexts. This avoidance is most probably because of the pathologised history of homosexuality (Meyer and Dean, 1998), and despite this, or perhaps directly in view of it, we are confronted with a variety of disturbing psychiatric scenarios. Homosexual persons are over-represented within certain diagnostic categories. For a start, Carlat *et al.* (1997) found that 42% of male bulimic patients self-identified as homosexual or bisexual. In a meta-analysis of clinical subjects who exhibit deliberate self-harm symptoms, Pattison and Kahan (1983) found that 26% of the sample reported being homosexual, of which 12 out of the 15 were male. Zubenko *et al.* (1987) found that 57% of 21 consecutive male patients with borderline personality disorder (BPD) who presented for psychiatric treatment were homosexual. In a sample of 80 male and female patients with BPD, 21% were homosexual and 5% were bisexual. In this sample, of the 19 males with BPD, 53% were homosexual. Dulit *et al.* (1993) found that 22% of the males with BPD in their in-patient sample were homosexual and 26% were bisexual. Paris *et al.* (1995) found higher rates of homosexuality in men with BPD than in non-borderline disordered men.

Now, although these findings are representative of homosexuals more broadly, rather than just of gay males, they certainly do suggest that gay men appear to be disproportionately represented among clinical samples of patients with borderline personality disorder, bulimia and self-harm syndrome. No doubt, these findings should be seen as suggestive and not absolute, given sample biases and methodological limitations. However, they do point to the fact that gay people, and gay males in particular, seem to be more likely to manifest these psychopathologies, resulting from the environmental stress or trauma experienced by virtue of being gay. Suicide and substance abuse are two other indicators of mental distress that have been greatly studied amongst gay people and in which they are likely to be disproportionately represented.

Similar results suggest that gay men and women have long been considered to be at a disproportionate risk of heavy or problematic drinking (Bux, 1996). Early studies suggested that a third of gay men and two thirds of lesbians have significant drinking problems, although more recent research indicates more conservative figures (Bux, 1996). From his overview on alcohol abuse Bux concluded that: 1) gays and lesbians are less likely to abstain from alcohol use; 2) gay men show little to no elevated risk of heavy drinking; and 3) lesbians are at a higher risk of alcohol abuse. Further yet, Gibson (1989 in D'Augelli, 1996b) speculated that gay youth are two to three times more likely to commit suicide, and that gay youth constitute up to 30% of all completed youth suicides. Various studies have found that between 20% and 42% of gay, lesbian and bisexual youth samples have attempted suicide (D'Augelli, 1996b; Hershberger and D'Augelli, 1995). This is clearly higher than general population high-school estimates that range between 6% and 16% and community sample estimates between 9% and 12% (Rotherham-Borus *et al.*, 1994). Widespread suicidal ideation has been found in various samples. D'Augelli and Hershberger (1993) found that in a gay and lesbian youth sample (under 21), 8% often thought about suicide, 21% sometimes, 30% rarely and 40% never. Bradford *et al.* (1994) found that 2% considered suicide often, 25% sometimes and 32% rarely, while only 41% never contemplated suicide. In Schneider *et al.*'s (1989) study of young gay males, 59% evidenced serious suicidal thinking.

In the absence of a clear understanding of the relationship between the life experiences of gay people and their mental health, the risk is high of inadvertently associating certain pathologies with homosexuality *per se*. In psychiatric evaluations, a person's homosexual orientation will be noted, whereas a heterosexual orientation is not commonly notable. The possibility hence arises for the unspoken association to be made between a person's homosexuality and their given psychopathology. Homosexuality in this case is constructed as an individual condition and not a particular relational experience within a heterosexist social context. The technologies of psychopathology may thereby implicitly pathologise homosexuality; e.g. day-to-day clinical practices and procedures may fail to address the complete reason for the presence or over-representation of gay males among certain pathologies. The person's sexuality will be noted without a thorough investigation of the various heterosexist stressors the person has been subject to, since no official typology of stressors exists. Researchers, and assumedly clinicians, counsellors and mental-health professionals more generally, therefore need to confront the current psychiatric vulnerability of people who self-identify as homosexual or gay. An increasingly important question is: 'What are the stressors that gay-identified people are experiencing?' and, following on from this, 'Do those potential stressors have any bearing on their vulnerability to certain psychopathologies?'

To address these questions, we need to first establish what gay-related minority stress is. Furthermore, we need to determine the severity of gay-related minority stress: is this phenomenon merely a stress, or can it be traumatic? Isaacs and McKendrick (1992) conceptualise gay-related stress within a crisis framework. They define a crisis as 'a period ... of psychosocial disequilibrium in which a traumatic, hazardous, or dangerous experience or event confronts an individual .... The danger or threat reduces ... the individual's capacity to deal with the situation by using his/her repertoire of familiar coping mechanisms. The crisis represents either an internal response to an external threat, or is a manifestation of a developmental ... process inside the individual' (1992: 42).

Isaacs and McKendrick speak of 'event stress' and 'developmental stress'. Developmental stress or crisis 'arises when the accomplishment of a task associated with a developmental phase of the lifecycle ... is disrupted, thwarted, or made excessively difficult' (1992: 44). Here the theorists are primarily referring to the task of identity development, which, seemingly, is not a specific event, but rather a gradual process. In developing a gay identity within a heterosexist context, subtle and overt forms of rejection, discrimination, threat or assault must be dealt with; but the experience of gay-related stress does not stop once an identity is developed. It is never-ending, as a person constantly deals with being marginalised, defending themselves against victimisation and overcoming fears that may arise in new contexts. Abolishing one's discomfort or disappointment in one's own sexuality may also be a constant battle when someone lacks access to effective counter-discourses, interactions or intimate relationships with other gay people or people holding gay-positive views.

## ■ Gay-related minority stressors

The experience of stress is therefore long-term, and bound to a heterosexist context. It is a product of what Heidegger (1962) referred to as 'throwness', i.e. a person's discursive and socially stratified locatedness that lies beyond their control. Gay-related stress is largely experienced contextually, as a set of circumstances, rather than as only an event or clearly identifiable incident (Isaacs and McKendrick, 1992). Various event-related stressors may be seen to contribute to this overall contextual-stress experience, but their effect cannot be viewed in isolation from that context.

Niesen (1993) has argued for the cumulative impact of the contextual experience of minority stressors. He refers to contextual stress as cultural victimisation that ranges from blatant discrimination and acts of violation to subtle forms of exclusion and a lack of acknowledgement, which may have pervasive effects. Niesen argues that the effects of cultural victimisation and sexual or physical abuse are similar. These symptomatic similarities are, blaming the self for the abuse, feeling shame and self-hate, a negative self-concept, feeling isolated, fear of being alone or overwhelming others, generalised fear, depression, anxiety and anger, self-destructive behaviour, victim mentality and difficulty in trusting. While this illuminates similarities in symptoms, Niesen omits investigating the similarities in stressors, which may be vastly different for gay people and victims of physical and sexual assault. How specifically is cultural victimisation similar to physical and sexual assault? The full range of symptoms resulting from physical and sexual assault may also not necessarily apply to gay people. Merely suggesting similarities in symptomatic outcomes does not offer a strong-enough argument for gay people's distress as being mostly caused by cultural victimisation. However, the comparison offers politically and clinically important hypotheses. Given that physical and sexual abuse may often lead to traumatic sequella, the question of interest is *whether or not heterosexist contextual stress and event-related stress may also give rise to trauma symptoms*. Investigating the relation of minority stressors to distress may be important in avoiding models that pathologise homosexuality, and offer new clinical sensitivities when working with gay and bisexual people, who may present with problems that are not immediately recognisable as stressor-related.

Using a contextual framework, the cumulative effect of insidious stressors may be postulated to be as severe or more so than the impact of singular victimising events. Ross (1996) notes that life hassles have been found to be more predictive of distress than major life events. Cumulative life-style stressors may therefore be important aspects of assessing the impact of minority stressors. In adult samples of gay males, gay-related life-style stressors have been found to make a significant negative impact on gay men's mental health as measured by the General Health Questionnaire (GHQ-28), with the most significant impact being on anxiety, insomnia and somatic symptoms (Ross, 1996). It was also found that gay youth who attempted suicide had experienced more gay-related stress than gay youth that made no such attempt (Rotherham-Borus *et al.*, 1994).

Gay-related contextual stress may also make people more prone to non-gay-related stressors. Correlations between non-gay-related life events and psychological functioning was considerably higher for gay males than in comparable studies of heterosexual people. Rotherham-Borus *et al.* (1994) similarly found that their sample of gay male youth had three to five times more negative non-gay life stress than comparable samples of presumably heterosexual youth. Contextual stressors may therefore impact on gay people through stressors particular to the minority, as well as by increasing vulnerability to general-life stressors. Social stratification may generate unequal exposure to stressful life events and greater vulnerability to stress in minority groups (Liem and Liem, 1984). Less access to supportive resources (friends, books, community services) combined with more stressors shape the context factors that determine the nature and extent of impact on mental health (Liem and Liem, 1984).

Gay-minority stressors should capture the breadth of the minority stress experience that a person becomes subject to when ascribing to a minority identity or feeling that one's being may implicate one within such an identity. This stress experience is long-term, spanning life development. It is characterised by a heterosexist context that may subject a person to specific stress events, such as public slander, social rejection and assault, as well as embed a person within a discursive context of devaluation, negative stereotypes and discrimination that may constantly weigh down on their cognition and emotions. It is further suggested by empirical findings that such a heterosexist context may increase the minority person's exposure to non-gay-related stressors as well. *What is required is an examination of the extent to which minority stress experiences impact on personal distress or mental health.* One means of doing so is to investigate whether gay-minority stressors may be traumatic.

## ■ DESNOS

One form of traumatic stress response that gay people may be more likely to be exposed to is that of complex post-traumatic stress disorder, alternatively named 'disorders of extreme stress not otherwise specified' (DESNOS), the latter label being a suggested DSM diagnostic category that was not included in the DSM-IV (Van der Kolk et al., 1996). DESNOS aims to capture the diversity of responses resulting from exposure to chronic traumatic stressors (Herman, 1992; Van der Kolk, 1996). The responses to chronic traumatic stressors are lost within more conventional trauma diagnoses like post-traumatic stress disorder (PTSD), which also obscures features associated with interpersonal stressors that DESNOS in turn is sensitive to (Brett, 1996). The chronic traumatic-stress reaction is thus not merely a long-term reaction to a particular trauma event, but may be a distinct reaction to a series of events or a context of oppression. DESNOS may provide an overarching framework with which the various subtle manifestations of chronic traumatic interpersonal stressors may be understood. The criteria for DESNOS do not require marked distress, but an overall endorsement of a pattern of specific symptoms (Newman et al., 1995). Newman et al. point out that this may cause DESNOS to be overinclusive, but also very sensitive, which is important, since a collection of mild DESNOS symptoms may together create a functional disturbance. There are two broad areas of disturbance in DESNOS that transcend simple PTSD (Herman, 1993). These include: 1) a more complex, diffuse and tenacious symptom picture; and 2) characterological changes (see Herman, 1993).

The diagnostic concept of DESNOS opens up a view of traumatic stress reactions as being responses to a context of stress and not merely singular events. This is applicable to gay people, where the experience of stress is not always a definitive event, but rather the experience of a heterosexist environment that enforces silence, discriminates and devalues same-sex desire, as well as the person who creates an identity based on it. DESNOS opens up the scientific imagination to the effects that long-term adaptations to contextual ongoing stress may have. Earl (1991) argued for perceived trauma as an experience of traumatic stress without a clearly identifiable event. DESNOS can recognise the possibility of such a reaction, given that long-term experiences of stress may create a Gestalt of trauma that cannot necessarily be pinned onto one event. The diffuse experience of contextual stress may collectively constitute trauma of the complex type.

DESNOS has been found to be co-morbid with PTSD, BPD, depression, mania, general and phobic anxieties, interpersonal sensitivity, paranoia, psychoticism, sexual dysfunction, eating disorders, anger, suicidality, and drug and alcohol addiction/abuse (Herman, 1992, 1993; McGorry, 1995; Jongedijk et al., 1995; Van der Kolk, 1996). Given the over-representation of self-identified homosexual people among sufferers of BPD, suicidality, eating disorders and substance abuse, it could be postulated that this is caused by the chronic traumatic stress experienced by gay people as a result of living in a heterosexist context.

Some preliminary evidence already suggests the possibility of gay-minority stressors leading to trauma reactions. Meyer (1995) found that stigmatic stress, internalised 'homo-negativity' and victimisation are associated with demoralisation. Harry Stack Sullivan developed the concept of demoralisation in order to account for the breakdown of morale among combat troops and civilian victims within the context of the Second World War (Link, 1987). Demoralisation indicates the erosion of self-esteem, feelings of helplessness and hopelessness, confused and less adaptive thought, dysphoric mood and pessimistic ruminations about the future. These have been found to empirically cluster together (Link, 1987). The factor theorised to lead to this condition was the breakdown of 'cherished beliefs about one's place in the world' (Link, 1987: 98). Through a highly stressful experience, expectations about the self and others become no longer tenable, the trusted universe collapses and the person's convictions, faith and beliefs appear to them to have been based upon self-deception (Link, 1987). The criteria for demoralisation are similar to those in victims of traumatic incidents, and may fall under the rubric of DESNOS, which includes a negative change in systems of meaning as one of its criteria. The breakdown of beliefs has also been observed in victims of traumatic incidents (Janoff-Bulman, 1992; McCann and Pearlman, 1990). Given Meyer's finding of the relation between gay-related stress and demoralisation amongst gay people, it seems that gay-related stress may be empirically related to trauma. The extent to which a person's relational world resembles that of active persecution and captivity, the greater the trauma can be expected to be (Herman, 1992). In its extreme form, such a traumatic relational world would be one devoid of social support and access to gay-positive views, consisting of a climate necessitating confession, policing of the self, policing by others and being actively punished by public shaming, ridicule or assault for deviating from the prescribed norm.

## ■ Clinical pragmatics

The DSM-IV makes allowances for the diagnosis of psychosocial stressors on Axis 4. Some minority stressors could be coded under this section, namely, problems with the primary support group, problems related to the social environment (discrimination), educational problems, occupational problems, housing problems (e.g. discord with a 'homo-negative' landlord), problems related to the legal system and crime (e.g. being a victim of crime or being incarcerated due to sexual orientation) and discord with homophobic caregivers (e.g. counsellors and social-service agencies). Yet the cardinal diagnostic problem at hand is determining the Axes 1 and 2 disorders that the person may be suffering from. The type of psychosocial stressors a person is subjected to are enquired into as an adjunct to understanding the nature of the presentation of the disorder and the route treatment may need to take. In practice, a diagnosis is mostly informed by a person's symptoms and not by the nature of their psychosocial stressors. The only diagnostic disorder where there is an exception to this rule is post-traumatic stress disorder. Here, a clearly identifiable psychosocial stressor must be present in order to inform a diagnosis of PTSD. Owing to the general diagnostic disjunction between stressors and disorders, the relations between various forms of disorders and stressors is tenuously noted and weakly considered. Where there is an unexceptional stressor, this may go unnoticed as contributive to a diagnosis. A lack of information as to the specific stressors certain persons within certain cultural milieu may be under further problematises the matter. Patients may not be aware of the stressors they are subject to, especially if these are minority stressors. A minority stressor is a force exerted on a marginal person that is deemed as appropriate by the dominant order. It is a stressor that is therefore viewed as part of the status quo, and may not qualify in the popular imagination as stressful, let alone traumatic. It therefore resides with the mental-health worker to be sensitised to the particular stressors a person with a minority identity may have. (The term 'minority' here does not necessarily refer to numerical minority, but to the marginal, powerless position ascribed to certain people.)

Without a clear idea of the possible relations between disorders and stressors, and the inter-relations between different disorders as a result of stressors, an incoherent and misleading diagnostic picture may emerge. Diagnoses such as BPD, eating disorders, suicidality, substance abuse, etc. may become more integrated within a patient profile if their relation to psychosocial stressors were more clearly realised. Our discussion of the relation between DESNOS and BPD has noted how a seemingly stressor-non-specific diagnosis such as BPD may in fact be insidiously related to certain interpersonal stressors.

The implicit pathologisation of homosexuality must be avoided, whereby a person's homosexuality and disorders are noted in the diagnostic profile without a clear picture of the relations between disorder and psychosocial stressors. It is not merely enough to notarise the different psychosocial stessors exacted upon a person as is done in Axis 4 of the DSM. This is beset with limitations, and does not address the relational nature of the manifestation of a disorder. Separate disorder and stressor diagnoses may miss the entrenched mutual constitution between the two. Research needs to move toward uncovering the ways in which psychosocial stressors are not merely *adjuncts* to disorders, but actually *constitute* them, as in PTSD. It is only by doing so that a complex understanding will be reached of the over-representation of certain minority groups (e.g. homosexually identified people, women, etc.) within psychiatric disorders. However, not only may social stressors make certain disorders among certain groups more likely, but also the psychosocial nature of the aetiology may affect the hermeneutics of the symptom. This means that a psychosocial stressor may not only make the experience of certain symptoms more likely, but may affect the way in which that symptom is experienced or the meaning given to the symptom. Without addressing the meaning of the symptom or the context from which it stems, the therapist may fail to help the person explore the effect or function of their symptom.

By noting the impact of stressors as integral to the characteristics of a disorder, the more relational and power-sensitive an understanding of the cause and cure of a disorder will be. It is necessary to associate Axis 1 and Axis 4 diagnoses as closely as possible, in order to distil the full picture of suffering, and it is the task of politically informed clinical research to establish these possible links. The co-morbid associations of DESNOS and PTSD may also further entrench the positioning of psychosocial stressors within Axis 1, rather than as a footnote to it. Greater effort must therefore be expended on not merely delineating and segregating diagnostic categories as self-contained, but on opening them up to more fluid and co-morbid understandings of the suffering person. What follows from these contentions is that the traditional idea of *individual* psychopathology should be reframed, loosened from its locus in the individual and recontextualised within a fuller socio-cultural and discursive milieu. Individual *intervention* may hence still remain important, but the individual will now be seen as the point of damage, rather than as the implicit *cause* and delimitation of psychopathology.

This has been a chapter of two halves. We have hoped, firstly, to critically problematise research regarding homosexuality, along with the related 'essentialisation' of gayness so frequently implicated by such work. Secondly, we have attempted to formulate a series of politically useful and clinically pragmatic positions with reference to both apprehending and treating psychopathology within minorities sufferers. This coupling of a seemingly post-structural position on knowledge production with such a priority on producing clinically relevant and utilisable forms of critique might be taken as something of an odd pairing. For us, this proves a useful, if somewhat unconventional, blending: one where a suspicion and awareness of the utility of critical knowledge production combine with the goals of needed forms of political activism and consciousness raising.

# Endnotes

1. Not all aspects of those discourses and practices associated with heterosexuality can automatically be assumed to be demeaning and/or antagonistic toward the discourses and practices of homosexuality. In this regard, the term 'heterosexist' should be distinguished as applying to those prejudiced and bigoted aspects of heterosexual discourse that actively seek to disqualify the legitimacy of gay discourses/practices.
2. This argument should not be misread as assuming that whereas gayness is fundamentally discursive, psychopathology is not. Psychopathology, like gayness itself, is undoubtedly discursively known and produced, and its effects and its experienced reality should not be seen as in any way less substantial for it.

## References

Altman, D. (1982). *The Homosexualisation of America, the Americanisation of the Homosexual.* New York: St. Martins Press.

American Psychiatric Association (1994). *Diagnostic and Statistical Manual of Mental Disorders* (4th edn).Washington, DC: American Psychiatric Association.

Bradford, J., Ryan, C. and Rothblum, E. D. (1994). National lesbian health care survey: Implications for mental health care. *Journal of Consulting and Clinical Psychology*, 62, 228–42.

Brett, E. A. (1996). The classification of posttraumatic stress disorder. In B. A. van der Kolk, A. C. McFarlane and L. Weisaeth (eds), *Traumatic Stress: The Effects of Overwhelming Experience on Mind, Body and Society*, pp. 117–28. New York: Guilford Press.

Butler, J. (1990). Gender trouble, feminist theory, and psychoanalytic discourse. In L. J. Nicholson (ed.), *Feminism/Post-modernism*, pp. 324–40. London: Routledge.

Bux, D. A. (1996). The epidemiology of problem drinking in gay men and lesbians: A critical review. *Clinical Psychology Review*, 16 (4), 277–98.

Carlat, D. J., Camargo, Jr., C. A. and Herzog, D. B. (1997). Eating disorders in males: A report on 135 patients. *American Journal of Psychiatry*, 154 (8), 1127–32.

Cass, V. C. (1979). Homosexual identity formation: A theoretical model. *Journal of Homosexuality*, 4 (3), 219–35.

Chauncey, G. (1994). *Gay New York: Gender, Urban Culture, and the Making of the Gay Male World, 1890–1940.* New York: Basic Books.

Coleman, E. (1982). Developmental stages of the coming out process. In J. C. Gonsiorek (ed.), *Homosexuality and Psychotherapy: A Practitioners' Handbook of Affirmative Models*, pp. 31–45. New York: Haworth Press.

D'Augelli, A. R. (1993). Preventing mental health problems among lesbian and gay college students. *The Journal of Primary Prevention*, 13 (40), 245–61.

D'Augelli, A. R. (1996a). Enhancing the development of lesbian, gay, and bisexual youths. In E. S. Rothblum and L. A. Bond (eds), *Preventing Heterosexism and Homophobia*, pp. 124–50. London: Sage.

D'Augelli, A. R. (1996b). Lesbian, gay, and bisexual development during adolescence and young adulthood. In R. P. Cabaj and T. S. Stein (eds), *Textbook of Homosexuality and Mental Health*, pp. 267–88. Washington, DC: American Psychiatric Press.

D'Augelli, A. R. and Hershberger, S. L. (1993). Lesbian, gay and bisexual youth in community settings: Personal challenges and mental health problems. *American Journal of Community Psychology*, 21 (4), 421–48.

Dulit, R. A., Fyer, M. R., Miller, F. T. and Sacks, M. H. (1993). Gender differences in sexual preference and substance abuse of inpatients with borderline personality disorder. *Journal of Personality Disorder*, 7 (2), 182–5.

Earl, W. L. (1991). Perceived trauma: Its etiology and treatment. *Adolescence*, 26 (101), 97–104.

Foucault, M. (1976). *The History of Sexuality: An Introduction*, Vol. 1. London: Allen Lane.

Foucault, M. (1977/1991). *Discipline and Punish: The Birth of the Prison.* Harmondsworth: Penguin.

Garnets, L., Herek, G. M. and Levy, B. (1990). Violence and victimisation of lesbian and gay men: Mental health consequences. *Journal of Interpersonal Violence*, 5 (3), 366–83.

Heidegger, M. (1962). *Being and Time.* London: SCM Press.

Herdt, G. (1993). Semen transaction in Sambia culture. In G. Herdt (ed.), *Ritualized Homosexuality in Melanesia*, pp. 167–210. Berkeley: University of California Press.

Herman, J. L. (1992). *Trauma and Recovery: From Domestic Abuse to Political Terror.* London: Pandora.

Herman, J. L. (1993). Sequela of prolonged and repeated trauma: Evidence for a complex post-traumatic syndrome (DESNOS). In J. R. T. Davidson and E. B. Foa (eds), *Post-Traumatic Stress Disorder: DSM IV and Beyond*, pp. 213–28. Washington, DC: American Psychiatric Press.

Hershberger, S. L. and D'Augelli, A. R. (1995). The impact of victimisation on the mental health and suicidality of lesbian, gay, and bisexual youths. *Developmental Psychology*, 31 (1), 65–74.

Isaacs, G. and McKendrick, B. (1992). *Male Homosexuality in South Africa: Identity Formation, Culture, and Crisis.* Cape Town: Oxford University Press.

Janoff-Bulman, R. (1992). *Shattered Assumptions: Towards a New Psychology of Trauma.* New York: Free Press.

Jongedijk, R. A., Carlier, I. V. E., Schreuder J. N. and Gerson, B. P. R. (1995). Is er een plaats voor de complexe posttraumatische stress stoornis? PTSS en DESNOS nader beschouwd. *Tydschrift voor Psichiatrie*, 37, 43–54.

Liem, R. and Liem, J. H. (1984). Relations among social class, life events, and mental illness: A comment on findings and methods. In B. S. Dohrenwend and B. P. Dohrenwend (eds), *Stressful Life Events and their Contexts.* New Brunswick: Rutgers University Press.

Link, B. G. (1987). Understanding labeling effects in the area of mental disorders: An assessment of the effects of expectation of rejection. *American Sociological Review*, 52, 96–112.

Martin, A. D. and Hetrick, E. S. (1988). The stigmatization of the gay and lesbian adolescent. *Journal of Homosexuality*, 15 (1–2), 163–83.

McCann, I. L. and Pearlman, L. A. (1990). *Psychological Trauma and the Adult Survivor: Theory, Therapy, and Transformation.* New York: Bruner-Mazel.

McGorry, P. D. (1995). The clinical boundaries of posttraumatic stress disorder. *Australian and New Zealand Journal of Psychiatry*, 29, 385–93.

Meyer, I. H. (1995). Minority stress and mental health in gay men. *Journal of Health and Social Behaviour*, 36, 38–56.

Meyer, I. H. and Dean, L. (1998). Internalized homophobia, intimacy, and sexual behaviour among gay and bisexual men. In G. M. Herek (ed.), *Stigma and Sexual Orientation: Understanding Prejudice against Lesbians, Gay Men, and Bisexuals.* London: Sage.

Minton, H. L. and McDonald, G. J. (1984). Homosexual identity formation as a developmental process. *Journal of Homosexuality*, 9 (2–3), 91–103.

Newman, E., Orsillo, M. S., Herman D. S., Niles, B. S. and Litz, B. T. (1995). Clinical presentation of disorders of extreme stress in combat veterans. *Journal of Nervous and Mental Disease*, 183 (10), 628–32.

Niesen, J. H. (1993). Healing from cultural victimisation: Recovery from shame due to heterosexism. *Journal of Gay and Lesbian Psychotherapy*, 2 (1), 49–63.

Paris, J., Zwieg-Frank, H. and Guzder, J. (1995). Psychological factors associated with homosexuality in males with borderline personality disorder. *Journal of Personality Disorders*, 9 (1), 56–61.

Pattison, E. M. and Kahan, J. (1983). The deliberate self-harm syndrome. *American Journal of Psychiatry*, 140 (7), 867–72.

Radkowsky, M. and Siegel, L. J. (1997). The gay adolescent: Stressors, adaptations, and psychosocial interventions. *Clinical Psychology Review*, 17 (2), 191–216.

Ross, M. W. (1996). Societal reaction and homosexuality: Culture, acculturation, life events, and social supports as mediators of response to homonegative attitudes. In E. D. Rothblum and L. A. Bond (eds), *Preventing Heterosexism and Homophobia*, pp. 205–18. London: Sage.

Rotherham-Borus, M. J., Hunter, J. and Rosario, M. (1994). Suicidal behavior and gay-related stress among gay and bisexual male adolescents. *Journal of Adolescent Research*, 9 (4), 498–508.

Savin-Williams, R. C. (1994). Verbal and physical abuse as stressors in the lives of lesbian, gay male, and bisexual youths: Associations with school problems, running away, substance abuse, prostitution, and suicide. *Journal of Consulting and Clinical Psychology*, 62 (2), 261–69.

Schneider, S. G., Farberow, N. L. and Kruks, G. (1989). Suicidal behavior in adolescent and adult gay men. *Suicide and Life-Threatening Behavior*, 19, 381–94.

Troiden, R. R. (1979). Becoming homosexual: A model of gay identity acquisition. *Psychiatry*, 42, 362–73.

Van der Kolk, B. A. (1996). The complexity of adaptation to trauma: Self-regulation, stimulus discrimination, and characterological development. In B. A. van der Kolk, A. C. McFarlane and L. Weisaeth (eds), *Traumatic Stress: The Effects of Overwhelming Experience on Mind, Body and Society*, pp. 182–213. New York: Guilford Press.

Van der Kolk, B. A., Pelcovitz, D., Roth, S., Mandel, F. S., McFarlane, A. C. and Herman, J. L. (1996). Dissociation, somatisation, and affect dysregulation: The complexity of adaptation to trauma. *American Journal of Psychiatry*, 153 (7), 83–93.

Weeks, J. (1985). *Sexuality and its Discontents: Meanings, Myths and Modern Sexualities*. London: Routledge and Kegan Paul.

Whitehead, H. (1981). The bow and the burden strap: A new look at institutionalised homosexuality in native North America. In S. Ortner and H. Whitehead (eds), *Sexual Meanings: The Cultural Construction of Gender and Sexuality*, pp. 80–115. Cambridge: Cambridge University Press.

Zubenko, G. S., George, A. W., Soloff, P. H. and Schulz, P. (1987). Sexual practices amongst patients with borderline personality disorder. *American Journal of Psychiatry*, 144 (6), 748–52.

# 'Race', ethnicity and the psychopathology of social identity

*George Ellison & Thea de Wet*

> *Narrow streets breed narrow minds*
> *Care for kin but not for kind*
> (Thorn and Watt, 1985)

## ▪ Introduction

Social identities come in all shapes and sizes, some based on ostensibly biological attributes, others on so-called 'cultural practices', most a combination of both. As such, all are socially constructed categories, or 'imagined communities' (Anderson, 1991), membership of which can be either self-ascribed or observer-assigned (Mason, 1990). Social identity is therefore flexible, multidimensional and context-specific – a complex, if somewhat nebulous, concept akin to a social 'niche' (which the ecologist Hutchinson (1957) famously described, in similarly elaborate terms, as an 'n-dimensional hypervolume'). However, those dimensions of social identity that most readily spring to mind (such as class, gender, 'race', ethnicity, sexual orientation and (dis)ability) also represent psychosocial fault lines, as is evident in contemporary political discourse on 'inequality' and 'diversity'. Indeed, social-identity theory provides a persuasive psychopathological explanation for the manifestation of social groups and the nature of relations between them (Worchel *et al.*, 1998). Drawing on a series of experimental studies, its principal proponent, Tajfel, concluded that in-group chauvinism reflected intrinsic individual needs for positive self-identity (Tajfel, 1970). Moreover, he claimed that categorisation alone, even when allocated arbitrarily, might be sufficient to create 'genuine awareness of membership in separate and distinct groups' (1978: 35). This view of social identity as the outward expression of internalised values sits comfortably alongside recent analyses of 'ethnicised' conflicts, both within and between nation states, where nationality, religion and political ideology are the pertinent dimensions of social identity (McGarry and O'Leary, 1993). It also supports the privileged position that competition theory and kin selection occupy in the types of explanations favoured by evolutionary psychologists for social discrimination and xenophobia (Crook, 1998). Competition theory lies at the heart of the neo-Darwinian project, and argues that the limited availability of shared resources should lead to selection for essentially competitive traits in any *individuals* capable of securing sufficient resources to reproduce faster (Gould, 1977). Kin selection seeks to modify competition theory at the level of the gene by arguing that competitive traits should not compromise the survival and reproduction of closely related individuals who share similar genes (Gould, 1977). Since competition for resources is most acute amongst individuals with exactly the same needs, the small bands of closely related hunter-gatherers thought to have characterised human existence for much of our 100 000 year history should have been subject to intense selection for traits that optimised their ability to out-compete neighbouring bands, while sharing resources amongst relatives (Van den Berghe and Peter, 1988).

However plausible such explanations might be, they may tell us more about the social contexts in which contemporary psychological theories arise than about the role of chauvinism, conflict and competition in the production of social identity. Indeed, the extent to which theoretical arguments based on empirical evidence of current human behaviour accurately represent the origins of that behaviour is a question that dogs the interface between positivist science and the post-modern condition (Lewontin, 1979). Between the two, critical realism distinguishes three very different theoretical domains, or layers of evidence: 1) on the surface are the 'empirical' (or the 'apparent'), i.e. phenomena that manifest as experiences; 2) underneath are the 'actual' i.e. events upon which experiences are based; and 3) at the core are the 'real', i.e. mechanisms leading to events that may, or may not, be experienced (Bhaskar, 1978). Within this analytical framework, *empirical* evidence drawn from experimental studies, 'ethnicised' conflicts and competition theory falls far short of that required to fully understand precisely how social identities might arise, even if it accurately reflects the *actual* nature of social identity as it is generally experienced. To fully understand the domain of the *real* (i.e. the mechanisms underlying the apparent psychopathological manifestation of social identity) requires an analysis capable of transcending those dimensions of social identity that manifest as group resources in times of conflict and those that do not. In so doing, any such analysis might help explain the peculiar salience of the former.

To address the first of these issues, it is worth adopting a deliberately abstract approach, in which social identity is simply an ecological measure of collective individual identities or, better still, an aggregate measure of those dimensions of individual identity that all community members share (Anthias et al., 1993). This approach accommodates the notion of social identities as signifiers of potentially benign rather than necessarily malign affiliations between communities, i.e. a perspective of social identity more in tune with the model of social tolerance favoured by multiculturalism (Fenster and Fenster, 1998). It also encompasses much of the contemporary discourse on 'social capital', which interprets voluntary organisations, mutual institutions and informal networks of reciprocal support between community members as evidence of 'healthy' civic societies (Wilkinson, 1996). In this sense, social identity might well be viewed as a prerequisite for the production of social capital, or at least one of its many purported benefits. This might seem tenuous, given the self-evident credibility of competition theory, but the plausibility of this view has been bolstered, somewhat unexpectedly, by the application of game theory to evolutionary biology (Lewontin, 1961). For example, within the game *The Prisoners' Dilemma*, in which the shared benefits of co-operating with an opponent (3 points each) exceed the average benefits of winning (5 points) and losing (0 points) or a tie (1 point each), the optimum outcome is one in which both opponents co-operate (Axelrod, 1984). Just as kin selection moderates unfettered competition between related individuals, so game theory extends the selective advantage of co-operation whenever the relatedness of individuals is uncertain.

## ■ Unpicking the psychopathological appearance of social identity

Whatever the analytical merits of multiculturalism, social capital or game theory (and there are many), their emphasis on social tolerance, reciprocal networks and co-operation as products of relations *within* communities seems to overlook the important role of relations *between* communities (be they conflicts *or* alliances) in the construction of communal (i.e. social) identities. Nevertheless, in the broader context of Anderson's (1991) 'imagined communities', encompassing disparate groups or isolated individuals sharing a common destiny or fate (Anthias *et al.*, 1993), these approaches do demonstrate the *possibility* that a palpable sense of social identity might occur in the absence of conflict. Yet this possibility is likely to be dismissed as wishful thinking by those who favour the empirical salience of experimental studies, 'ethnicised' conflict and competition theory. There is certainly a tendency among those aspiring to a pluralist vision of social identity to 'enshrine the notion with a kind of utopianism whose naivety will assure its elusiveness' (Williams, 1997: 2). But the plausibility of both *mechanistic* explanations (i.e. pathological and beneficent) should caution against any bias towards competition over co-operation that the *apparent* psychopathological manifestation of social identity might seem to dictate (Fenster and Fenster, 1998). However much social identity *appears* pathological in the experiential accounts of social commentators, 'it ain't necessarily so', i.e. the apparent ubiquity of 'ethnicised' conflict *does not* reflect its inevitability (Williams, 1997).

To avoid the emptiness of utopian rhetoric, it is necessary to unpick the psychopathological *appearance* of social identity, while eluding any tendency to see this as sufficient or adequate grounds for *mechanistic* explanation. This is more difficult than it may seem. Within the domain of the empirical, experiential accounts of social identity are preoccupied (if not preconditioned) by notions of in-group chauvinism, 'ethnicised' conflict and competition – past and present, explicit and implied. But the extent to which these experiential accounts reflect *actual* events is far from certain, and ultimately depends upon the context in which they are 'experienced' and narrated: 'The recognition that ... [social] identity is a discursive production impels the analyst ... to examine the process of articulation through which elements of everyday experience come to connote the presence of a thing which is never actually evidenced in full' (Bowman, 1994: 140). It is therefore important to examine the role that professional, scientific and popular discourse plays (either deliberately or subconsciously) in reproducing the views and interests of particular individuals or particular social groups – thereby promulgating one particular experiential account, if not interpretation, of 'events'. Just as characterising the natural state of humanity as 'solitary, poor, nasty, brutish, and short' (Hobbes, 1962) validates the necessity of central authority, so characterising 'other' as 'inferior' validates the superiority of 'self' (Murray, 1900). Both of these accounts serve the views and interests of very particular constituencies, i.e. those seeking approbation for authority and control, and those seeking justification for exploitation and oppression. In unpicking the psychopathological appearance of social identities as discursive objects within such quasi-empirical accounts, it should be possible to identify the constituencies whose views and interests are served by essentialising (i.e. 'naturalising') chauvinism, conflict and competition.

## ■ The role of 'race' and ethnicity in the psychopathology of social identity

Contemporary discourse on social identity is so inculcated with the idiom of ethnicity that it is almost impossible to consider one without the other. Indeed, ethnicity is increasingly viewed as the definitive essence of social identity, rather than one of its many different dimensions (Lay and Verkuyten, 1999). To some extent, the extraordinary salience of ethnicity reflects the application of ethnic categorisation to authenticate social identity, as is evident in the growing tally of ethnic categories included in the US census (Office of Management and Budget (OMB), 1997). In this, ethnic categorisation is being used in much the same way that early formulations of 'race' were applied to recognise the legitimacy of nation states and national identities. So in his somewhat prescient rejection of European economic union, Alfred Mond, the first Lord Melchett, concluded: 'obviously the differences in language and race would make it a very remote possibility in the political sense' (1930: 19). Both of these approaches to social identity reflect a belief in the legitimacy of rights accrued on the basis of descent, kinship, origin or heritage – a belief that appears to have a long and vibrant history in human cultures (albeit in the quasi-empirical ethnographic accounts of Eurocentric anthropologists (Carrithers, 1992)). The earliest constructions of 'race' (i.e. '"race" as lineage') were therefore used without any presupposition of innate or permanent typological distinction (Banton, 1998), and it is in this sense that ethnicity is often invoked in contemporary parlance. However, for some time before, and long after, Alfred Mond's day, 'race' was used to legitimise a very different approach to social identity. The concept of '"race" as lineage' was co-opted by scientists searching for a term around which to classify human biological diversity. Socially constructed notions of descent, kinship, origin and heritage meant that '"race" as lineage' offered a convenient and ostensibly natural proxy for *biological* relatedness (just as ethnicity does today). But it is also true that the use of '"race" as lineage' to authenticate national identities (just as ethnicity authenticates social identities today) offered a convenient guise in which to naturalise, and thereby justify, national chauvinism. This transformation of '"race" as lineage' into '"race" as type' was flawed from the outset, as is evident in the use of subjective typologies to compile deliberately physiognomic and hierarchical taxonomies of *social* groups. In so doing, the anthropologists involved (Georges Cuvier, Samuel Morton and Johann Blumenbach, amongst others) laid the foundations of a new discipline, i.e. racial science, which changed forever the nature of social identity. So much so that while the quasi-scientific tenets of physiognomic typologies have long been discredited (Unesco, 1950) and invalidated (Gould, 1981), racial science has 'continued to scar contemporary social arrangements with the transcendent urgency of their hand-me-down grief' (Williams, 1997: 11). In part, this reflects the past application, and current manifestation, of 'racialised' identities in the unequal allocation of rights and property. In part, it is reproduced and entrenched by policies and activities that claim to redress the injustice caused.

While the contemporary rationale for collecting information on social identity may be explicitly therapeutic, Blumenbach's (1865) racial typologies, and the phenotypic characteristics used to define them, remain largely unchanged in the racialised ethnic categories of social identity presented in the US census (OMB, 1997; see below) – an approach that can also be seen in the presentation of social identity as racialised ethnicity by censuses and population surveys elsewhere (Smaje, 1995). On the face of it, racialised ethnic categories do appear to be the most appropriate (if not the most transparent and thereby 'honest') mechanisms for 'monitoring and enforcing' the impact of civil-rights legislation (OMB, 1997) and similar statutes that prohibit discrimination on the grounds of 'race' and ethnicity elsewhere. At the same time, however, the sheer diversity of social identities and the ability of individuals and communities to adopt flexible and multiple social identities means that alternative (i.e. non-categorical) approaches are likely to be constrained by the ability and willingness of respondents to offer comparable, consistent or pertinent responses (Bartlett and Fiander, 1995). Yet standardising social identity by presenting respondents with prescribed ethnic categories (or collapsing whatever alternatives respondents offer into predetermined categories (Aspinall, 1995)) authenticates a *very particular* and, in the approaches used, explicitly racialised view of social identity. It is a process that *encourages* if not *requires* respondents to conceptualise social identity as ethnicity in a very particular way – one that is very different to the accounts they might otherwise offer, and one that some may find impossible to contrive (Bartlett and Fiander, 1995).

In acknowledging that social identities have been thoroughly contaminated by racial science, the use of racialised ethnic categories as measures of social identity attempts to reconcile the fallacy of '"race" as type' with the reality of 'race' as pernicious manifestation of social identity. The extraordinary significance of 'race' among those for whom 'race' symbolises the injustice of racism (both past and present, explicit and implied), makes it untenable to ignore – even when rejecting 'race' outright might suppress the views of those for whom 'race' symbolises the legitimacy of racism. Indeed, 'the very notion of colour-blindness constitutes an ideological confusion at best, and denial at its very worst' (Williams, 1997: 2). Yet measuring social identity using racialised ethnic categories imbues unrelated (and hitherto 'un-raced') dimensions of social identity with symbolic connotations similar to those attached to 'race'. So recognising all five of Blumenbach's (1865) original racial categories (*American* – 'American Indian or Alaskan Native'; *Caucasian* – 'White'; *Ethiopian* – 'African American'; *Malay* – 'Pacific Islander'; and *Mongoloid* – 'Asian American') as legitimate social identities within the US census implies that others (authenticated as 'Hispanic', 'Middle-Eastern', 'Western Asian' or 'Cape Verdean' (OMB, 1997)) are also racial in character. Whenever racialised ethnic categories are operationalised as a strategy for authenticating social identity, they become mechanisms for extending the insidious irrationality of 'race' way beyond the fault lines originally invoked by racial science. The approach appears to be a Pyrrhic compromise between the views and interests of contradictory constituencies – those seeking to redress injustice (progressive anti-racists) or celebrate diversity (liberal multiculturalists) on the one hand, and those seeking to mitigate demands for restitution (elitist conservatives) or entrench discrimination (chauvinist nationalists) on the other. In reproducing the hierarchical and xenophobic products of racial science by authenticating social identity through ethnic categorisation, and operationalising ethnicity through racialised categories, the psychopathological *appearance* of social identity is itself authenticated and essentialised.

## ■ In the land of the colour-blind the blue-eyed Caucasian is (still) king

The insatiable public appetite for the 'just so' stories invoked by evolutionary psychology demonstrates the appeal of naturalised (and thereby normalised) explanations for social dispensations. While it is less clear whose interests might be served by essentialising the psychopathological manifestation of social identity in this way, it is plainly facile to dismiss the racialisation of ethnic and social identity as an unfortunate, regrettable and indelible product of the past, or the result of reprehensible attitudes among those labelled above as 'elitist' or 'chauvinist'. Indeed, within this discourse lies an exemplary demonstration of self-approbation through the authentication of social (or in this instance, socio-political) identities as competitive dichotomies (progressive versus conservative; multiculturalist versus nationalist). Although 'elitist' and 'chauvinist' are undoubtedly pejorative when set against the values espoused by an ostensibly meritocratic and egalitarian Western democratic tradition, the choice of these labels was not entirely contrived. If when we examine our own empirical analyses (as critical realism insists we must) we find them so insidiously contaminated by such cosy discursive habits, then whose *experiential* accounts of social identity can we trust? The answer may lie in what is *left out* of *all* such accounts – what is *not* said. As Williams explains:

> Perhaps one reason that conversations about race are so often doomed to frustration is that the notion of whiteness as 'race' is almost never implicated. One of the more difficult legacies of slavery and colonialism is the degree to which racism's tenacious hold is manifested not merely in the divided demographics of neighbourhood or education or class but also in the process of what media expert John Fiske calls the 'exnomination' of whiteness as racial identity. Whiteness is unnamed, suppressed, beyond the realm of race. Exnomination permits whites to entertain the notion that race lives 'over there' on the other side of the tracks, in black bodies and inner-city neighbourhoods, in a dark netherworld where whites are not involved (1997: 4–5).

This explanation presents a radical yet compelling possibility: radical because it suggests that some ('un-raced') social identities may no longer require, nor respond to, authentication using racialised ethnic categories as other ('raced') social identities do; and compelling because it implies that these ('un-raced') social identities may only be able to exist by continuing to authenticate other social identities (if not 'other' *per se*) as 'raced', using racialised ethnic categories. Essentialising the psychopathological manifestation of social identities that are authenticated using racialised ethnic categories therefore serves the interests of the 'un-raced' precisely because it perpetuates the denigration of those who are 'raced', and those who are 'race-able'.

In the past, racial discrimination and colonial exploitation were required to secure the unequal advantages enjoyed by those 'of the ruling colour' (Murray, 1900: 156). But in contemporary Western democracies, scarred by 'legacies of slavery and colonialism', those 'of the ruling colour' (henceforth ostensibly 'un-raced') are able to retain their privileged social positions, while espousing egalitarian and meritocratic values. This is because such values pose little threat to advantage inherited posing as advantage accrued on the basis of equal opportunity and merit. In this way, the status quo is maintained without the need for *overt* racist policies, and the 'un-raced' are immune from allegations of racial chauvinism – after all, how can they be 'race' supremacists if they have no 'race'? Indeed, the 'un-raced' elite can even make a virtue out of necessity by suppressing supremacist ideologies within their own ranks (which would otherwise threaten the peculiar status of their social identity as 'un-raced'), and in as much as these ideologies reflect the resurgence of 'race' as social identity among the 'un-raced' working class, their suppression also enables the 'un-raced' elite to denigrate the class struggle within their own community (Lipsitz, 1998).

The 'exnomination' of 'male' in the lexicon of contemporary discourse on gender, and the 'exnomination' of 'upper class' in discourses on class, have many parallels with the '"exnomination" of whiteness'. All conceal the origins of advantage and privilege, and all establish 'white', 'male' and 'upper class' as unspoken norms against which 'disadvantaged' and 'underprivileged' are defined.[1] Just as the suffrage movement and class struggle were resolved by co-opting sufficient numbers of emancipated women and the working-class majority into the ranks of the male middle-class elite (Evans, 1992), so assimilating 'raced' minorities into an 'un-raced' elite serves to diffuse racial agitation. In the US census, the unconditional assimilation of 'Irish' and 'Jewish' categories (both of which have been, and continue to be, experienced as 'raced' social identities (Lewis, 1998)) into the category 'White' was possible because their inclusion did not threaten the '"exnomination" of whiteness'. However, the conditional assimilation of the 'Mexican' category (which was given full racial status in the 1930 census (Bates *et al.*, 1996)) into the category 'White Hispanic' (OMB, 1997) excludes those with 'African American' or 'Native American' origins whose inclusion would contaminate the 'un-raced' purity of 'White'. This approach broadens the constituency of those whose social identities are 'un-raced', while fragmenting the constituency of those whose social identities are 'raced'. A similar interpretation might be drawn from the addition of a national prefix or suffix (i.e. 'American') to census categories (as in 'African American', 'American Indian' and 'Asian American'), in what appears to be an attempt to imbue fragmented social identities with a sense of national unity common to all communities. In this, the absence of a prefix or suffix from just one category ('White') and the continuing use of geographical affinities in all of the remainder (along similar lines to those adopted by Blumenbach in 1865), presents 'White' as not only synonymous with 'American' (hence in no need of a suffix), but also as *the definitive* national identity – 'un-raced' by any aspersions cast upon it by alternative geographical affinities (such as

'European'). Given the central role that respondent preference occupies in the design of census categories (Bates *et al.*, 1996; OMB, 1997), these interpretations might seem to malign the best intentions of those involved. Yet in the provision of pre-coded categories and 'multiple answer(s)', the OMB (1997) advocates an approach that does more than 'reduce ... misunderstanding about the information being asked', it *teaches* respondents what answers are required, and supplants any alternative taxonomies of social identity.

## ■ Challenging the psychopathological manifestation of social identity

In configuring the changing manifestation of racialised ethnic categories as a cipher for communal power relations, this analysis tends to favour the empirical salience of experiential accounts situated in competition and conflict over those situated in reciprocity and co-operation. This is not to say that alternative constructions of (therapeutic, benign or beneficent) social identity do not exist or should be excluded from any such analytical framework; it is simply that these are likely to have limited relevance to understanding the psychopathology of social identities authenticated by racialised ethnic categories. In unpicking the psychopathological *appearance* of social identity, it is the salience of empirical evidence drawn from power relations, competition and conflict that *must* be addressed. The reason these *appear* essential (or natural) in the psychopathological manifestation of social identity is precisely because their observation justifies and reifies their own existence. If we are to overcome our appetite for 'just so' stories, and expose their idle, tautological complacency, we have to reject the tendency to accept things for what(ever) they (might) *appear* to be, i.e. social experiences of 'natural', 'essential' phenomena. Only then might it be possible to examine these phenomena dispassionately and identify potential solutions.

The historical and contemporary injustice underlying the psychopathological manifestation of social identities as 'raced' and 'un-raced' suggests that two potential solutions present themselves: the 'exnomination' of all social identities that remain 'raced'; *or* the 're-nomination' of those that have become 'un-raced'. The first involves eliminating 'colour-consciousness' by adopting 'un-raced' social identities across the board in a world that is genuinely, not just officially, 'colour-blind' (Williams, 1997). The second involves eliminating the unequal (dis)advantage of official 'colour-blindness', by adopting 'raced' social identities across the board in a world that is openly, but fairly, 'colour-conscious'. The first is equivalent to the policies advocated by 'liberal multiculturalists', who set out to supplant the unequal dichotomy of 'un-raced' and 'raced' social identities by celebrating the diversity of separate but equal social identities across a variety of alternative (and primarily cultural) dimensions (Sue *et al.*, 1999). The second is equivalent to the policies advocated by 'progressive anti-racists', who set out to expose 'un-raced' privilege and (re)distribute (dis)advantage equally across all social identities using corrective (i.e. affirmative) action (Soni, 1999) and/or redistribution on a grand scale (Marais, 1998).

Both approaches face difficult obstacles. The likelihood that 'colour-conscious' policies, invoked to exact restitution, thereby entrench (if not enflame) social identities along racial lines, undermines the legitimacy of *anti*-racism, however much the end might justify the means. At the same time, popular (Evans, 1992) and commercial opposition (Marais, 1998) to redistributive policies, and the constraints placed on pursuing these within a globalised economy, make such policies unsustainable (at least within 'free-market' democracies where the 'tyranny of the majority' suppresses the rights and aspirations of minorities (Guinier, 1994)). Yet as long as the historical products of past racial (dis)advantage remain visible in the 'divided demographics of neighbourhood or education or class', policies to promote colour-blindness create what Williams calls the 'dilemma of the Emperor's new clothes' (1997: 3), i.e. society becomes so invested in maintaining the fiction that 'colour doesn't matter' that it neglects the daily experience of those who inherited disadvantage and continue to suffer discrimination. For this reason, any tendency to classify social identities along (multi)cultural lines relegates these to the same fate as social identities authenticated using racialised ethnic categories: dominant cultures tend to manifest as an invisible norm, against which alternative cultures are 'raced'. In this way, cultural categories of social identity are viewed as analogous to, if not euphemisms for, racialised notions of ethnicity.

## Conclusion

The psychopathological manifestation of social identity depends upon the essentialisation of in-group chauvinism, 'ethnicised' conflict and unbridled competition evident in the authentication of social identities as racialised ethnic categories. However unpalatable 'colour-conscious' policies may be in the short-term, and however politically and commercially difficult they may be to sustain, the long-term legitimacy of the anti-racist tradition lies in its goal of creating equality of opportunity, and thereby the possibility for 'colour-blindness' to exist (Soni, 1999). 'When we face up to our inheritance – of a society still beset by racial injustice – we find that some color conscious policies and some kinds of color consciousness may minimize injustice today and make it possible to be both fair and colour blind in the future. This vision of the future is one that, despite our differences, we can all share' (Gutmann, 1996: 178). Psychologists and other social scientists have an important role to play in deconstructing the psychopathological *appearance* of social identity and addressing the twin challenges that anti-racist policies face, i.e. 1) substantiating the putative benefits of social tolerance, reciprocal support and co-operation to overcome the argument that redistributive fiscal policies incur 'unsustainable' personal, social and commercial costs; and 2) targetting restitution at those who are 'raced' without reproducing the chauvinism, aggression and xenophobia that accompanied the allocation of advantage to those whose social identities are 'un-raced'.

## Acknowledgements

Our thanks to Laurel Baldwin-Rageven, Ian Rees Jones, Ann Oakley, Paul Allsop and Chris Bonell for taking time to discuss many of the ideas contained in this chapter, and to Patricia Williams, whose magical prose inspired us to look for them. This work was supported by grant 057182 from the Wellcome Trust's Biomedical Ethics Programme.

## Endnote

1  This phenomenon extends across all dimensions of social identity, such as the 'exnomination' of the heterosexual and able-bodied in discourse on sexual orientation and disability.

## References

Anderson, B. (1991). *Imagined Communities: Reflections on the Origin and Spread of Nationalism*. London: Verso.

Anthias, F., Yuval-Davis, N. and Cain, H. (1993). *Racialized Boundaries: Race, Nation, Gender, Colour and Class and the Anti-racist Struggle*. Johannesburg: Routledge.

Aspinall, P. J. (1995). Department of Health's requirement for mandatory collection of data on ethnic groups of inpatients. *British Medical Journal*, 311 (7011), 1006–9.

Axelrod, R. (1984). *The Evolution of Co-operation*. New York: Basic Books.

Banton, M. (1998). *Racial Theories* (2nd edn). Cambridge: Cambridge University Press.

Bartlett, A. and Fiander, M. (1995). Psychotic illness in ethnic groups. Census categories of ethnic group are limited. *British Medical Journal*, 310 (6975), 332.

Bates, N., Martin, E. A., De Maio, T. J. and De la Puente, M. (1996). Questionnaire effects on measurements of race and Spanish origin. *Journal of Official Statistics*, 11 (3), 433–59.

Bhaskar, R. (1978). *A Realist Theory of Science* (2nd edn). Brighton: Harvester Press.

Blumenbach, J. F. (1865). *The Anthropological Treatises of Johann Friedrich Blumenbach*. London: Anthropological Society of London.

Bowman, G. (1994). 'A country of words': Conceiving the Palestinian nation from the position of exile. In E. Laclau (ed.), *The Making of Political Identities*, pp. 138–70. London: Verso.

Carrithers, M. (1992). *Why Humans Have Cultures: Explaining Anthropology and Social Diversity*. Oxford: Oxford University Press.

Crook, P. (1998). Human pugnacity and war: Some anticipations of socio-biology. *Biology and Philosophy*, 13 (2), 263–88.

Evans, G. (1992). Is Britain a class-divided society? A reanalysis and extension of Marshal *et al.*'s study of class consciousness. *Sociology*, 26 (2), 233–58.

Fenster, A. and Fenster, J. (1998). Diagnosing deficits in 'basic trust' in multiracial and multicultural groups: Individual or social psychopathology? *Group*, 22 (2), 81–93.

Fowers, B. J. and Richardson, F. C. (1996). Why is multiculturalism good? *American Psychologist*, 51 (6), 609–21.

Gould, S. J. (1977). *Ever since Darwin*. New York: W. W. Norton.

Gould, S. J. (1981). *The Mismeasure of Man*. New York: W. W. Norton.

Guinier, L. (1994). *The Tyranny of the Majority: Fundamental Fairness in Representative Democracy*. New York: Free Press.

Gutmann, A. (1996). Responding to racial injustice. In K. A. Appiah and A. Gutmann, *Color Conscious: The Political Morality of Race*, pp. 106–83. Princeton: Princeton University Press.

Hobbes, T. (1962). *Leviathan*. New York: Collier Books.

Hutchinson, G. E. (1957). Concluding remarks. *Cold Spring Harbour Symposium on Quantitative Biology*, XX, 415–27.

Lay, C. and Verkuyten, M. (1999). Ethnic identity and its relation to personal self-esteem: A comparison of Canadian-born and foreign-born Chinese adolescents. *Journal of Social Psychology*, 139 (3), 288–99.

Lewis, G. (1998). Welfare and the social construction of 'race'. In E. Saraga (ed.), *Embodying the Social: Constructions of Difference*, pp. 91–138. London: Routledge/Oxford University Press.

Lewontin, R. C. (1961). Evolution and the theory of games. *Journal of Theoretical Biology*, 1 (2), 382–403.

Lewontin, R. C. (1979). Sociobiology as an adaptationist program. *Behavioral Science*, 24 (1), 5–14.

Lipsitz, G. (1998). *The Possessive Investment in Whiteness: How White People Profit from Identity Politics*. Philadelphia: Temple University Press.

Marais, H. (1998). *South Africa, Limits to Change: The Political Economy of Transformation.* Cape Town: University of Cape Town Press.

Mason, D. (1990). A rose by any other name ...? Categorisation, identity and social science. *New Community*, 17 (1), 123–33.

McGarry, J. and O'Leary, B. (1993). *The Politics of Ethnic Conflict.* London: Routledge.

Melchett, Lord (1930). *Imperial Economic Unity.* London: Harrap.

Murray, G. (1900). The exploitation of inferior races in ancient and modern times. In F. W. Hirst, G. Murray and J. L. Hammond (eds), *Liberalism and the Empire*, pp. 118–57. London: Johnson.

OMB (Office of Management and Budget) (1997). Recommendations from the Interagency Committee for the Review of the Racial and Ethnic Standards to the Office of Management and Budget concerning changes to the standards for the classification of federal data on race and ethnicity. *Federal Register*, Part II, 36873–946.

Smaje, C. (1995). *Health, 'Race' and Ethnicity: Making Sense of the Evidence.* London: King's Fund.

Soni, V. (1999). Morality vs. mandate: Affirmative action in employment. *Public Personnel Management*, 28 (4), 577–94.

Sue, D. W., Bingham, R. P., Porche-Burke, L. and Vasquez, M. (1999). The diversification of psychology: A multicultural revolution. *American Psychologist*, 54 (12), 1061–9.

Tajfel, H. (1970). Experiments in intergroup discrimination. *Scientific American*, 223 (5), 96–102.

Tajfel, H. (1978). Interindividual behaviour and intergroup behaviour. In H. Tajfel (ed.), *Differentiation between Social Groups: Studies in the Social Psychology of Intergroup Relations*, pp. 69–119. London: Academic Press.

Thorn, T. and Watt, B. (1985). *Any Town.* London: Blanco Y Negro/WEA.

Unesco (United Nations Educational, Scientific and Cultural Organisation) (1950). *Statement on Race.* New York: Unesco.

Van den Berghe, P. L. and Peter, K. (1988). Hutterites and Kibbutzniks – a tale of nepotistic communism. *Man*, 23 (3), 522–39.

Wilkinson, R. G. (1996). *Unhealthy Societies: The Afflictions of Inequality.* London: Routledge.

Williams, P. J. (1997). *Seeing a Colour-Blind Future: The Paradox of Race.* London: Virago.

Worchel, S., Morales, J. F., Páez, D. and Deschamps, J. (1998). *Social Identity: International Perspectives.* London: Sage.

# SECTION 3

# SOUTH AFRICAN PATHOLOGIES

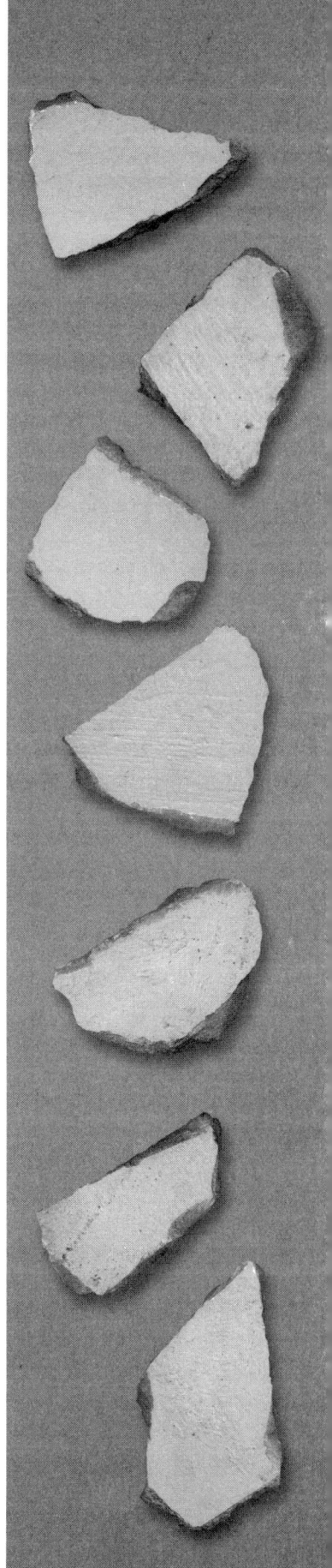

# Unsettling meanings of madness: Competing constructions of South African insanity

*Carol Long & Estelle Zietkiewicz*

## ■ Introduction

The past three decades have seen an exponential growth in interest in the relationship between culture and mental health. Further, the status of indigenous healing in a reformed health system has been the focus of much debate in South Africa (e.g. Freeman, 1990; Seedat, 1997; L. Swartz, 1986, 1987, 1996). Many writers have called for the inclusion of indigenous healing in mental-health considerations (Freeman, 1991; Seedat, 1997; L. Swartz, 1996), although a recent mental-health policy document (see Pillay and Freeman, 1996) is notably silent on the issue of indigenous healing as well as on understandings of the explanatory frameworks clients draw upon in order to make sense of their experiences (see Kleinman, 1988). The general consensus appears to be that inclusion of indigenous healing into Western frameworks of treatment can only be beneficial (Seedat, 1997; L. Swartz, 1996), although L. Swartz (1996) notes that there is little evidence to support the efficacy of indigenous healing and that many have failed to consider the political implications of dialogue between the two paradigms or to approach the debate critically.

In spite of a massive accumulation of data regarding culture and mental health, Western psychiatry has, for the large part, continued to ignore the articulation of socio-cultural factors in its theoretical and applied approaches to the problem. These perspectives are now the subject of growing criticism and debate, and cross-cultural studies have provided extensive data challenging the adequacy of the disease models used for understanding psychological distress (Marsella and White, 1989). It has been argued that transcultural psychiatry would inform us of the pathoplastic effects of culture on mental illness. Instead, data from virtually every continent are suggesting that culture is not simply incidental to mental health and therapy. Rather, it is a basic variable that interacts with biological, psychological and environmental variables in determining the causes, manifestations and treatment of the entire spectrum of mental disorders.

Studies have suggested that many South Africans draw on both biomedical and traditional taxonomies and treatments in order to address their 'madness'[1] (e.g. Letlaka-Rennert, Butchart and Brown, 1991 in Seedat, 1997; Lund and Swartz, 1998), but, as appears to be the case with biomedical explanations, there has been little critical analysis of what indigenous taxonomies bring with them or of how biomedical and indigenous explanatory frameworks intersect in the lived experience of those drawing upon them. Seedat, for example, maintains that 'liberatory psychologists will enhance their discourse if they remain sensitive to *ordinary*, other-than-western discourses of illness' (1997: 264; our emphasis). This elides possibilities that 'other-than-western' taxonomies are as able to participate in sites of power as biomedical taxonomies, constructing such 'ordinary' taxonomies as simple, unproblematic and unitary. Such conceptualisations of indigenous taxonomies contain a host of uncritical assumptions of indigenous healing as pure, natural, but, ultimately, nonetheless 'other'. Further, the possibility that individuals may incorporate such taxonomies as discourses into their subjectivity in contradictory and conflictual ways has been inadequately explored, particularly regarding experiences of the interface between biomedical and indigenous discourses of madness.

This chapter takes as its starting point theories such as those of Foucault (1967) that undermine truth values in any available taxonomy of madness. In terms of this framework, we argue that taxonomies construct madness in different ways and offer different discourses for people to position themselves within. Taxonomies intersect with discourse because they provide ways of constituting knowledge and offer sets of social practices that construct the insane object. For Weedon, discourses are 'ways of constituting knowledge, together with the social practices, forms of subjectivity and power relations which inhere in such knowledges and the relations between them' (1987: 505). Further, this construction is not understood as neutral. Constructions of madness set up power relations between 'sane' and 'insane', allow the justification of certain practices, offer possibilities for inclusion and exclusion, and offer constructions of 'truth' and 'expertise', all of which may be incorporated into subjectivity and lived experience and which support certain institutions (Foucault, 1967).

In suggesting that madness is socially constructed, we do not intend to discount the personal pain experienced by those labelled as 'mad', but we do argue that 'madness' does not exist purely in the realm of the personal, unaffected by discourses and practices. We follow Parker et al. in eroding or deconstructing the relation between taxonomies and discourses: 'Deconstruction looks at things askew, seeing things that do not at first glance seem to be there, it is very suspicious, and it breaks the rules to show that what is usually treated as normal is really rather odd' (1995: 3). Through deconstructing biomedical and indigenous taxonomies of madness in South Africa, we will argue that neither are value-neutral, and that both need to be considered in a more critical light. Because of the broad availability of both taxonomies, we examine more closely the intersection of the two contradictory discourses, drawing on a case study in order to illustrate the complexities involved in being located at the intersection of competing discourses of madness.[2] The aims of presenting this case study are to deconstruct emergent contradictions of lived experience in relation to discourse and to introduce complex and, no doubt, controversial debates regarding the status of the various taxonomies of madness dominant in South Africa at the present time.

## ■ Meanings of madness: a post-structuralist account

A number of accounts of psychopathology (Foucault, 1967, 1986; Parker et al., 1995; Ussher, 1991) aim to provide an historical account of the construction of madness in order to problematise the boundaries that separate madness from normality, to undermine static understandings of madness through tracing changes in construction over time and to deconstruct the truth values and power relations implicit in conceptualisations of psychopathology. Deconstruction of the universality of such conceptualisations offers us ways of tackling the inherent contradictions in psychiatric texts. The task of deconstruction is not only to explore medical conceptualisations of mental disorder, but to move beyond them and to offer alternate ways of thinking about mental disorder by locating it in a broader social context and analysis of social relations. One of the aims is to disrupt, unsettle or explode the neat taxonomies of madness. Foucault (1967, 1986) illustrates that taxonomies of madness are not fixed or objective, but rather participate in productive and exclusionary practices in the exercise of power. He states, for example, that: 'man became a "psychologizable species" only when his relation to madness made a psychology possible, that is to say, when his relation to madness was defined by the external dimension of exclusion and punishment and by the internal dimension of moral assignation and guilt' (Foucault, 1986: 73).

Further, much of the recent work conducted in the area of transcultural psychiatry has shown that the illness experience is an *interpretive* enterprise that is constructed in social situations according to the premises of cultural theories about illness and social behaviour generally. In the past decade, it has become clear that apparently similar illness events may be interpreted in highly variable ways, depending on the cultural theories (or discourses) available for reasoning about them.

## Myths of transhistoricity and transcultural validity in the social construction of madness

Many critical understandings of madness critique the biomedical psychiatric model's conception of madness as universal, ahistorical and clearly demarcated in terms of neat diagnostic categories (Kaplan and Sadock, 1991; Wetherell, 1996). They argue that current Western conceptualisations of madness as static and definable offer particular constructions that facilitate a web of power relations and institutional claims. Foucault suggests that such static definitions reinforce the power of professional discourse: 'Madness is a redoubtable danger precisely in that it is not foreseeable by any of those persons of good sense who claim to be able to recognise it. Only a doctor can spot it, and thus madness becomes exclusively an object for the doctor, whose right of intervention is grounded by the same token' (1980: 205). Foucault contests the existence of such dimensions of madness, arguing instead that madness is an active concept constituted by culturally and socially relative categories whose precise boundaries and meanings vary over time and are highly contested (1967).

Specifically, the charge that madness is historically located and not universal is illustrated by Foucault in *Madness and Civilization* (1967), where he traces a radical disjuncture between conceptualisations of madness in the Middle Ages (when it was possible for madness to be constructed as the voice of genius or divine inspiration, and when insanity was in dialogue with sanity) and conceptualisations that influence our current understandings. He argues that current taxonomies are based on notions of binary opposition between sanity and insanity, and particularly reason and unreason: oppositions that police the boundaries of society and justify the exclusion of problematic members through the compelling logic of scientific truth and through the simultaneous subjectification of the self to moral guilt. Although it is not possible here to provide an exposition of this work that does justice to its complexity, *Madness and Civilization* represents a seminal illustration of the historicity of conceptualisations of madness. The historicity argument has been explored through other work, and is confirmed by the observation that the ICD (a method for coding diagnoses to receive reimbursement) is in its 10th revision and the *Diagnostic and Statistical Manual of Mental Disorders* (DSM) in its 4th, and that categories have not remained stable over time (Busfield, 1996).

The argument that madness is culturally specific is stated in its milder form in terms of the notion of 'culture-bound syndromes' (American Psychiatric Association, 1994; Littlewood and Lipsedge, 1986). The argument here is that madness cannot be universal because different cultures exhibit different manifestations – madness takes on a distinct symptomatology that is only found in a particular culture. Marsella and White (1989) have shown through a rigorous comparative analysis that mental disorders have personal meanings and social significance *only* within specific cultural contexts, and that the very notion of 'mental disorder' is located within an ethnocentric Western cultural and historical tradition.

A South African example would be the condition *amafufunyana* (Edwards *et al.*, 1982), which has been described as violent, uncontrollable behaviour understood to be caused by spirit possession and often resulting in the sufferers speaking in languages not their own (Lund and Swartz, 1998). Thus the diagnosis of *amafufunyana* retains assumptions that static, clearly definable disorders exist. A stronger form of the cultural-specificity argument would suggest that madness differs culturally not only in terms of manifestation, but also at the level of basic underlying assumptions influencing issues of explanation and treatment. This is often articulated in terms of Western-traditional differences, in which Western conceptualisations are understood as ostracising, whereas traditional systems include the mad within the system. While it will be suggested later that this version may be oversimplified, there does seem to be indication that madness is not universal at symptomatic or explanatory levels (Parker *et al.*, 1995).

In addition to myths of transhistoricity and transculturality, the imprecise and ill-defined nature of madness can also be seen in the nebulous distinctions between mental disorder and 'normality'. Russell (1995) shows that a major epistemological concern is that the objects of study, namely *mental illnesses* or *mental disorders,* are by no means conceptually clear. Nor is this epistemological concern diminishing as taxonomies shift and change with each new edition of the major classificatory systems (Russell, 1995). The categorical thinking currently adopted in psychiatric and medical taxonomies (and typical of modernist thought) has an implicit assumption that clear boundaries exist between sickness and health, and between various categories of mental and physical disorder. Critical theorists have argued for a dimensional view, where there are gradations of health and sickness, on a multivariate continuum, and hence only an arbitrary cut-off between the two (Busfield, 1996; Goldberg and Huxley, 1992; Russell, 1995).

This view appears to be confirmed by the historical shifting of systems of classification, which have illustrated the permeability and fluidity of boundaries. Some authors (e.g. Busfield, 1996) have shown that psychiatric diagnoses merely constitute practical devices, in that they serve as intellectual lenses attempting to impose clarity and order on the complexity of human experiences, structuring thought and practice and providing recipes for action. What is clear is that the constructions of psychiatrists and other mental-health professionals change – and that professionals develop and improve their skills better to monopolise the territory (Busfield, 1996).

## The personal, social and political construction of madness

Madness has most often been constructed as a personal trajectory that the individual negotiates through a web of social resources – in most of the traditional literature it has been constituted as highly individual, personal and private (S. Swartz, 1996). Critics of the construction of psychopathology such as Rose (1989) have argued that discourses of madness become incorporated into subjectivity, such that the subject's personal experience is appropriated by the dominant discourse. For example, S. Swartz (1996) argues that despite the observation that *patients* are described in stereotypical ways, they may begin to see themselves in ways that conform to institutional expectations. Critical commentators have argued that the construction of madness as personal both eclipses and acts to conceal the workings of the social. In particular, Western discourses, both popular and professional, have tended to locate the causes of mental disorder within the individual, particularly within the self as a unitary social actor. In contrast, comparable Asian, Pacific and African models give proportionately greater weight to interdependent somatic processes, supernatural forces and social relations as causative agents (Marsella and White, 1989). Beliefs in supernatural forces and beings have important implications for the attribution of responsibility in cultural explanations of mental disorder, i.e. the perception of agency entails significant social consequences, particular for the nature of the response of others to the afflicted individual.

In terms of the personal and social construction of madness, it may be argued that the person who is deemed psychiatrically ill will behave and function in ways that reflect his/her individual construction or personal theory of illness (Marsella and White, 1989). Moreover, it may be speculated that his/her preparedness to seek and accept specific interventions will be influenced by this theory. The extent to which significant others share the individual's representations and attributions regarding the 'illness' and the extent to which harmony and support are generated will inform this personal theory. Marsella and White argue that the personal theories of the inflicted individual and the perceptions of others may mitigate social and psychological functioning. Similarly, the extent to which the individual representations or attributions overlap with those of care providers informs the extent to which they seek orthodox care, comply with medical regimen and are influenced positively by medicines and procedures that such providers have available to them (Marsella and White, 1989).

Foucault (1986) argues that expressions of *psychiatric* illness in thought and behaviour are of necessity mediated by the symbolic forms of language and culture. In general, however, interest in how personal or social meanings of illness are constituted through linguistic and social processes has been secondary to more direct research on the behavioural manifestations of behaviour and ethnopsychoses. Researchers have tended to treat cultural constructs as an independent variable that can be used to explain observable differences in behaviour or psychiatric phenomena. Much of this cross-cultural research to date has proceeded with quite simple assumptions about the role of ordinary language in 'labelling' forms of psychological disturbance, with little recognition of the creative power of language used in the social context and the extent to which illness terms and concepts may be embedded in the wider power relations of cultural systems and may provide particular constructions of reality (L. Swartz, 1996).

One argument that has been put forward suggests that madness can be understood as a symptom not of personal distress but of social distress. Ground-breaking critical theorist Chesler (1972), and later Irigaray (1985), began to argue that the high rates of mental disorder among women could be explained through social repression. Their argument suggested that women were oppressed by their gender roles and that this oppression may give rise to 'madness', since women are necessarily alienated from their female role. Irigaray argued that identity is tied up with sexuality, and that under patriarchy, women's sexuality has been conceptualised in male terms and that women had not been allowed to speak for themselves about their desire and their pleasure. Furthermore, this silence was held in place by the linguistic and logical processes that structure thought (Irigaray, 1985). Similarly, it has been suggested that *amafufunyana* can be understood as a 'symptom' of racial inequality (Weiss, in Swartz, 1986). This is supported by the fact that *amafufunyana* first appeared in the 1920s, when intergroup conflict began to escalate in South Africa (Wessels, 1985).

Simultaneously, authors such as Szasz (1974) and Foucault (1967) propounded even more radical externalist (social) explanations, which implied that the mad identity has little to do with the distressed person's own problems, hopes and fears and much to do with the purposes (professional, policing, governmental) of the groups and agencies wielding the labels. An oft-quoted example of this is the identification of homosexuality as a diagnosable disorder in the DSM until 1973.

A third understanding of madness is that it exemplifies resistance to the social. Goffman (1961) notes that despite the stereotyping of patients, many still retain a sense of their own uniqueness and are able to resist and form oppositional decodings of institutional structures by choosing when to conform and when not to. Some have suggested that a diagnosis may offer spaces for resistance previously not available to a person, and as such may have adaptive qualities. For example, *ukuthwasa*, a form of ancestor possession that signifies a calling to become a healer, may offer the sufferer opportunities to change role and to ensure wider support from his/her family network (Mills, 1985). When one examines the restrictions placed on a *thwasa* sufferer (most of whom are women), one can understand that it may represent a way out for women in oppressive situations. Such women must remove themselves from public life and live away from their homes with the *igqirha*.[3] This means an unhappy home life or an abusive husband can be left behind. Because they remove themselves from their previous social settings, many of the restrictions of those settings fall away. For example, the system of *hlonipha*, whereby a woman may not say any word containing the name of her husband, or any word that sounds like it or has a similar meaning, or any word relating to procreation (Buhrmann, 1977), restricts a woman's speech markedly. By taking on a new and superior role, subscription to this system falls away. A further restriction placed on a *thwasa* sufferer is that she must avoid all sexual contact in order to remain 'clean'. A woman who suffers from *thwasa* can thus legitimately leave her husband's house, kitchen and bed without fear of retribution. Additionally, many black women have limited participation in the economy and few opportunities to earn a living. *Ukuthwasa* may hold financial advantages. Being a sufferer may thus be empowering, as one of O'Connell's respondents implies: 'A female diviner can do anything a man can do. She is a man. I am a man'(1980: 21).

Further labelling theorists have shown that the ascription of mental disorder evokes culturally prescribed (social) responses from others that structure the experience of the afflicted individual as he/she moves about in the social system. The study of conceptions of mental disorder becomes important as a means of determining what kinds of social reality are likely to be created by the interpretation of behaviour as mentally disordered.

## ■ Social, political and financial institutions that inform the construction of madness

Parker (1992), following Foucault, stresses the need to analyse the relation between discourses and social institutions. Western conceptualisations of madness have increasingly become the domain of the psychiatric institution and of medical discourse, but also participate in penal institutions and influence/inform other interest groups such as various mental-health-care professions and the psychopharmacology industry (see Breggin, 1993 for an extended discussion). Similarly, it could be argued that indigenous belief systems keep indigenous healers in business and also contribute in complex ways to the survival of cultural distinctiveness. Understandings of madness are thus not value-neutral, but are constructed in line with the needs of institutions, including the need to take ownership of areas of knowledge in order to promote professional survival (Rose, 1989).

In South Africa, psychiatrists, as medical experts, still have prime responsibility for the care and treatment of the 'mentally disturbed', although the world of community care and other professionals compete with them for influence and power. As such, several authors (e.g. Busfield, 1996) would argue that psychiatrists still monopolise the formal construction of the dominant social discourses through which mental disorder is constructed and imbued with meaning. Busfield (1996) shows that, from a medical perspective, mental disorder is viewed as a distinctive type of illness to be understood, as with other types of illness, first and foremost in physical terms, and is to be treated through physical intervention. It can be argued that these strong, although varying, emphases on physical causes and treatments of mental disorder are indicative of assimilatory tendencies (Rose, 1989). Foucault (1967) and others have argued that this trend can be traced historically and that psychiatry survived the 19th century by laying claim to mental disorder as distinctive.

The role of institutions in a post-structuralist critique can also be illustrated through the ways in which madness has developed in relation to the three contested and changing boundaries of social deviance, physical illness and mental health. Busfield (1996) notes that mental disorder stands in a difficult and precarious position between bodily illness and social deviance, and there is an ongoing struggle between various professionals and social theorists as to where the boundaries should be set.

The location of the boundary between physical illness and mental disorder has long been contested both within the medical profession and without (Ussher, 1991). It has been shown, for example, that whether a particular constellation of symptoms is deemed a mental or a physical illness depends largely on the interests of the institutions, professionals and lay people involved (Busfield, 1986). While disputes over the boundary between mental disorder and physical disorder have been dominated by professional rivalries within medicine, the boundary between mental disorder and social deviance has been a matter of rivalry between the medical profession and the law (Smith, 1980; Walker, 1968 in Ussher, 1991). Decisions on cases of this nature are not just a matter of the power and potential of competing discourses and attendant values, but are also linked to service provision. Authors such as Kleinman (1988) have harshly critiqued those traditional psychiatric views that present biology as the basis of mental disorder and psychological and social structures as epiphenomena or superstructural layers to be stripped away in order to address the infrastructural physiological level.

Therefore, while psychiatrists may find it relatively straightforward to offer a formal definition of the concept of mental disorder through their listing of specific types of disorder, determining the precise boundaries is far from easy in practice. The comment made by Parker *et al.* that 'notions of madness and abnormal psychology as we understand them are particular and peculiar to our culture and our time' (1995: 4) is becoming a more widely accepted and a less controversial view as the precariousness of boundaries around madness becomes more apparent.

## Power relations are inextricable from constructions of madness

In many ways, it is artificial to proclaim that the construction of madness is related to power in a separate point in our argument, since the workings of power infiltrate all levels of explanation. The relation between power and madness therefore forms an overarching theme of this chapter. Theories of the relation between madness and power have a long history. A number of issues will be highlighted here, including the relation between madness and political/professional power, between patriarchy and power and, following Foucault (1967), between knowledge and power.

Psychiatry, psychology and the study of the *abnormal* is one of the primary ways in which power relations are established in society. When abnormality and its corresponding norms are defined, it is always the *normal* that defines the *abnormal* (Parker *et al.*, 1995). It has been argued that political and professional power serves to police those who do not conform (Foucault, 1967) and to separate deviants or misfits from the rest of society (Rose, 1989). In *Discipline and Punish*, Foucault (1975) shows how disciplinary power operates not through physical force but through a hegemony of norms, political technologies and the consequent shaping of body and soul. As Rose points out:

> At stake was more than the simple imposition of a moral code under the threat of punishment, more than blind obedience to an arbitrary set of doctrines. The existence of a space of regulated freedom depended upon the generalization of a set of ethical

techniques for self-inspection and self-evaluation in relation to the code, a way of making the feelings, wishes, and emotions of the self visible to itself, a way in which citizens were to problematize and govern their lives and conduct, to find a way in which, as free subjects, they could live a good life as the consequence of their own characters (1989: 224).

The workings of professional power, it has been argued, operate through calling upon the subject to participate in forms of (often scientific) knowledge that are constructed as truth. Thus S. Swartz (1996), for example, argues that the professional practice of rendering patients' histories as linear sequences of events that produce current symptoms is not a neutral technology. Through this, 'patients are narrated into spaces which psychiatric knowledge has the power to explain' (S. Swartz, 1996: 150). In the case study presented below, it could be suggested that professional institutions vie for markets (both monetary and ideological) through laying claim to bases of expertise and world-view.

Against modern theories that see knowledge as neutral and objective, Foucault has emphasised that knowledge is indissociable from regimes of power, and that there is a circular relationship between knowledge and power (Best and Kellner, 1991). Foucault (1986) stresses that power is multiple and dispersed, such that different kinds of knowledge are related to multiple kinds of power. This analysis of the power/knowledge complex has come to influence a range of perspectives in the study of mental health, in that it has exposed the epistemology of disease taxonomies as an element of the moral control of individuals and populations, and of the regulation of individuals through regulating their bodies. Foucault (1986) argues that the whole historical development of psychology and psychiatry could be seen in terms of the generation of forms of knowledge related to an extension of power over the subordinate populations of suburban Europe. Having emerged within the contexts of relations of power through practices and technologies of exclusion, confinement, surveillance and objectification, disciplines such as psychiatry in turn contributed to the development, refinement and proliferation of new techniques of power (Best and Kellner, 1991). Psychiatric institutions came to function as laboratories for the observation of individuals, experimentation with correctional techniques and acquisition of knowledge for social control. Foucault (1967, 1986) argues that a principal technology of power within psychiatry is the professional *gaze*, which is concerned with gathering information to inform and elaborate the discourses of madness. He argues that the examination, including the mental-health examination, combines the techniques of the observing hierarchy with those of normalising judgements: 'It is a normalising gaze, a surveillance that makes it possible to qualify, to classify and to punish. It establishes over individuals a visibility through which one differentiates them and judges them' (Foucault, 1986: 184). In so doing, normalisation becomes a primary instrument of professional power.

Foucault's (1967) historical exploration of madness has been drawn upon elsewhere in this chapter. One of his central arguments is that the separation of 'reason' from 'unreason' into binary opposition is a fairly recent phenomenon, and that the division of 'reason' has become associated with 'normal' in a way that becomes increasingly difficult to deconstruct. For Parker *et al.* (1995), Foucault's primary argument is that madness is *irrational otherness*. Foucault (1967) argues that the sequestration of 'unreason', partly through technologies of subjectivity, has highlighted normality through obsessive study and thought about the historically recent division between mad and sane. For him, pathology is constructed around the policing of a firm distinction between the normal and the pathological. For those who diagnose others as pathological, a position of normality is secured, as are the grounds for questioning the legitimacy of the views of others (Parker *et al.*, 1995).

Foucault (1986) suggests that the link between madness and unreason is not a logical, natural one, but one in which a number of troublesome groups in society can be labelled as mad. Ingleby (1982) argues that if we go back to first principles, what the 'mentally ill' have lost is not their bodily health, nor their virtue, but their *reason*, and so their conduct simply does not make sense. Insanity ascriptions, in this view, are made when behaviour does not seem accountable to any plausible motive, or seems to be quite unfounded; such ascriptions may be ruled out simply by providing a credible motive for action or a reasonable ground for belief.

It should be borne in mind that knowledge about mental health and medicine is not simply formulated by mental-health professionals and disseminated to the public, who passively accept such knowledge as a matter of course. Rather, the knowledge that is generated around discourses of madness provides a valuable tool of government at the levels of political discourse, institutions and individual subjectivity, where it forms a critical dimension to the exercise of power. However, Foucault stresses that an understanding of power as operating from 'dominator' to 'dominated' is too simple, and does not recognise that 'there are no relations of power without resistance; the latter are all the more real and effective because they are formed right at the point where relations of power are exercised' (1980: 142).

We have discussed a number of inter-related issues through which it may be asserted that madness is a social construction, that it is an active and changing concept, that it is not purely located within the individual, that institutions are influential in forming and maintaining conceptions of madness and that processes of power imbue every aspect of the construction of madness. We will now introduce a case study in order to illustrate some of these ideas and to provoke thinking regarding broader use of taxonomies of madness in South Africa.

## A case study: ancestors and aetiology

X, a young university student, presented at a local psychiatric hospital requesting therapeutic intervention after a confusing experience he was struggling to make sense of. The previous year, his family had pressured him to undergo ritual circumcision. He felt this conflicted with his Christian beliefs and so refused, triggering family conflict. At about the same time, he failed his university exams. Soon after this, he left on a journey to his home village. Before he arrived, he found himself naked in a misty forest on a hill. He relates that he could see figures and shapes, but no more detail than that. These figures spoke to him, but he could not understand what they were saying. He remembers feeling confused and then does not remember anything else until finding himself bruised and sore in a village near his own. Apparently he had arrived at this village and had been aggressive and incoherent. Some of the villagers had beaten him up, after which a friend of his family had taken him in. This friend then sent him home to his family.

His parents decided that these events had been caused because X had angered the ancestors in some way. According to X, they forced him to go to a *sangoma*, who confirmed the diagnosis and prescribed circumcision. He resisted the *sangoma*, and eventually managed to return to his university town. Once back there, he says he felt completely normal, ceased hearing voices, but was plagued by conflict regarding how to understand his recent experience. He felt that perhaps God had been trying to communicate with him, but was also plagued by guilt for having experienced something that might have been related to his ancestors. In this sense, he concurrently interpreted his experience in terms of his religion and in terms of his family's explanation. He decided to approach the biomedical institution for answers.

This case evoked heated debate in a subsequent case conference. Initially, this was centred around how to deal with 'cultural explanations' of X's experience, coupled with a reluctance to label him as 'schizophrenic'. It was suggested that he be allocated a black therapist who would be able to understand his world-view. Little reference was made to his fragmented relationship to his world-view. Discussion then shifted to focus on what 'precipitated' his 'breakdown'. We suggest that the availability of this biomedical language, framed as a universally important question, opened space for a slippage into biomedical discourse. This may have facilitated the next discursive manoeuvre. One person stated that, since this had clearly been a schizophrenic and possibly dissimulating episode, the probability was high that X would remit, and that therefore it was dangerous for him not to be maintained on drug therapy. This became the focus of the rest of the case conference. X's complex experience had been reduced to the need for psychopharmacology. Interestingly, X only attended a few sessions of therapy, and then left. No information is available about his subsequent experiences.

## Voices competing for discursive space: discourse and subjectivity

X's complex experiences and understandings present rich possibilities for analysis of the discourses at play. He is graphically positioned within and between contradictory and powerful discourses, both of which have strong institutional bases with which to locate him. It is not possible here to undertake a full analysis. Rather, we will use the case study to briefly highlight sites of conflict and contradiction and the relation between discourse and subjectivity. We will then address issues of power and resistance, in order to explore broader relations between biomedical and indigenous discourses.

Three dominant and competing discourses can be identified relating to biomedical, religious and indigenous institutions. Each offers alternative opportunities for creating meaning and different possibilities for action. X's reason for referral can be related to his being caught between the various discourses and being unsure as to where to position himself in relation to their contradictions. It is possible to understand his experience as a symbolic expression of his conflict regarding the different requirements of religious and indigenous discourses. Religious discourses require him to reject traditional values and therefore the values of his family, while indigenous discourses require actions and belief systems he feels unable to incorporate into his subjectivity exactly because they contradict the requirements of religious discourse. Within this interpretation, it is interesting to note that his experience in the forest could represent the influence of the indigenous discourses he is trying to reject. This particular geographical location is culturally accepted as a burial ground for the ancestors, and is therefore a holy place in indigenous discourse. Conversely, then, religious discourse may locate this as a place of 'evil'. This provides some indication of how discourses may vie for power, not only at the level of language and institution, but also at the level of subjectivity.

An examination of the truth claims offered by indigenous over against biomedical discourses punctuates the different constructions of the person and different production of 'facts' offered by each. Positioned in relation to Christian religious discourses, X felt unable to participate in indigenous practices, but nonetheless experienced conflict between the competing demands of each. His attempt to cohere his experience (by approaching a psychiatric hospital) represented an invocation of biomedical discourse as a channel for reaching truth. It may be argued that this discourse required an equal refutation of indigenous African and religious discourse. In order to accept the truths offered by biomedical discourse, X would have needed to re-story his experience in terms of illness and deficit. Perhaps the fact that X turned to science for answers to a question about the meaning of his experience underlines the power of biomedical discourse. In the ultimate analysis, he was given a simplified answer (schizophrenia), but it could be argued that this foreclosure could not adequately account for all his subject positions. While he turned to biomedicine for answers, he also exited biomedical discourse once answers had been given, possibly as a result of the label's lack of explanatory power for him. His lack of compliance could therefore be understood as yet another rejection of a discourse that he was unable to reconcile with his construction of his experience, and that did not offer the payoffs he needed to cohere his experience into his discursive net.

For X, the argument presented by some South African authors that biomedicine and indigenous taxonomies should be used in conjunction (Freeman, 1991; Seedat, 1997) would not have been satisfactory. X did not incorporate either discourse unproblematically. This case may highlight how both discourses require self-policing and management of subjectivity. Both require discursive action that implies subjugation to the truth claims of the discourse. Prescription of drugs in biomedicine is akin to prescription of circumcision in indigenous taxonomies, in the sense that both treatments demand that the subject submits to the truth claims at work. While this may be so for discourse in general (and therefore not any more problematic than many of the discourses we participate in), the absolute commitment demanded of X was problematic for him. This illustrates how simple claims of whether indigenous or biomedical taxonomies should be used discount the conflict and complexity of the experience involved.

This brief analysis of the discourses operating for X raises a number of points regarding the theoretical conceptualisations of madness discussed above. His personal experience of madness was clearly mediated through a number of social expectations and practices. It could even be argued that his experience in the forest was a form of negotiation with social expectations (to be a good son; to be circumcised; to be a good Christian; to be a good student). Further, his personal experience became subject to social meanings and requirements. It is important to stress that it was not merely a case of different stakeholders offering him different explanations. Each explanation came with a social imperative to participate or to suffer the loss of subjective rewards offered by each discourse. While X describes feeling these imperatives on a subjective level, he also clearly illustrates that people are not passive to the social demands of the category of madness. In line with theory arguing that madness is a form of resistance, X's experience may have been an enacted resistance to the contradictory demands placed upon him.

For X, the claim that madness is an active process was experienced at the level of subjectivity, as he struggled to negotiate the available discourses in order to make sense of his experience. Definitional boundaries were fluid for him, and not static. The claim that psychiatric labels are reductive, for example, was possibly experienced by him in relation to the inadequacy of the term 'schizophrenia'. A number of more general points seem to arise from this case study. In it we witness in action the contestation of boundaries between the realm of indigenous taxonomies (which place his experience in the realm of the spiritual) and biomedical taxonomies (which call upon the realm of the physical). It could be said that the two discourses compete for legitimacy and commitment, and that the requirements of each demand an exclusion of participation in the other. Biomedical discourse may tolerate indigenous explanations, but is much less likely to tolerate 'non-compliant' drug use. Similarly, indigenous taxonomies may not openly exclude biomedical taxonomies, but require commitment that may more insidiously exclude the possibility of the subject's participation in both discourses.

The fiction of cultural and temporal universality is further highlighted by this case, raising pertinent questions regarding understandings of the various taxonomies in South Africa. We suggested earlier that a trend in South Africa is to uncritically romanticise indigenous taxonomies as natural, fixed and wholesome. Critical psychiatric literature has similarly noted a reification of psychiatric taxonomies as static, transhistorical and imbued with scientific truth. The case study highlights that understandings are not necessarily shared within a particular culture, even less between cultures. While it is more accepted that biomedical taxonomies ignore cultural specificity and historicity, it could be argued that so too do indigenous taxonomies. Indigenous discourses may imply that there is one culture that is shared by all those sharing ancestors. This formulation is unable to account for the varied experiences of people. Further, indigenous discourses may call upon a notion of timeless wisdom passed down in untainted form from many generations ago. To think that indigenous taxonomies have not been influenced by the profound social changes of the last century seems naive, and is dismissive of the influence of current social configurations on the presentation, understanding and treatment of madness.

## ■ The road to truth: power and resistance

Issues of power have been highlighted through the case study and the chapter: such issues are central to a post-structuralist analysis of madness. A Foucauldian analysis of power emphasises the bidirectional and pervasive nature of power, and reconceptualises power as productive rather than oppressive (Foucault, 1975; Parker, 1989). This framework examines the intersection between power and issues of subjectivity, discourse and the institution. We analysed the case study in terms of contradictory discourses competing for power and, concurrently, different stakeholders exercising power in different ways. We can therefore analyse power on a number of levels. For example, the power of the *sangoma* to hold X against his will is linked with the power of his discourse to give legitimacy to his prescriptions and actions in the eyes of X's family. Similarly, members of the medical profession have the power to commit X to an institution, but here power also works at the level of the case conference, through which his experience can be transformed into a medicalised category through medicalised language. On a more diffuse level, it is noted that, while X was relatively clear on which discourse he wanted to position himself in relation to (religion being a primary discursive influence), the power of indigenous, biomedical and a range of other (e.g. family) discourses was such that he experienced conflict on the level of subjectivity. A Foucauldian explication of power has the further advantage of avoiding the portrayal of X as a helpless victim. His resistance first to the *sangoma* and then to the psychiatric team represented an important and shaping exercise of power, although it appears to have been gained at some cost to himself.

Therefore, some of the dominant institutions involved in X's situation participated in the power matrices that emerged, i.e. indigenous healing system, psychiatric team and church (of which we know little – it could be speculated that X's next choice would be to approach the church for meaning). In addition, we have illustrated the complex interactions between institutions and subjectivity on the level of lived experience. Many more institutions are at play (e.g. institutions of the family and of education). Focus on the two institutions most clearly represented in this case study – the biomedical and the indigenous – and their systems of discourse highlights their conflictual relationship. In conjunction with available literature, this case study illustrates their competition for legitimacy on the level of discourse as well as on the level of subjectivity. Our final task will be to examine this competitive relationship more carefully, returning to Foucault's (1967) historical analysis of madness.

At first glance, it might be said that Western and traditional taxonomies represent co-existing correlates of Foucault's historical analysis of differences in world-view between modernity and pre-modernity. Such notions have entered popular discourse through metaphors such as the 'noble savage'. In this (naive) understanding, it might be said that biomedical taxonomies represent the pinnacle of the binary and socially valued division between reason and unreason (Foucault, 1967), where unreason is vilified and constructed as 'to be rectified' by those who possess reason. Indigenous taxonomies, then, may be seen as a harkening back to pre-modernity, where reason and unreason were in dialogue and the language of the mad stood to hold meaning. Therefore, we might say that the psychiatric staff aimed to chemically straitjacket that which is not acceptable in society and label it as 'chronic', while the indigenous healer's aim was to prescribe a way to enter into dialogue with the social (in the form of appeasing the ancestors), with the aim of reincorporation of the mad person into the social network.

Besides the paternalistic overtones of this formulation, it appears problematic when one explores the implications of the fact that both metaphysics are linked by shared historical location and cultural availability. Such a formulation would only hold if the two were completely ostracised from each other and held no mutually constructing influence whatsoever. Further, because intersecting social discourses and practices overlap between the two metaphysics, it becomes possible that they are both, at least in part, subject to similar social imperatives. Upon reflection, this implies a new binary opposition between the biomedical and the indigenous, an opposition in which both are constructed as transhistorical. Post-structuralism would treat this, like other binary oppositions, as an artificial system of power and difference that serves to undermine the power relations between biomedical and indigenous systems, and it becomes an opposition to be critically deconstructed. Through the maintenance of such a binary opposition, both conceptions resist change and therefore constrain the subject through the terms of participation in that particular discourse, be it biomedical or indigenous. Both are also competing for legitimacy. We have aimed to illustrate that both participate in power relations and that both demand conditions of inclusion and exclusion. If one is positioned in relation to possible access to either, the binary opposition (which implies that values are attached to each taxonomy) undermines the option of a simple choice between them. By calling on one discourse, one must also negotiate the other discourse set in relation to it. Both taxonomies are important and dominant in the lives and meanings of many South Africans, and we suggest that to sequester the one from the other or to accept either uncritically is to ignore the complexity of the issues at play.

# ■ Conclusion

In this chapter we called for a more critical approach to all available taxonomies of madness, and focused particularly on the complex relations between biomedical and indigenous discourses. The case study we drew upon portrays a person caught between competing discourses who is struggling to find meaning. Other people may have very different experiences. The location of this story within an institutional setting, and subsequently within this chapter, within yet another complex web of power/knowledge relations, echoes with irony Foucault's argument regarding the simultaneous exclusion and moral subjectification of the madman: 'Th[e] turning of real lives into writing is no longer a procedure of heroization; it functions as a procedure of objectification and subjectification. The carefully collated life of mental patients or delinquents belongs, as did the chronicle of kings or the adventures of the great popular bandits, to a certain political function of writing; but in a quite different technique of power' (1975: 192).

We have, however, hoped to show through the case study and theoretical discussion that, in order to understand constructions of madness, it is necessary to understand the person's narration of self as well as the intersection of this with available discourses and power dynamics. We call particularly for a recognition that the narration of meaning is not a categorical process, nor one removed from broader discursive struggles and networks.

Deconstructive approaches have been criticised as potentially nihilistic and paralysing (Burman, 1990), leaving few strategies to negotiate a way forward. Our aim has been to demonstrate the usefulness of deconstruction in critically examining taken-for-granted knowledge in order to open opportunities for more sophisticated understandings that are able to recognise discourses at play. This has practical utility for South Africa at a point of transition and, more specifically, at a point where mental-health policy is being radically reformulated. Deconstruction offers opportunities for reconstruction, which in turn offers opportunities for movement and change in how we understand madness, how we position ourselves in relation to our own discursive imperatives and how we interact with the discursively constructed experiences of others.

## Endnotes

1 The term 'madness' is used in this chapter in order to avoid drawing on either biomedical or traditional taxonomies and in order to highlight the problematics and shifting meanings of this term.
2 The purpose of using this case study is to use a specific example to discuss broader issues of discourse and the broad interaction between discourses and institutions. We in no way wish to imply that the specific interventions involved in the case were inappropriate. The focus is on the case and not on the specifics of intervention. Details have been changed in order to preserve confidentiality. It should also be noted that one of the authors (Long) gained access to this case study through the secondary source of participating in the case conference referred to in the chapter. As such, the interpretations offered rely heavily on the subjective experiences and reconstructions (from clinical notes) of the author concerned. The case study presented here has been offered for verification to fellow participants at this case conference. This chapter does not claim to offer objective truths, which we, along with others (e.g. Giddens, 1976; Hollway, 1989; Parker, 1992), regard as an unattainable methodology for the social sciences. Rather, our aim is to enter debate around interpretations, using these as a starting point for future critical thought around the issues raised in this chapter.
3 This is a Xhosa word signifying a type of indigenous healer.

## References

American Psychiatric Association. (1994). *Diagnostic and Statistical Manual of Mental Disorders* (4th edn). Washington, DC: American Psychiatric Association.
Best, S. and Kellner, D. (1991). *Postmodern Theory: Critical Interrogations*. London: Macmillan.
Breggin, E. (1993). *Toxic Psychiatry*. London: Fontana.
Buhrmann, M. (1977). Western psychiatry and the Xhosa patient. *South African Medical Journal*, 51, 464–7.
Burman, E. (1990). Differing with deconstruction: A feminist critique. In I. Parker and J. Shotter (eds), *Deconstructing Social Psychology*. London: Routledge.
Busfield, J. (1986). *Managing Madness: Changing Ideas and Practice*. London: Hutchinson.
Busfield, J. (1996). *Men, Women and Madness: Understanding Gender and Mental Disorder*. Basingstoke: Macmillan.
Chesler, P. (1972). *Women and Madness*. New York: Avon.
Edwards, S., Cheetham, R., Majozi, E. and Lasich, A. (1982). Zulu culture-bound psychiatric syndromes. *South African Journal of Hospital Medicine*, 8, 82–6.
Foucault, M. (1967). *Madness and Civilization: A History of Insanity in the Age of Reason*. London: Tavistock.
Foucault, M. (1975). *Discipline and Punish: The Birth of the Prison*. Harmondsworth: Penguin.
Foucault, M. (1980). *Power/Knowledge: Selected Interviews and Other Writings by Michel Foucault, 1972–1977*. Worcester: Harvester Press.
Foucault, M. (1986). *Mental Illness and Psychology*. Berkeley: University of California Press.

Freeman, M. (1990). *Is There a Role for Traditional Healers in Health Care in South Africa?* Johannesburg: Centre for Health Policy, University of the Witwatersrand.

Freeman, M. (1991). Mental health for all: Moving beyond rhetoric. *South African Journal of Psychology*, 21 (3), 141–9.

Giddens, A. (1976). *New Rules of Sociological Method.* London: Macmillan.

Goffman, E. (1961). *Asylums.* Harmondsworth: Penguin.

Goldberg, D. and Huxley, P. J. (1992). *Common Mental Disorders: A Biosocial Model.* London: Routledge.

Hollway, W. (1989). *Subjectivity and Method in Psychology.* London: Sage.

Ingleby, D. (1982). *Critical Psychiatry: The Politics of Mental Health.* Harmondsworth: Penguin.

Irigaray, L. (1985). *The Sex which is not One.* Ithaca: Cornell University Press.

Kaplan, H. I. and Sadock, B. J. (1991). *Synopsis of Psychiatry.* Baltimore: Williams and Wilkins.

Kleinman, A. (1988). *Rethinking Psychiatry: From Cultural Category to Personal Experience.* New York: Free Press.

Littlewood, R. and Lipsedge, M. (1986). The 'culture-bound syndromes' of the dominant culture: Culture, psychopathology and biomedicine. In J. L. Cox (ed.), *Transcultural Psychiatry.* London: Croom Helm.

Lund, C. and Swartz, L. (1998). Xhosa-speaking schizophrenic patients' experience of their condition: Psychosis and *amafufunyana*. *South African Journal of Psychology*, 28 (2), 62–70.

Marsella, A. and White, G. (1989). *Cultural Conceptions of Mental Health and Therapy.* Dordrecht: D. Reichel.

Mills, J. (1985). The possession state *intwaso*: An anthropological re-appraisal. *South African Journal of Sociology*, 16 (1), 9–13.

O'Connell, M. (1980). The aetiology of *thwasa*. *Psychotherapeia*, 6 (4), 18–23.

Parker, I. (1989). *The Crisis in Modern Social Psychology – and how to end it.* London: Routledge.

Parker, I. (1992). *Discourse Dynamics: Critical Analysis for Social and Individual Psychology.* London: Routledge.

Parker, I., Georgaca, E., Harper, D., McLaughlin, T. and Stowell-Smith, M. (1995). *Deconstructing Psychopathology.* London: Sage.

Pillay, Y. and Freeman, M. (1996). Mental health policy and planning: Continuing the debates. *Psychology in Society*, 21, 60–71.

Rose, N. (1989). *Governing the Soul: The Shaping of the Private Self.* London: Routledge.

Russell, D. (1995). *Women, Madness and Medicine.* Cambridge: Polity Press.

Seedat, M. (1997). The quest for liberatory psychology. *South African Journal of Psychology*, 27 (4), 261–70.

Smith, M. L. (1980). *The Benefits of Psychotherapy.* Baltimore: Johns Hopkins Press.

Swartz, L. (1986). Transcultural psychiatry in South Africa, Part I. *Transcultural Psychiatric Research Review*, 23, 273–303.

Swartz, L. (1987). Transcultural psychiatry in South Africa, Part II. *Transcultural Psychiatric Research Review*, 24, 5–30.

Swartz, L. (1996). Culture and mental health in the rainbow nation: Transcultural psychiatry in a changing South Africa. *Transcultural Psychiatric Research Review*, 33, 119–36.

Swartz, S. (1996). Shrinking: A postmodern perspective on psychiatric case histories. *South African Journal of Psychology*, 26 (3), 150–6.

Szasz, T. (1974). *The Myth of Mental Illness.* London: Routledge.

Weedon, C. (1987). *Feminist Practice and Post-structuralist Theory.* Oxford: Basil Blackwell.

Wessels, W. (1985). Understanding culture-specific syndromes in South Africa – the Western dilemma. *Modern Medicine of South Africa*, September, 51–63.

Wetherell, M. (ed.) (1996). *Identities, Groups and Social Issues.* London: Sage.

Ussher, J. (1991). *Women's Madness: Misogyny or Mental Illness?* New York: Harvester Wheatsheaf.

# Xenophobia: A new pathology for a New South Africa?

*Bronwyn Harris*

## ■ Introduction

In 1994, South Africa became a new nation. Born out of democratic elections and inaugurated as the 'Rainbow Nation' by Nelson Mandela, this 'New South Africa' represents a fundamental shift in the social, political and geographical landscapes of the past. Unity has replaced segregation, equality has replaced legislated racism and democracy has replaced apartheid, at least in terms of the law. Despite the transition from authoritarian rule to democracy, prejudice and violence continue to mark contemporary South Africa. Indeed, the shift in political power has brought about a range of new discriminatory practices and victims. One such victim is 'The Foreigner'. Emergent alongside a new-nation discourse, The Foreigner stands at a site where identity, racism and violent practice are reproduced. This paper interrogates the high levels of violence that are currently directed at foreigners, particularly African foreigners, in South Africa. It explores the term 'xenophobia' and various hypotheses about its causes. It also explores the ways in which xenophobia itself is depicted in the country. Portrayed as negative, abnormal and the antithesis of a healthy, normally functioning individual or society, xenophobia is read here as a new pathology for a 'New South Africa'. This chapter attempts to deconstruct such a representation by suggesting that xenophobia is implicit to the technologies of nation-building and is part of South Africa's culture of violence.

The chapter will provide a brief history and critique of the ways in which xenophobia has been understood in South Africa. Building on these understandings, it will contextualise xenophobia as a current and arguably socially located phenomenon, one which is framed as pathological. It is important to mention that, within the chapter, xenophobia is not understood as a typical form of psychopathology. This is because psychopathology is usually constituted as an individual rather than social difficulty and is usually located in terms of disjuncture with society rather than vice versa. Both of these premises are contestable in an examination of xenophobia. Despite this, there is political value in framing xenophobia as a pathology, even if it is not properly psychological (i.e. psychopathological), because it allows for critical reflection on the discursive tropes that construct pyshopathology and the implications that these have at a social, as well as individual, level.

## ■ Xenophobia: a violent practice

In the dictionary, the term 'xenophobia' is defined as a 'hatred or fear of foreigners' (*South African Pocket Oxford Dictionary of Current English*, 1994). More commonly, the term is used to denote a 'dislike of foreigners'. In this understanding, xenophobia is characterised by a *negative attitude* towards foreigners, a *dislike*, a *fear*, or a *hatred*. By framing xenophobia as an attitude, however, there is no comment on the *consequences* or *effects* of such a mind-set. This is misleading, because xenophobia in South Africa is not restricted to a fear or dislike of foreigners. Rather, as the following interview extracts reveal, it results in 'intense tension and violence by South Africans towards immigrants' (Tshitereke, 1999: 4).

> A man from the Congo was attacked and he cried but no-one helped him. And after the thief had gone, the people on the sides said that 'because you are crying in English, we didn't help you. If you are crying in Zulu, we will help you'. Then he went to the police and was told that 'you are not our brother, we can't help you' (Focus Group with foreign students, 99/10/25).

> Four guys put a gun to my head and told me to get in the car. They told me that *makwerekwere*[1] have got bucks and that I must give them money. They took my three hundred rand and those shoes I bought. And then they were beating me. And one stabbed me here [points to scar on left side of the abdomen]. Then they told me that they would let me live on one condition: 'each and every month we gonna come and fetch three hundred rand ...'. I went to the police but they didn't even ask me questions. They just took my refugee papers and tore them up. Then they arrested me, saying that I'm illegal in the country, that I don't have a paper. They put me in jail for the weekend. They told my friends to bring money so that I can be freed .... And those men came every month for the money. They threatened me that they would kill me and I did it for three years (interview with Rwandan refugee, 99/11/30).

Kollapan (1999) warns that xenophobia cannot be separated from violence and physical abuse. In this sense, a rewriting of the dictionary definition of xenophobia is necessary. 'Xenophobia' as a term must be reframed to incorporate *practice*. It is not just an attitude: it is an activity. It is not just a dislike or fear of foreigners: it is a violent practice that results in bodily harm and damage. More particularly, the violent practice that comprises xenophobia must be further refined to include its specific target, because, in South Africa, not all foreigners are uniformly victimised. Rather, black foreigners, particularly those from Africa, comprise the majority of victims. It is also important to explore why 'the unknown' represented by (largely black) foreigners should necessarily invite repugnance, fear or aggression. These questions and a revised definition of xenophobia must be borne in mind throughout the chapter. They must inform an explanation for the phenomenon and must underpin issues regarding why, how and whom xenophobia targets.

## ■ Hypotheses of xenophobia

Various explanations for xenophobia have been offered in the literature and popular culture (magazines, speeches, documentaries, etc.). For the purposes of this chapter, these explanations have been grouped into three hypotheses, namely, 'the scapegoating hypothesis', 'the isolation hypothesis', and 'the biocultural hypothesis'. It is important to recognise that these hypotheses are not mutually exclusive, but rather offer different levels of explanation for xenophobia within contemporary South

Africa. They operate as straightforward theoretical descriptions that do not interrogate the term 'xenophobia' itself, as much as look at its background, symptoms and indications. Through their presentation, I consequently note with irony that the following sections serve much the same purpose as a textbook discussion of 'schizophrenia' or some other diagnostic syndrome.

## The scapegoating hypothesis of xenophobia

The scapegoating hypothesis has largely emerged through sociological theory. It locates xenophobia within the context of social transition and change. Hostility towards foreigners is explained in relation to limited resources, such as housing, education, health care and employment, coupled with high expectations during transition (Morris, 1998; Tshitereke, 1999). Tshitereke suggests that

> In the post-apartheid epoch, while people's expectations have been heightened, a realisation that delivery is not immediate has meant that discontent and indignation are at their peak. People are more conscious of their deprivation than ever before .... This is the ideal situation for a phenomenon like xenophobia to take root and flourish. South Africa's political transition to democracy has exposed the unequal distribution of resources and wealth in the country (1999: 4).

In this context, Tshitereke notes, 'people often create a "frustration-scapegoat"' (1999: 4), i.e. they create a target to blame for ongoing deprivation and poverty. Foreigners, this theory suggests, often become such scapegoats. This is because they are interpreted as a threat to jobs, housing, education and health care (Morris, 1998; Tshitereke, 1999). Morris comments that 'Research and historical events have indicated that if a majority group is in a perilous economic position they are more likely to feel threatened by minorities, especially if they are foreign' (1998: 1125).

Generally, scapegoating theory explains xenophobia in terms of broad social and economic factors. Tshitereke (1999) introduces a psychological level of explanation to supplement this sociological interpretation. He conceptualises xenophobia in terms of frustration and relative deprivation. Relative-deprivation theory suggests that 'a key psychological factor in generating social unrest is a sense of relative deprivation. This arises from a subjective feeling of discontent based on the belief that one is getting less than one feels entitled to. When there is a gap between aspirations and reality, social discontent is likely to result' (De la Rey, 1991: 41). Tshitereke states that violence is not an inevitable outcome of relative deprivation:

> The anger caused by deprivation and perceived or real threats from immigrants as it relates to resources does not directly cause the nationals to commit violence, but it frustrates them. Political scientist Annette Seegers says, 'frustration breeds anger, yet angry people do not always commit violence'. They could turn their anger inwards and commit suicide. Alternatively, people release their anger on that 'frustration-scapegoat', usually non-national minorities (1999: 4).

Here, Tshitereke draws on psychological theories of aggression and frustration to explain that there is a 'causal link between relative deprivation, xenophobia and collective violence' (1999: 4). This link is forged through scapegoating the foreigner.

Relative-deprivation theory offers a psychological explanation for scapegoating. Concepts of frustration and aggression are interpreted as subjective, intrapsychic processes. In this way, the theory understands xenophobia from the inside out. Psychoanalytic theory similarly offers an intrapsychic explanation of scapegoating as a projective and defensive process. For both these theories, De la Ray points out that 'The cause of social unrest cannot be simply located within subjective perceptions of reality. The search for causes of social action must extend beyond the subjective psychological realm to include its complex inter-relatedness with objective social reality' (1991: 41).

Tshitereke's (1999) psychological interpretation of scapegoating must not be divorced from the socio-economic realities of contemporary South Africa. He reminds us that the psychological process of relative deprivation rests on social comparison. This takes place at the level of jobs, houses, education and even women, such that foreigners are scapegoated for taking our jobs, taking our houses and stealing our women. Politics, economics and patriarchy impact on the scapegoating process.

### The isolation hypothesis of xenophobia

The scapegoating hypothesis of xenophobia states that the foreigner is used as a scapegoat, someone to blame for social ills and personal frustrations. In this way, the foreigner becomes a target for hostility and violence. Here, however, there is an implicit assumption that foreigners automatically become scapegoats. The hypothesis does not clarify why *the foreigner*, and not another social group or individual, comes to signify unemployment, poverty and deprivation. It does not explain why nationality is the determining feature of such scapegoating. In contrast, the *isolation hypothesis of xenophobia* situates foreignness at the heart of hostility towards foreigners.

The isolation hypothesis understands xenophobia as a consequence of apartheid South Africa's seclusion from the international community. Morris (1998) argues that apartheid insulated South African citizens from nationalities beyond Southern Africa. In this hypothesis, foreigners represent the unknown to South Africans. With the political transition, however, South Africa's borders have opened up and the country has become integrated into the international community. This has brought South Africans into direct contact with the unknown, with foreigners. According to the isolation hypothesis, the interface between previously isolated South Africans and unknown foreigners creates a space for hostility to develop: 'When a group has no history of incorporating strangers it may find it difficult to be welcoming' (Morris, 1998: 1125).

The isolation hypothesis suggests that suspicion and hostility towards strangers in South Africa exists due to *international* isolation. The hypothesis also explains contemporary xenophobia by recourse to *internal* isolation, the isolation of South Africans from South Africans, as a consequence of apartheid: 'There is little doubt that the brutal environment created by apartheid with its enormous emphasis on boundary maintenance has also impacted on people's ability to be tolerant of difference' (Morris, 1998: 1125).

Due to the creation of strict boundaries between South African citizens, as well as between the country and other nations, South Africans are unable to accommodate, and indeed, *tolerate* difference. According to the theory of isolation, South Africans find difference threatening and dangerous (Morris, 1998). In this theory, xenophobia exists because of the very foreignness of foreigners. It exists because foreigners are different and unknown.

Complementing the hypothesis of South African isolation is Hobsbawm's attempt to explain xenophobia in contemporary European societies. He conceptualises the phenomenon in terms of change, as something that works parallel to rapid social transition. For him, the 'old ways of life [in Europe] have changed so drastically since the 1950s that there is very little of them left to defend' (1996: 264). Because old, traditional ways of life have corroded, he argues, xenophobia, separatism and fundamentalism 'are comprehensible as symptoms of social disorientation, of the fraying, and sometimes the snapping, of the threads of what used to be the network that bound people together in society. The strength of this xenophobia is the fear of the unknown ... ' (1996: 264–5). In Hobsbawm's reading, 'xenophobia' is understood as the product of social transition, as a defence against the anxiety induced by 'the unknown'.[2] This applies directly to the isolation hypothesis, which situates xenophobia in the South African context of change and a large 'unknown world out there'. However, it must be acknowledged that this hypothesis does not explain why 'the unknown' produces anxiety and why this automatically results in aggression.

### The biocultural hypothesis of xenophobia

The isolation and scapegoating hypotheses of xenophobia provide a general explanation for the phenomenon. In the latter, foreigners are scapegoats for social ills, and the difference (or foreignness) engendered by foreigners accounts for violence and hostility. In both theories, the foreigner is treated as a homogeneous category, and there is no scope for differentiation between various types of foreigner. However, xenophobia in South Africa is not applied equally to all foreigners. Some foreigners are at greater risk than others. African foreigners seem to be particularly vulnerable to violence and hostility (Human Rights Watch, 1998; Human Rights Commission, 1999). The biocultural hypothesis of xenophobia offers an explanation for the asymmetrical targeting of African foreigners by South Africans.

The biocultural hypothesis locates xenophobia at the level of visible difference, or otherness, i.e. in terms of physical biological factors and cultural differences exhibited by African foreigners in the country. For example, Morris suggests that Nigerians and Congolese, 'are easily identifiable as the "Other". Because of their physical features, their bearing, their clothing style and their inability to speak one of the indigenous languages, they are in general clearly distinct and local residents are easily able to pick them out and scapegoat them' (1998: 1125).

In this example, Nigerian and Congolese foreigners are scapegoated due to biocultural factors such as physical appearance and the 'inability to speak one of the indigenous languages'. These factors apply to the identification of Africans from Southern Africa too. Consider, for example, the identificatory methods used by the Internal Tracing Units of the South African Police Service:

> In trying to establish whether a suspect is an illegal or not, members of the internal tracing units focus on a number of aspects. One of these is language: accent, the

pronouncement of certain words (such as Zulu for 'elbow', or 'buttonhole' or the name of a meerkat). Some are asked what nationality they are and if they reply 'Sud' African this is a dead give-away for a Mozambican, while Malawians tend to pronounce the letter 'r' as 'errow' .... Appearance is another factor in trying to establish whether a suspect is illegal – hairstyle, type of clothing worn as well as actual physical appearance. In the case of Mozambicans a dead give-away is the vaccination mark on the lower left forearm ... [while] those from Lesotho tend to wear gumboots, carry walking sticks or wear blankets (in the traditional manner), and also speak slightly different Sesotho (Minaar and Hough, 1996: 166–7).

The biological-cultural features of hairstyles, accents, vaccination marks, dress and physical appearance can be read as indexical markers or signifiers. They signify difference and point out foreignness in a way that is immediately visible. As signifiers, these features do play a common role in prompting xenophobic actions. For example, a report by the South African Human Rights Commission on the arrest and detention of persons in terms of the Aliens Control Act observes that 'at least ten percent' of the subjects[3] interviewed in the study were apprehended 'on the basis of appearance, with nothing more' (1999: xxii). Similarly, Boullion reports that for French-speaking Africans *language* is a 'handicap, as they feel hostility in the way people react when they realise their inability to speak any African South African languages .... *Dress and hair* are [also] handicaps in the context of rife street crime on the one hand and the "sniffing out" methods adopted by the Internal Tracing Units of the South African Police ... on the other hand' (1996: 10; my emphasis).

Reading physical features as signifiers of foreignness offers a valuable framework for understanding the significance of these features in xenophobic actions. Biological-cultural markers are significant in generating xenophobia because they point out *whom* to target, i.e. they indicate which particular group of foreigners the South African public dislikes and initiates violent practice against. However, *what* they signify and *how* they have come to signify this must also be explained in order to comment on reasons for xenophobia and its asymmetrical application to certain (black) foreigners. Although the visible otherness of foreign Africans seems to be an important factor behind local hostility, this is not a sufficient explanation for the asymmetrical xenophobia directed towards this group. Biological-cultural factors may stand as indexical markers of difference, but then so do the language, accent, clothing and physical features of white and Asian foreigners. This is not to suggest that these groups are automatically immune to xenophobia, but, relative to African foreigners, they do appear to be at a lower risk for violence.

While the three hypotheses discussed above offer important insights into xenophobia, they do not properly account for why the (black) foreigner – as the unknown other – evokes violence and aggression in South Africa. Similarly, unless they are read as an interconnected series of explanations, they risk presenting xenophobia as uniform or monolithic, whereas it is usually black foreigners who bear the brunt of this phenomenon. They do not allow for degrees of hostility or foreignness. Taken together, these hypotheses do not explain the 'whys' of xenophobia.

One possible way of understanding why black foreigners are targets of violence is to postulate a new hypothesis, one that situates xenophobia within South Africa's transition from a past of racism to a future of nationalism. At a most basic level, this involves looking at the role of broad social institutions, such as the media, in generating specific images of African foreigners in the country. More theoretically, this involves looking at the mechanisms of nationalism and the ways in which xenophobia itself has been represented.

## ■ Representations of Africa and African foreigners

To understand why African hairstyles, accents and vaccination marks take on xenophobic significance, i.e. why African foreigners are specific targets of violence, it is important to consider how foreign Africans are represented in society. The generalisations and stereotypes that are commonly offered regarding Africa and African immigrants offer insight into the hostility that meets this group. Consider the following media representations:

- Illegal immigrants from war-torn and poverty-stricken parts of Africa are flooding into most SA cities (*Natal Witness*, 94/11);
- In one of the biggest apartment blocks in Jo'burg, notices in English and Afrikaans have taken a second place to signs in French and Portuguese as thousands of new migrants from Africa pour into the city ... (*Sunday Times*, 93/06/06);
- Foreign influx: citizens fear for their job prospects after hordes descend on the country from the troubled north (*Sowetan*, 93/07/29);
- Xenophobia rife as Africans flood SA ... (*Sunday Times*, 94/08/28);
- City haven for victims of Africa's wars and woes (*Argus*, 97/04/26);
- As citizens of neighbouring countries flood the home affairs department with applications for legal residence ... (*Sunday Independent*, 96/09/29);
- [F]low of job-seekers from neighbouring countries (*Electronic Mail and Guardian*, 97/02/05);
- Illegals are helping to turn SA into a banana republic ... I want to say that even under the most oppressive conditions we endured under apartheid, our economic conditions were never as bad as in the rest of Africa (*Weekend Star*, 95/02/19, letter: S. Modise).

In these newspaper extracts, Africa and the foreign African are represented negatively. 'Africa' appears as a homogeneous, undifferentiated place. There is no recognition that this is a large continent consisting of many different interests and nations, including South Africa. Rather, it is seen as 'the troubled north', a vague space marked by wars, woes and poverty. In this way, South Africa is divorced from the rest of the continent. Africa appears as a negative space 'out there', totally separate from the space 'in here'. This affords an interesting link back to the scapegoating hypothesis and the notion of 'the unknown', because Africa is portrayed as a negative collective force without specific form or identity thereby representing an easy object of blame and anxiety.

Similarly, African foreigners are pictured as masses *flooding* into South Africa illegally. Words such as 'flood', 'descend' and 'pour' create the impression of an uncontrollable, unstoppable process (Sontag, 1988). Here, African foreigners are linked to chaos and disorder. They are also presented as illegal and therefore, as criminal. Peberdy suggests that

> the depiction of African migrants as 'illegals', 'illegal aliens', and 'illegal immigrants' implies both criminality and difference. The persistent use of 'illegals' to describe undocumented migrants suggests a close connection with crime and criminal acts. The SAPS [South African Police Service] also provide the number of 'illegal aliens' arrested in crime swoops, or stop and search operations. Although these figures may improve the arrest rates of the SAPS, the conflation of arrested criminals and arrested undocumented migrants creates spurious links between crime and undocumented migrants (1999: 296).

Alongside representations of criminality and illegality, the quotes from the newspapers given above also paint African foreigners as a disease or a plague descending on the country. Peberdy explains that the language of 'contamination' permeates national discourse: 'The state's negative attitudes to both immigrants and migrants is most evident ... in the ways it argues non-South Africans threaten the nation by endangering its *physical health*, its ability to provide resources, employment and levels of crime. The language of the department is replete with images of Africans as carriers of disease' (1999: 298; my emphasis).

This language expands beyond the state and the Department of Home Affairs to include the media and the public. Through the image of contamination, Peberdy suggests, the African foreigner is generated as a disease, a physical threat to the body politic. As an example of this, she highlights the ongoing HIV/AIDS scare surrounding foreign mineworkers as carriers and spreaders of the disease.

In this process, the African foreigner is represented as a physical disease that literally threatens the body politic with contamination. The African foreigner also represents a symbolic threat to the South African nation. Peberdy links the images of physical contamination and criminality to a threatened nation state:

> The focus of the state on what it sees as the parasitical relationship of non-South Africans to the nation's resources, and the way that the state criminalizes them, suggests that the state sees immigrants, and particularly undocumented migrants, as a threat to the nation and the post-1994 nation building process. The language of the state, which rarely attaches the pre-fix African, shows that it conceptualizes most immigrants as Africans, and Africans as potentially the most dangerous of all 'aliens' (1999: 296).

Peberdy makes two important points here. Firstly, she comments that foreigners in South Africa are represented as a threat to the nation. Secondly, she explains that these threatening, dangerous foreigners are African, even although this is rarely stated explicitly in public discourse.

A similar position is adopted by Morris, when he claims that 'foreign black Africans, especially those originating from countries north of South Africa's neighbours, are being portrayed as a major threat to the success of the post-apartheid project' (1998: 1117).

## ■ The post-apartheid project

The term 'post-apartheid project' is a general, blanket term that covers a range of policies, objectives and discourses in post-1994 South African society. Due to its breadth and all-encompassing nature, it can be read in a variety of ways and in relation to many aspects of society. One such way involves considering the post-apartheid project through two monolithic discourses, namely discourses of the 'New South Africa' and the 'African Renaissance'.

Broadly, a discourse of the 'New South Africa' involves concepts such as democracy, deracialisation, reconciliation and unity. Economically, it conveys notions of reconstruction, development and upliftment. Socio-politically, it is aligned with building the nation, and nationalism is a vital element of the discourse. Indeed, the 'New South Africa' is often used interchangeably with the term 'Rainbow Nation' (Durrheim, 1997; Hook and Harris, 2000). By contrast, a discourse of the 'African Renaissance' underplays national boundaries and emphasises regional and pan-African cohesion in terms of economics, culture, growth and development (cf. Makgoba, 1999).

Both discourses have economic, political and social development at their roots. However, they contradict each other at the point of nationalism. The 'New South Africa' is defined in terms of national borders, as the new nation. Nationality is a fundamental feature of this discourse and a *South African* identity prevails. In contrast, the 'African Renaissance' is defined in terms of continental borders, rather than national barriers. In this discourse, an *African* identity, and not a South African identity, predominates.

Discourses of the 'New South Africa' and the 'African Renaissance' offer but one way to describe the post-apartheid project. They are significant for this chapter because both are in common circulation and yet they contradict each other at the point of nationalism. This is important for understanding the post-apartheid phenomenon of xenophobia, particularly because it is the *African* foreigner who appears most vulnerable to hostility and violence. To understand xenophobia in relation to these discourses, it is important to introduce the way in which *xenophobia itself* has been represented in South African literature and media.

## Xenophobia as a pathology

The word 'xenophobia' describes violent actions against foreigners, as well as negative social representations of immigrants, refugees and migrants. Through the application of this word, it is possible to develop hypotheses, such as the scapegoating, isolation and biocultural hypotheses, regarding relations between South Africans and foreigners. While these hypotheses suggest certain reasons for xenophobia, they do not interrogate the term itself. That is, they accept and present the term as a given, as a neutral term of description. Contemporary language theory teaches that words and texts are not, however, neutral (Wilbraham, 1994; Fairclough, 1995). Rather, words are 'multifunctional, always simultaneously representing the world (ideational function) and enacting social relations and identities (interpersonal function)' (Fairclough, 1995: 25). In Fairclough's (1995) terms, the scapegoating, isolation and biocultural hypotheses of xenophobia function at the 'ideational' level. They engage with the phenomenon as representative and descriptive of the South African world. To better understand xenophobia, however, it is also necessary to consider the social relations and identities that are reproduced in the term itself.

Reflect on the following media representations of xenophobia:

- Cosatu and ANC are determined to stem the rising tide of xenophobia (*Mail and Guardian*, 94/09/29);
- Unknown irrational fear of 'uitlanders' is not new to SA (*Sunday Independent*, 97/05/04);
- The old laager mentality is raising its ugly head again in the form of xenophobia (*Mail and Guardian*, 95/02/09);
- Learning to cope with the irresistible human tide .... Violent public outbursts and the constant arrest-and-repatriation routine of the government illustrate the rise of a xenophobic mentality in SA and the failure of current immigration policy – rooted in a 'fortress SA' mentality – to deal with the issue (*Financial Mail*, 97/10/03);
- SA must not develop a hatred of foreigners because of the illegal immigrant problem, Acting President Thabo Mbeki said ... (*Argus*, 94/11/03);
- Alien has become almost a swearword in this country, used by xenophobes to describe those who have come to take our jobs, our homes, our women; conmen from Nigeria who've come to steal our money and feed us drugs ... (*Star*, 95/08/14);
- We did not expect national chauvinism and xenophobia as the outcome of the national liberation struggle (*Star*, 94/09/27; letter).

There are two striking features in these media headlines. Firstly, xenophobia is presented as something negative, ugly and unwanted. It is a cause of worry and concern, and it is something that must be eradicated from South African society. Secondly, xenophobia is presented in the same way as that which it denotes. This means that xenophobia, as a term, is described with the same language and images that are used to describe foreigners in xenophobic language. Indeed the word 'xenophobia' is easily substitutable for the word 'foreigner' in many of these representations. For example, a xenophobic portrayal of the foreigner reads as 'stemming the tide of illegals', while a depiction of xenophobia itself reads as 'stemming the tide of xenophobia'. There are close parallels between the xenophobic depiction of foreigners and the depiction of xenophobia *per se*.

Just as African foreigners are criminalised and tainted, so xenophobia is presented as a contaminant in South African society. It appears as an unstoppable and irrational fear or plague, sweeping across the country. Through metaphors of disease, floods and the laager mentality, xenophobia is pathologised. That is, it is represented as a pathology, as something abnormal and unhealthy. This notion of pathology is strengthened by the phonetic confusion of xenophobia with the psychological phobias. The suffix 'phobia' is regularly used in the *Diagnostic and Statistical Manual of Mental Disorders* (4th edition) (DSM-IV) by psychology and medical practitioners (American Psychiatric Association (APA), 1994). In this manual, a range of anxiety-depression disorders are listed under the phobias, e.g. agoraphobia, social phobia, and simple phobias such as claustrophobia and arachnophobia. A psychological 'phobia' is diagnosed if exposure to the object of phobia results in 'intense anxiety' (APA, 1994). Xenophobia, as a violent practice, does not have the characteristics of psychological phobias. Yet, although it is not listed in DSM-IV, it has the phonetic potential to be associated with the phobias, as a psychological pathology (V. Dutton, 1999; personal communication).

Xenophobia is portrayed as something abnormal and unhealthy: in other words, it is presented as something separate from the normal, healthy South African nation. In the light of such a position, I would like to speculate on the political interests that are served by treating xenophobia as a pathology. For example, it is important in light of the 'New South Africa' discourse. This discourse privileges concepts of tolerance, harmony and diversity. Although it rests on national barriers, it does not entertain intolerance, violence or chauvinism. Consequently, the hostile practice of xenophobia finds no place in this discourse. By pathologising xenophobia, the phenomenon is effectively quarantined from the healthy 'New South Africa'; it is isolated from the ideals that comprise the discourse. Similarly, the pathologising of xenophobia serves the 'African Renaissance' discourse. This discourse underplays nationalism and does not allow for hostility towards African foreigners. As a pathology, xenophobia is neatly separated from the healthy objectives of the 'African Renaissance'.

It is postulated that the pathologisation of xenophobia serves to disguise the implicit contradiction that exists at the point of nationalism between the 'New South Africa', on the one hand and the 'African Renaissance', on the other hand. Xenophobia, and not this implicit contradiction, stands as *the* obstacle to realising national ideals, including the ideal of the African Renaissance. This makes it possible for an 'African Renaissance' to co-exist with a nation-building project. It also makes it possible for an 'African Renaissance' discourse to exist while African foreigners are being victimised through xenophobia.

As a pathology, xenophobia is portrayed as a major threat to the success of the post-apartheid project. It is a scapegoat for the intolerance and disunity that threatens the health of the nation. It is represented as a disease and something that must be cured in order for the 'New South Africa' and the 'African Renaissance' to function in harmony. But what if xenophobia is not as easily separable from the strategies and practices that reproduce the 'New South Africa'? What if xenophobia is implicit to the technologies that create South African nationalism?

Wetherell and Potter proclaim that 'patriotism and pride are the "positive" face, and xenophobia and chauvinism the unacceptable face of nationalism' (1992: 141). Here, xenophobia is conceptualised directly in relation to nationalism, and is seen as one side of a nationalism coin.[4] This argument is important because it ties xenophobia to the process of nation-building; it interprets xenophobia as a negative consequence of nationalism and nation-building (1992). As such, xenophobia is not totally divorced from national processes and discourses, as the previous hypotheses have done. However, because they separate the positive face from the negative face of nationalism, Wetherell and Potter (1992) cannot escape the pathologising of xenophobia. It is still seen as negative, unhealthy and different from the positive, healthy functioning of a nation. This approach does not allow for the possibility that xenophobia is part of the 'New South Africa', rather than a parasitic pathology or a negative consequence of nation-building. Such a possibility must, however, be entertained, as the following section on South Africa's culture of violence reveals.

## South Africa's culture of violence

By presenting xenophobia as negative and abnormal, a contrasting comment is made on the normal functioning of the nation. In the South African context, the normal society is *not*, however, divorced from violence. A solid body of research highlights what has been termed South Africa's 'culture of violence' (Simpson *et al.*, 1992; Hamber, 1997; Hamber and Lewis, 1997). The culture of violence can be described as a situation in which social relations and interactions are governed through violent, rather than non-violent, means. This is a culture in which violence is proffered as a normal, legitimate solution to problems: 'violence is seen as a legitimate means to achieve goals particularly because it was legitimised by most political role-players in the past' (Hamber and Lewis, 1997: 8).

The culture of violence is a legacy of apartheid. It finds its roots in the 1980s, when violence was predominantly political in nature, i.e. 'where the dominant motivation [for violence was] based on political difference or the competing desire for political power' (Simpson *et al.*, 1992: 202). During this period, violence was utilised and sanctioned across the political spectrum (Hamber, 1997). The politics of the 1980s effectively laid the foundation for an ongoing culture of violence in the 1990s. According to analysts, the form of violence has altered across this period. Hamber explains that 'whilst levels of political violence have generally dropped ... the transition has been characterised by dramatic increases in violent crime' (1997: 3). Hence, violence today is described as criminal rather than political in nature. So, although the form of violence may have altered across time, violence itself still persists as the dominant means to solve problems in South Africa. It is in this context of a culture of violence that xenophobia in South Africa must be conceptualised.

Despite the pervasiveness of South Africa's culture of violence, it is ironic that xenophobia has been represented as something abnormal or pathological. Xenophobia *is* a form of violence and violence *is* the norm in South Africa. Violence is an integral part of the social fabric, even although the 'New South Africa' discourse belies this. Indeed, by belying and excluding xenophobia, the 'New South Africa' discourse is able to define itself as peaceful and tolerant. It is similarly able to co-exist with the 'African Renaissance' discourse and to perpetuate ideals of harmony and diversity. But in order to do this, it is necessary that xenophobia is created and represented as a pathology. Consequently, xenophobia as a pathology is central to national discourse. It must be recognised as part of the new nation, and is not separate from the 'New South Africa', even although it is pathologised within and by the discourse. It is also not a negative consequence of nationalism. Rather, it functions within the culture of violence to give definition to the 'New South Africa' and the forms of identity that accompany this discourse. Xenophobia can thus be understood as a central feature of nationalism. This point is borne out by looking at the experiences that black foreigners have had in South Africa, which suggest that xenophobic violence is an integral feature of their daily lives here.

## ■ Migrant voices

Sinclair's (1998, 1999) work engages with the impact of xenophobia on foreign identity in post-apartheid South Africa. Drawing on interviews with seventy-seven African foreigners, she notes that 'hostility towards foreigners has become one of the most significant features of post-apartheid South African society' (1999: 466). Hostility and abuse are reported throughout her sample, spanning a range of institutions and interactions, from the police and the Department of Home Affairs to employers and neighbours. She comments that 'All migrants interviewed mentioned hostility towards them as their over-riding concern; surpassing even issues of legal status, job security and financial difficulty' (1999: 471).

As a consequence of this hostility, social networks and support structures have developed among non-South Africans during the post-apartheid era. Sinclair (1998, 1999) explains that these communities have been established largely along national lines, and do not span nationality divisions. Rather, they exist as discrete networks, representing particular nationalities, such as 'Nigerians', 'Angolans' and 'Mozambicans'. These local communities have developed as safe havens and comfort zones for migrants.

Company and mutual protection, rather than long-term assimilation, are the central criteria for these local migrant communities. There is no permanence or long-term stability about them. Indeed, the element of transience impacts directly on foreign identities here and this, Sinclair explains, is a direct response to xenophobia. For many migrants 'permanence has become untenable, given the realities of the harsh life in South Africa' (1999: 471).

South African hostility encourages foreigners to leave South Africa, and to feel impermanent while living here. Another response to xenophobia is that of resentment and hostility on the part of foreign migrants: 'Many migrants respond with anger and indignation [to the hostility that they face]' (Sinclair, 1999: 469). Morris notes this from Nigerians and Congolese living in South Africa: 'the antagonism and prejudice experienced has resulted in an unfortunate cycle. It has encouraged a strong sense of nationhood among the Congolese and Nigerian immigrants .... The harsh treatment has also encouraged a tendency to view South Africans as the inferior "Other"' (1998: 1126).

He comments further that South Africans are viewed through negative stereotypes. Besides the feeling that South Africans are prejudiced and parochial, a prominent perception was that South Africans, especially black South African men, are extremely violent: 'Informants often depicted South African men as lazy, adulterous and not nurturing of their partners .... Often, laziness and crime were interlinked .... South Africans were portrayed as unenterprising and wasteful ... poorly educated and ignorant' (Morris, 1998: 1127–8). In contrast, Morris' respondents portrayed themselves as hard-working, enterprising, caring, educated and cultured (1998).

It must be recognised that responses to xenophobia may manifest in hostility, and possibly violence, from foreigners themselves. Indeed, the potential for violence rests within the *actions and interactions* that develop at the point of national identity. Morris comments that identity is caught up in a cyclical and complex relationship at the border of nationality: 'The Nigerians and Congolese interviewed generally exuded self-confidence and were often disparaging about the local Africans. There is little doubt that this combination further alienates the local black population from them' (1998: 1126).

Ironically, the experience of hostility may generate further hostility through the deployment of coping strategies such as isolation, superiority and bitterness. As Kristeva comments, 'just because one is a foreigner does not mean one is without one's own foreigner .... As enclave of the other within the other, otherness becomes crystallized as pure ostracism: the foreigner excludes before being excluded, even more than he is being excluded' (1991: 24).

Exclusion, alienation and hostility operate in a complex, ongoing spiral across the line of nationality, i.e. between South Africans and foreigners, particularly African foreigners. Studies such as those conducted by Sinclair (1998, 1999) and Morris (1998) reveal that xenophobia impacts directly on foreign identity. It cannot be separated from the normal foreign individual in South Africa. Through xenophobia, foreigners feel foreign. This effect, in turn, alienates and excludes foreigners further from South African society. It also contributes to foreign hostility, and possibly violence, towards South Africans. This understanding of the impact of xenophobia on identity, together with the culture of violence that pervades ordinary South African life, suggests that xenophobia is not the pathology it is represented to be. Rather, it is a key component of the 'New South African' nation. To read xenophobia as a pathology is to contest traditional, normal understandings of psychopathology. It is not individually located and is not counter-normative, but rather operates through the social, for the social, serving to disguise relations of power and discursive contradictions. It is for these very reasons that such a reading is valuable, as its seeming incongruence with psychopatholgy highlights the subtle ways in which certain pathologies are problems of political control, representing the failure of regulatory systems to fully govern particular aspects of the individual.

At the level of the social, instead of accepting xenophobia as something abnormal and separate from the ideals of nationalism, it is vital to interrogate *why* it has been represented in this light. It is also crucial to uncover *what* such pathologisation does in order to understand the consequences of seeking a cure. This is particularly important in light of the inherent contradiction between the 'New South Africa' and 'African Renaissance' discourses at the point of nationalism. While contemporary emphasis is on stabilising the continent and bringing peace to the region, Billig reminds us that 'it should be remembered that violence is seldom far from the surface of nationalism's history. The struggle to create the nation-state is a struggle for the monopoly of the means of violence. What is being created – a nation-state – is itself a means of violence. The triumph of a particular nationalism is seldom achieved without the defeat of alternative nationalisms and other ways of imagining peoplehood' (1995: 28).

# ▪ Endnotes

1 The word '*makwerekwere*' is derogatory. It purportedly depicts the phonetic sound of foreign African languages.
2 The psychoanalytic overtones of this interpretation are apparent. And while Hobsbawm's (1996) work attempts to draw on 'social' dynamics, he ultimately cannot escape the level of the 'individual' in his explanations of xenophobia.
3 The subjects in question were 149 detainees at Lindela.
4 'Nationalism' is a hotly debated concept. A vast field is dedicated to defining and critiquing the term (cf. Bjorgo and Witte, 1993; Billig, 1995; Reitzes, 1995). For the purposes of this

literature review, 'nationalism is identified as the ideology that creates and maintains nation-states' (Billig, 1995: 19). It is tied directly to the process of nation-building that marks the 'New South Africa' discourse and is generated through the everyday practices that constitute the nation.

# References

American Psychiatric Association (1994). *Diagnostic and Statistical Manual of Mental Disorders* (4th edn). Washington, DC: American Psychiatric Association.
Billig, M. (1995). *Banal Nationalism*. London: Sage.
Bjorgo, T. and Witte, R. (1993). Introduction. In T. Bjorgo and R. Witte (eds), *Racist Violence in Europe*, pp. 1–16. Basingstoke: Macmillan.
Boullion, A. (1996). 'New' African immigration to South Africa. Unpublished paper presented at the Conference of the South African Sociological Association, Durban, 7–11 July.
De la Rey, C. (1991). Intergroup relations: Theories and positions. In D. Foster and J. Louw-Potgieter (eds), *Social Psychology in South Africa*, pp. 27–56. Isando: Lexicon.
Durrheim, K. (1997). Peace talk and violence: An analysis of the power of 'peace'. In A. Levett, A. Kottler, E. Buman and I. Parker (eds), *Culture, Power and Difference: Discourse Analysis in South Africa*, pp. 31–43. Cape Town: University of Cape Town Press.
Fairclough, N. (1995). *Media Discourse*. New York: Edward Arnold.
Hamber, B. (1997). Dr Jekyll and Mr 'Hide': Problems of violence prevention and reconciliation in South Africa's transition to democracy. In E. Bornman, R. van Eeden and M. Wentzel (eds), *Perspectives on Aggression and Violence in South Africa*, pp. 3–20. Pretoria: Human Sciences Research Council.
Hamber, B. and Lewis, S. (1997). *An Overview of the Consequences of Violence and Trauma in South Africa*. Johannnesburg: Centre for the Study of Violence and Reconciliation.
Hobsbawm, E. J. (1996). Ethnicity and nationalism in Europe today. In G. Balakrishnan (ed.), *Mapping the Nation*, pp. 255–66. London: Verso.
Hook, D. and Harris, B. (2000). Discourses of order and their disruption: The texts of the South African Truth and Reconciliation Commission. *South African Journal of Psychology*, 30 (1), 14–22.
Human Rights Commission (1999). *Report on the Arrest and Detention of Persons in Terms of the Aliens Control Act*. Johannesburg: South African Human Rights Commission.
Human Rights Watch (1998). *'Prohibited Persons': Abuse of Undocumented Migrants, Asylum Seekers, and Refugees in South Africa*. New York: Human Rights Watch.
Kollapan, J. (1999). Xenophobia in South Africa: The challenge to forced migration. Unpublished seminar, Graduate School, University of the Witwatersrand, 7 October.
Kristeva, J. (1991). *Strangers to Ourselves*. New York: Columbia University Press.
Makgoba, M. W. (ed.) (1999). *African Renaissance: The New Struggle*. Cape Town: Tafelberg.
Minaar, A. and Hough, M. (1996). *Causes, Extent and Impact of Clandestine Migration in Selected Southern African Countries with Specific Reference to South Africa*. Pretoria: Human Sciences Research Council.
Morris, A. (1998). 'Our fellow Africans make our lives hell': The lives of Congolese and Nigerians living in Johannesburg. *Ethnic and Racial Studies*, 21 (6), 1116–36.
Peberdy, S. A. (1999). Selecting immigrants: Nationalism and national identity in South Africa's immigration policies, 1910–1998. Unpublished doctoral thesis, Queens University, Canada.
Reitzes, M. (1995). *The Reconstruction of Citizenship in South Africa*. Johannesburg: Centre for Policy Studies.
Simpson, G., Mokwena, S. and Segal, L. (1992). Political violence: 1990. In M. Robertson and A. Rycroft (eds), *Human Rights and Labour Law Handbook 1991*, Vol. 2, pp. 193–219. Cape Town: Oxford University Press.
Sinclair, M. R. (1998). Community, identity and gender in migrant societies of southern Africa: Emerging epistemological challenges. *International Affairs*, 74 (2), 339–53.

Sinclair, M. R. (1999). 'I know a place that is softer than this ...' – emerging migrant communities in South Africa. *International Migration*, 37 (2), 465–81.
Sontag, S. (1988). *AIDS and its Metaphors*. Harmondsworth: Penguin.
*South African Pocket Oxford Dictionary of Current English* (1994). Cape Town: Oxford University Press.
Tshitereke, C. (1999). Xenophobia and relative deprivation. *Crossings*, 3 (2), 4–5.
Wetherell, M. and Potter, J. (1992). *Mapping the Language of Racism: Discourse and the Legitimation of Exploitation*. Hemel Hempstead: Harvester Wheatsheaf.
Wilbraham, L. A. (1994). Confession, surveillance and subjectivity: A discourse analytic approach to advice columns. Unpublished masters dissertation, University of Cape Town.

# CHAPTER 10
# Stigma in the social construction of sexually transmitted diseases

*Kopano Ratele & Tamara Shefer*

## ■ Introduction

Sexually transmitted diseases (STDs) are one of the most enduring health issues in South Africa. Despite what are now recognised as their alarming social, medical and economic costs, STDs have, historically, been largely neglected as a public-health matter, until, that is, the local and international emergence of HIV/AIDS. Empirical evidence of a link between STDs and HIV/AIDS has lead to a greater focus on the classic sexually transmitted infections (Laga *et al.*, 1991; Legion, 1992; Wasserheit, 1992; National AIDS Research Programme of the Medical Research Council, 1993). This link has elevated the profile of other STDs, and has pointed to the urgency of the need to speak more about sexuality generally, and safe sex in particular and, perhaps most urgently, about efforts to control the spread of all STDs, specifically HIV/AIDS. The need to stem the tide of sexually transmitted infection is all the more urgent given the recent figures pertaining to contraction of STDs in South Africa. This country is believed to have one of the highest infection prevalence rates of 'classic' STDs in the world (Buve *et al.*, 1993; Block and Dehaeck, 1987; Leiman, 1976). Though no rigorous national surveillance studies on the prevalence or incidence of these types of STDs have been conducted to date, estimates are that about 4 000 000 episodes of STDs occur yearly (Pham-Kanter *et al.*, 1996). In respect of HIV/AIDS, South Africa is considered to have the fastest-growing epidemic in the world (Department of Health, Directorate of HIV/AIDS and STDs, 1996). A survey of HIV sero-prevalence in antenatal public-health facilities estimated that 22.8% of women attending these clinics were HIV-infected at the end of 1998, a 33.8% national increase in the prevalence rates from 1997 (Pham-Kanter *et al.*, 1996).

One of the reasons why STDs, including HIV/AIDS, remain a major health problem in South Africa is that despite the recent upsurge of sexual education there continues to be widespread lack of knowledge, resistance, lack of understanding, or popular misconceptions regarding the aetiology and epidemiology of STDs. The same reasons go for control and preventative measures to use against sexually transmitted infections. A part explanation for this is the conservatism of large segments of the population, which has meant that open and frank talk on sexuality in general and STDs specifically continue to be taboo in many South African communities. Furthermore, it is clear that the stigmatisation of STDs, particularly HIV/AIDS, is still very central in the social construction of these illnesses and necessarily acts as an inhibiting factor in respect of seeking health care. Given such a context, it is not surprising that tackling STDs, both in terms of prevention and treatment, is then still an uphill battle, as the problem continues to be marginalised (McNiel, 1999).

## The social construction of STDs

An exploration of the social construction of STDs cannot be viewed outside the way in which HIV/AIDS has been constructed over the last two decades. While HIV/AIDS may have its own unique set of constructions, these constructions might usefully be used as a way of informing the social construction of 'other' STDs. Despite that it may seem an obvious point, it is worth reiterating the fact that social constructions of AIDS powerfully reflect dominant aspects of current social contexts, in particular norms and constraints with respect to sexuality. Weeks sums up:

> AIDS has become the symbolic bearer of a host of meanings about our contemporary culture: about its social composition, its racial boundaries, its attitudes to social marginality; and above all, its moral configurations and its sexual mores. A number of different histories intersect in and are condensed by AIDS discourse. What gives AIDS a particular power is its ability to represent a host of fears, anxieties and problems in our current post-permissive society (1989: 2).

Plummer (1988) describes two central discourses operating in the construction of AIDS, one that is overtly medical and scientific, and one that is characterised by social and moral meanings. Both no doubt also play a large role in the broader social construction of STDs. The first and most dominant of these is a medicalising discourse, which constructs AIDS as an epidemic, with powerful notions of illness, plague and death. Central to this discourse are military metaphors such as notions of invasion and battle (cf. Brandt, 1988; Sontag, 1988). These are images that are powerfully evident in the media, and that serve to create an emotional context of fear, anxiety and panic (Kitzinger and Miller, 1991; Patton, 1990; Watney, 1987; Wellings, 1988).

The second central means of stigmatising HIV/AIDS, following Plummer (1988), relies on those discourses, historically familiar, within the realm of STDs, centring around moralistic and punitive social constructions of sexuality. As was the case in the history of syphilis, 'AIDS was seen as the result of sexually excessive and degenerate individual behaviour, which originated among aliens' (Strebel, 1993: 17). This 'othering' process had much to do with the way in which the first cases of HIV/AIDS were identified *amongst gay men* in the USA; this was a categorical association that fuelled homophobia and contributed immeasurably to the pathologisation of homosexuality. The fact that it was gay men who were infected allowed for the reproduction of the stigmatisation of homosexuality more broadly, with gay men constructed as sexually promiscuous, and traditional notions of homosexuality as inherently deviant and pathological, both in practice and consequence (Patton, 1990; Plummer, 1988; Treichler, 1987). Such constructions served to distance the illness from heterosexuals and facilitated a process of 'othering' that was reinforced by the spread of HIV to other 'deviants', including sex workers and drug users (Gilman, 1988; Holland *et al.*, 1990). HIV-stigmatising discourses quickly incorporated racist discourses too, as the illness began emerging among minorities in the USA and then quickly reaching large numbers in Africa, accompanied by racist 'othering' notions such as the claim of the virus originating in Africa and the reinforcement of the old racist link between promiscuity and blackness (Kitzinger and Miller, 1991; Sabatier, 1988; Sontag, 1988).

Arguably, much of the progress that had been made with respect to the liberalisation of sexuality and sexual practices by the late 1900s suffered a major regression with the 'moral panic' that ensued following the emergence of HIV/AIDS. Theorists argue that 'new permissive' discourses on sexuality were viewed as a threat to the nuclear family and 'traditional' values and moralities. It is not surprising, then, that the stigmatising discourses on HIV/AIDS, and probably STDs more broadly, were seized on and served to destabilise any ground won by those outside of the narrow constraints of heterosexist traditional norms and practices of sexuality. In this way, one might suggest that the stigmatising discourses that frame STDs emerged most powerfully in the realm of HIV/AIDS, and function to serve as a powerful constraint on an open expression and practice of diverse 'sexualities'. The historic stigmatisation and pathologisation of forms of sexuality lying outside of the normalising realm of the nuclear, monogamous, heterosexual dyad are hence given a powerful boost by the currently popularised talk of STDs, with the spectre of AIDS serving all the while as 'divine' proof of and retribution for subversive sexualities.

## ■ The study

The work arises out of a 1999 national study commissioned by the National Department of Health on factors influencing those seeking help with and treatment for STDs in South African communities. The study, conducted over slightly more than a year, involved a team of seven researchers and numerous fieldworkers, working in diverse communities across four provinces of South Africa: the Eastern Cape, Mpumalanga, the North West and the Western Cape. The focus of the larger study was on four inter-related categories: general perceptions of STDs (knowledge, attitudes, beliefs); sexual behaviour; health-care-seeking behaviour for STDs; and the quality of care received when treated for an STD at a primary health-care clinic. That study incorporated a variety of methods, quantitative and qualitative, along with multiple modes of data-gathering and analysis. This particular chapter is a qualitative analysis of 10 focus groups working with community members across the four provinces. Participants for the groups were recruited with the help of local contacts and were self-selecting. Although there was some attempt to target those more 'at risk', which included groups such as mineworkers, sexworkers, youth and male prisoners, it is important to emphasise that these group discussions do not represent statistically the views of all South Africans, or even those of all South African mineworkers, sexworkers, youth or male prisoners.

Given the widespread acknowledgement that knowledge of the nature, causes and ways of controlling STDs does not necessarily or readily translate into safer sex practices, it has become especially important to study specifically *how meaning is constructed* in respect of STDs, HIV/AIDS and sexuality more broadly. Grasping these constructions as closely as possible might afford us something of an explanation as to why people do not practise safer sex, even when they have the necessary knowledge of why and how to do so. In the South African context, this focus on constructions of meaning has been increasingly implemented through qualitative studies on sexuality, especially among groups believed to be at greatest risk (for example, Abdool Karim *et al.*, 1992; Buga *et al.*, 1996; National Progressive Primary Health Care Network, 1995;

Shefer, 1999; Strebel, 1993; Wood and Foster, 1995; Wood and Jewkes, 1998; Wood *et al.*, 1996; Varga and Makubalo, 1996). This chapter is primarily concerned with the kinds of discourses participants drew on to talk about and explain STDs. More specifically yet, this chapter is concerned with how participants constructed the prospective *causes, controls and treatments* of STDs.

Through participants' talk, it became abundantly clear that the overriding construction of these illnesses was one of stigmatisation and pathologisation. This type of construction operated at a number of levels, and ultimately served to inhibit both the prevention and treatment of sexually transmitted infections. Such discourses were in evidence not only in the way in which participants constructed the causes and effects of STDs, but also, and perhaps more worryingly, in the ways in which participants discussed preventative and curative interventions. Particularly striking were the ways in which female sexuality and physiology were viewed as inherently pathological. The sexuality of men, by contrast, was not viewed in such overtly pathologising or problematising terms. In fact, both males and females posited (other) female bodies and behaviours to be integrally related to, or lying at the root of, the onset and spread of STDs.

## The construction of STDs

Stigmatising, pathologising and 'othering' discourses were omnipresent in the ways in which participants spoke about what it meant to have an STD. It was clear that there were very powerful stigmas attached to having an STD, with those inflicted almost inevitably constructed as 'other' and/or deviant in some or other respect. In particular, the popular association of STDs with sexual promiscuity was very strong:

I: Are there certain types of people who are prone to have STDs?
P: Yes there are. These are the people who are promiscuous. If a person has one partner the likelihood of getting STDs is very slim (Butterworth prisoners).

P1: I think one gets this problem when one comes into contact with a wrong person. A person who sleeps around and that kind of thing ... .
P2: So, like people who do it for money. They come into contact with many people and when one comes into sexual contact with them, one may get this problem from dirty blood (Rustenberg mineworkers).

Generally, typical and stereotyped perceptions of, and attitudes towards, STDs were used as a means of distancing those without such diseases from the likelihood of contracting them. This strategy of distancing appeared as an integral part of stigmatisation. Stigmatisation of STDs has been described as a primitive reaction to disease that divides people into mutually exclusive categories of 'us' and 'them'. Other well-worn discursive strategies that were part of this process, and that lead to the same outcome, were discrimination, stereotyping and scapegoating (Gilmore and Somerville, 1994). When the prevalence of an infection is increased in a minority group, a marginalised community or an already stigmatised community, they were likely to be singled out as the object of a stereotyping/stigmatising response in relation to the infection. The most pervasive form of stigma label associated with STD was one of 'promiscuity'. This included images of sexual licentiousness, prostitution, immorality and sexual 'dirtiness'.

By contrast, participants *who were* sufferers of STDs, expressed emotions of humiliation, fear and discomfort in relation to having contracted such a disease. These emotions evidentially acted to inhibit the help-seeking behaviour of these participants, as shown in the following excerpts:

> I: [H]ow did you feel about going to the hospital?
> P: Well I at first, I did not like the idea. I just did not feel like telling anyone about it because I was embarrassed.
> I: Why were you embarrassed? If I recall clearly, when one has a sore hand they can easily go to the hospital. So what was the problem then?
> P: I was just scared but then when I saw it becoming worse I knew it was going to cause complications (Butterworth prisoners).

> P: But then you also get people, the girls... that are shy.... Mmm and they walk around with the disease as they are too shy to go to the doctor (Western Cape sexworkers).

Euphemistic and distorting labelling practices were commonly used to highlight the stigmatisation and discomfort associated with STDs:

> I: So ... are there particular words they give to people who have STD?
> P1: Ja, there are, if Phindi is having STD and tells one that she has this illness and she also tells Nomhle, they will call her PZZ, there is a name they use, PZZ.
> P2: (*laughs*)
> P1: 'Phindi *Zifo Zonke*' ('Phindi All Diseases').
> (*laughter*)
> P1: SZZ, you will hear them calling you 'all diseases'.
> (*several voices at once*)
> P2: This makes difficulty even to share this with your friends that you've got this illness because of the labels they give to people (Standerton volunteer healthworkers).

> P1: Or they call [you an] 'HIV case' ..... They do not call you with your name, they do not take you as human being they name you 'the case' (Standerton volunteer healthworkers).

Both of these quotes illustrate the way in which STDs and HIV were given obfuscatory labels. Rather than protecting the patient, these labels served to dehumanise and objectify them, frequently, and understandably, creating discomfort around disclosure. Some of the labels for STDs functioned to highlight the negative construction of these illnesses as dirty, such as the popular term '*vuilsiekte*' (Afrikaans for 'dirty illness') and the common notion of 'dirty blood'. Another example of the negative construction of STDs emerges in the following quote that associates STDs with negative emotions, such as volatile moods and aggression:

> P: I notice that my attitude was no longer the same. I was aggressive, tense and so on. And then I realised that I had to go to the clinic (Mossel Bay community group).

In general, it was felt that there was much secrecy surrounding sexually transmitted diseases, on the part of both community and professional healthworkers:

> P: ... I can tell you in Zulu that these diseases are not known and they are secretive ... even the doctors are not telling them (White River church group).

> P: People are not open about this sex, about this sickness ... people are very secretive (Western Cape sexworkers).

The last quote highlights the way in which the repression of sexuality more broadly impacts on attitudes towards STDs. Similarly:

> P: Nowadays people are taught in the rural areas about safe sex which was ... never done before ... you mustn't speak about sex, you mustn't speak about periods. No man must hear that you got your periods ... not even your friends .... It was something very secret and when we were sick we are given herbs, not taken to a doctor (Western Cape sexworkers).

Frequently, a cultural discourse was used to explain the secrecy surrounding sexuality:

> P: It's because we blacks ... like us women, we don't want openness with our children. We don't allow them that space and they grow up with a notion that there is a need for secrecy. If there's an issue, it's mine alone (Katlehong residents group).

> P: I think another thing is this, in our culture ... there are certain things I mean that you don't say ... in our culture we are not talking, we are not talking openly about sex (University of the Western Cape (UWC) female students).

Discourses of culture emerged regularly in the study, especially in relation to talking about sex and gender. These discourses usually served to legitimate certain practices, such as male power in relationships and society (Shefer, 1999; Shefer et al., 1999). Furthermore, such discourses served to reproduce and reify certain cultural notions in an ahistorical and determinist manner. This recourse to discourses of culture also often acted to privilege historically dominant cultures over marginalised and oppressed groups.

Participants often spoke about the difficulties in being honest about having an STD in a community, and about the ways in which those with STDs became stigmatised and alienated from the community, for example:

> P: I think what causes the problem is – if say a certain man has this kind of a problem, he will of course think of tell[ing] friends about it. But the problem is that one tends to think that if you tell one of your friends about this problem he will go about telling others that Mr so-and-so has this kind of problem. So this thing will spread ... (Rustenberg mineworkers).

While the stigmatisation of STD patients was spoken about throughout the groups, it was also evident that there were gender differences in the way in which STDs were perceived and experienced. Frequently STDs appeared to be constructed in more positive ways for men, with the occurrence of such an illness seen as representative of successful masculinity. For men, an STD may therefore have been seen as a source of pride or a proof of their masculinity, rather than a humiliation:

*P1:* With men, let me speak [on] behalf of men, with men we do really not hide. If I have, maybe gonorrhoea I will go to men and say, 'Hey men, I've got gonorrhoea can you try me an *imbiza*?' Then men will refer me to a traditional healer, then they will cure me, it is easy with us, we can talk, with women, it is where the stigma lies to … is mostly with women, with men no … .

*P2:* And a man … can have pride to call other men to look at his penis if it is sore, a man has guts to do that but [this is not the case] with women … (Standerton volunteer healthworkers).

This experience was in line with the popular construction of masculinity as driven by inherent sexual urges, what has been termed the 'male sexual drive' in the literature on heterosexuality (Hollway, 1989). Male sexuality was explained as follows:

*P1:* Is there a guy who does not want sex? … If you want to buy a shoe what do you do? … You do not look for the size … .

*P3:* You try it on … .

*P1:* I mean, let us look here … let us not betray each other. The real fact is that women will always be women, let's put it like that … .

*P4:* Men will be always men (Standerton volunteer healthworkers).

For women, the stigma of having contracted an STD was far more derogatory, far more demeaning and far more indicative of 'loose' or questionable morals. Such discourses appear to have emerged out of the gendered construction of sexuality, i.e. out of the system of double standards that has been applied to male and female promiscuity, where men are frequently rewarded for active sexuality, whereas women, by contrast, are punished and stigmatised. There are many examples of this:

*P1:* I do not think that we can interpret [the sexuality of men and women] … in the same way … they will think that Jabu [as a man] has a right … with the woman [but] she will be seen as having no right. The woman deserves what she has [that is an STD], but Jabu, in a case with Jabu they will … [interpret] it differently in different communities … .

*P2:* I have seen that women and men are given different names, the other [the woman] is seen as sleeping around and deserves to get illness because of behaving in that way, but if it is a man … [that] person will be seen differently … .

*P3:* Er … in other words, the woman would be called prostitute, bitch. A male will be called 'a man' so the issue is with man … . We … as men, we undergo this disease and finish up the course … but women do not [leave behind this stigmatising experience] … they are insulted although we have the same illness, gonorrhoea (Standerton volunteer healthworkers).

STDs were constructed as basically 'female' illnesses, and were as such blamed on women, particularly in the view of male participants, who generally maintained that women were responsible for starting and spreading them:

*P:* It's mostly women who commonly have these STDs. You do talk to your partner, but sometimes they don't listen. The thing is what they have is like compost – you do not really know what's happening (Butterworth prisoners).

## The construction of cause

While some participants appeared to be familiar with relatively accurate understandings of STDs – at least with reference to their underlying causes – there were still many areas of mystification, confusion and distortion surrounding such accounts. Participants' understandings of the causes of STDs further highlight the way in which these illnesses were negatively constructed in communities. For a number of participants, popular non-medical explanations were expressed alongside medical explanations. Causative accounts were often constructed as mystical and extra-human, or were imbued with supernatural explanations:

> I: Okay, are there any other ways of contracting STDs beside having had sex with an infected person?
> P: Yes, there things like pubic lice which are seen as STD but these come through bewitchment. I agree you can get them through your partner but the main cause is bewitchment (Butterworth prisoners).

As we have mentioned, there was a common perception that women were at the root of, and therefore to blame for, STDs, for example:

> I: Okay, how did you get this Drop and what did you do?
> P1: I got it from my girlfriend. I'm not sure as to what really happened but as soon as I noticed there was something wrong, I went to the hospital.
> I: Gentlemen, as you hear, he says it's his girlfriend; how does one really get Drop?
> P2: You get it through having sexual intercourse with a girl who is not clean on the inside (Butterworth prisoners).

> P: A woman can get this kind of a problem from a man, but it is rare. It is rare, really. Usually this kind of problems are gotten from women (Rustenberg mineworkers).

The construction of woman as being to blame for STDs appeared to centre around their particular physiology, typically constructed by men as inherently prone to illness and as a 'fertile ground' for infection, hence one participant's comment that 'like compost – you do not really know what's happening'. This pathologisation of women's bodies has been well documented in feminist literature and is powerfully evident in contemporary society through a range of discourses on the female body as enacted through the mass media (cf. Wood, 1997). Some of these include the pathologisation of the reproductive capacities of women, such as the construction of PMT and menopause as diseases (Greer, 1992; Richmond-Abbot, 1992; Tavris, 1992). This pathologisation is continued in the overall scrutiny of women's bodies through stringent bodily regimes to achieve idealised (yet largely unattainable) images of femininity (Bartky, 1990; Coward, 1984). Northrup, for example, suggests that there is a strong contemporary belief in the 'fact' that there is something basically 'wrong' with women's bodies. As she asserts: 'Women are socialised to think that their bodies are essentially dirty – requiring constant surveillance for "freshness" so that we don't "offend"' (1995: 10). Several of the participants within the study reiterated such discourses of the 'pathological female body', typically accusing women of not keeping themselves 'clean' enough. Quite clearly here, the sexual physiology of women was constructed as dirty, and as particularly prone to infection:

> P: I believe it's females who cause these STDs. You find that the person only wipes the vagina instead of washing properly. This then resembles bread with mould ... [hence] the charges ... of uncleanliness (Butterworth prisoners).

Another of the frequent reasons given for women's responsibility for STDs centred around their use of 'potions' to increase male pleasure, specifically by creating the pretence of virginity and/or a 'tighter', dry vagina. Some of the substances that were frequently mentioned included Zambuk, snuff and various 'cleansing' pills (such as laxatives). For some, any medication taken by a woman was viewed as potentially responsible for the creation of an STD:

> P1: Maybe Jabu has sex with [his] ... girlfriend and the girlfriend is not having another affair ... is honest with him ... but the girlfriend had used one of the things they put on the vagina like snuff, Zambuk, all those things ... .
>
> P2: I think, maybe Jabu's girlfriend was cleaning herself by taking pills to purify herself.
>
> P3: On that point I think the woman was going to say 'Jabu, I have used tablets, so I think we should not have sex today because we both do not use the condoms. I've taken the pill' – even disprin can cause gonorrhoea (Standerton volunteer healthworkers).

> P: Ja, I am saying that when L [participant's name] has taken laxative and I slept with her, definitely by sleeping with L I am going to have STD. Does it not happen like that? (Standerton volunteer healthworkers).

Women's promiscuity, rather than men's, was further cited as a cause of STDs, as in this example, which also highlights the discourse of 'unclean blood' in understandings of STDs:

> P: What I think is the problem is that you find that there are women who have sexual intercourse with several men. For instance, today she sleeps with me and we have sex. The following day she meets another man and they do the same thing we did a day before. So, she comes into contact with ... different blood and it mixes with her blood. So, in her is a mixed blood. Therefore, when yet another man sleeps with her (perhaps the third man or so) he will get a problem because he finds mixed blood in her. That is how one can get such a problem (Rustenberg mineworkers).

Furthermore, some women were believed to consciously *create* an STD as way of revenging prior injustices committed upon them by their partners. Such notions again draw on discourses of the supernatural, associating women with witchcraft and with the magical propensity to 'mix potions' to damage men:

> P: At times it happens that people do it deliberately, like women. Say you have a relationship with her. Sometimes they think that they are clever. They drink all sorts of things. These things mix up in her body and they make her blood dirty. It is like that (Rustenberg mineworkers).

STDs were also seen as being caused by women's contraceptives, and as such women are again constructed as blameworthy, ironically, *despite* the fact that they are acting in a sexually responsible manner:

> P: My boyfriend said that I gave him this disease and I got it from the family planning method I am using ... because he doesn't want me to use it (UWC female students).

Whereas men put much of the blame on women, some women resisted this construction and pointed to men's role in the cause of STDs:

> P1: ... a lot of the time women get blamed, that they are rotten there – maybe they're having other sexual relationships ... but in fact men bring the disease to their wives ... .
>
> P3: Ja, these men are the problem. Most of the time they bring diseases to the family (Katlehong student group).

Another constructed cause of STDs was that of an abusive or problematic sexual relationship. In the following example, a young woman's sexual experience with an older man is viewed as a physically negative experience for her, and as such, the cause of an STD. This is an important example, not only because it powerfully demonstrates the influence of a normalising discourse of sexual practice, but also because, perhaps incidentally, it suggests the notion of healthy female sexuality and desire. This is unusual in the present context, particularly given the extent to which such positive constructions of female sexuality are so typically marginalised. (This marginalisation of a healthy and productive female sexuality has been highlighted both locally (cf. Shefer, 1999; Wood and Foster, 1995) and internationally (cf. Holland *et al.*, 1991; Holland *et al.*, 1996).)

> P: We do not think she is enjoying sex with an older man. When she reaches climax she surely does not get an orgasm. [Her] ... burning urine is caused by the sperms she does not omit ... . These sperms then cause complications inside and results in the bad discharge. This all happens because the girl did not enjoy sex with the older man (King William's Town rural community group).

Nutritional causes for STDs were also provided by some participants. Again the belief of women's inherent vulnerability to STDs is reproduced together with restraints on women's eating behaviours:

> P1: She stopped eating potatoes and pap because she had a discharge .... I've heard that it's potatoes ... if you eat too much ... .
>
> P2: Older people say that you mustn't use a lot of vinegar, and you must not allow female children to use a lot of it ... .
>
> P3: ... There's this woman who used to eat fish. I bought some of this fish for a friend of mine, but she said she doesn't eat fish. When I asked her why, she said it will come out down there ... (Katlehong residents group).

In some groups, a racialised discourse emerged in the discussion on the causes of STDs, with STDs viewed as a predominantly 'white' illness. The following quote highlights the deep embeddedness of a discourse of sexualised racism, which clearly has its roots in the apartheid taboos on sexual relations across 'races':

> *P1*: You get these diseases from running around with white men.
> *P2*: Black men don't seem to give us problems (Standerton sexworkers).

## The construction of sexuality in relation to STDs

Participants' discussions of STDs were generally so enmeshed with social constructions of male and female sexuality and with differential sexual rights and prerogatives that it ultimately became impossible to view discussions beyond the broader politics of gender and heterosexuality. Insights into the nature of typical gender relations and heterosexual practices emerged significantly in discussions about ways of preventing STD infection. Particularly prevalent here were issues of resistance to condom usage, particularly by men, but also, for other reasons, by women:

> *P*: It's true men do not want these condoms. I think what's also important is the way we speak to them about these condoms. They will think we don't trust them if we started using the flesh to flesh method then all of a sudden we want them to use condoms (Standerton volunteer healthworkers).

> *P*: Men do not easily accept things. They are always having responses for everything. They always project their filthy doings onto you as a woman. They will question you about your own behaviour whilst they are not at home. The argument will be based on the fact that since you came up with the suggestion [to use condoms], it shows that you've used them with someone else in his absence (King William's Town rural community group).

Women also spoke of male violence and coercion as playing a significant role in constraints on using condoms:

> *I*: What makes it difficult for a woman to insist on men using a condom?
> *Multiple voices*: Because she's scared of him ....
> *P1*: Some will beat you up. Once you start on the subject, he is quick to get to the stick, you see.
> *P2*: These kids go out in the early evening to see their boyfriends, not carrying any condoms. And when they get there the boy coerces them to go away with them. When they get there the girl has no way of protecting herself and because the boy wants what he wants, they have sex (Katlehong residents group).

Male control over women and sexuality was also put forward as a barrier to condom usage, and in some cases cultural discourses were drawn on as well:

> *P1*: Men, you know, men decide when to have sex, and where to have sex and how to have sex. So if he's not gonna [use a condom], if he tells you 'I'm not gonna use that', it's very difficult.
> *P2*: It's mostly the men from rural areas who insist on not using condoms .... They said 'I paid lobola, I paid so much, so I have every right to do whatever I want to do'. So woman is their property (UWC female students).

Male groups were very open about their resistance to using condoms:

> I:  Gentlemen, we have not spoken of condoms. Are these condoms commonly used?
> P:  Some people use them but they have their problems as well.
> I:  What are those problems?
> P:  Well, when using condoms the job you are doing takes forever. You end up sweating as if you were busy doing hard work. You don't sweat much when not using it. (*background laughter*) But now because the world is like this we are forced to use it (Butterworth prisoners).

Physiological reasons for disapproving of condoms are frequently cited, for example:

> P1: Condoms are a disturbance. It constantly works on your mind whilst you are busy having sex. As a result you just cannot wait to take it out and throw it away. Whilst you are busy you can really feel this thing which is an obstruction. Maybe if we had grown up using them, things would be different.
> P2: To me it seems as if it cuts the blood circulation, as a result you don't really climax properly (Butterworth prisoners).

Participants, especially men, also expressed the sentiment that women too resist condoms in certain contexts:

> P1: Well, I have a problem. Actually my girlfriend complains that she does not want to use condoms. Since I don't want to have these STDs again, I end up hiding it from her and using it. Sometimes she catches me and we end up fighting – she says these condoms can slip off whilst we are still busy. I now end up not knowing what to do. Women don't want them.
> P2: My girlfriend also told me that if I insist on using condoms then we had better terminate the relationship. She gave me an example by saying nobody can eat a wrapped sweet.
> P3: I also encountered a similar problem whereby on two occasions the condom slipped off inside my girlfriend. So now she also does not want me to use them. On another occasion, I used a condom which was very tight. It seemed to cut off my circulation because I could not ejaculate (Butterworth prisoners).

Women's resistance to condoms appeared to be mostly related to issues of trust in their men, and how long-term and committed the relationship is:

> P1: In other cases, this is when a man is going to use a condom, then a woman will say 'You do not trust me' or 'Do you think I am sleeping with other man or I am having some illness, or sick?' sort of, then condom will not be used. So [we] will still really have a problem in both categories, the women and men … .
> P2: It was going to be better if from the beginning with your partner you have used condoms from the first time the affair starts, if you are going to have a relationship, long-term relationship, then after some time you come up with an idea of using condom, trust is not there, no one is honest. Those who manage to use condom are those who have started from the beginning of the relationship to use condom – maybe they've got a problem that is known by only both of them, then they will continue (Standerton volunteer healthworkers).

> *P1*: You see, with regards men who are married, it is not necessary to use a condom. Condoms are for those who are still going around. Those people should use condoms. But for married man to wear such a thing (*chuckles*) … .
> 
> *P2*: … this gentleman's statement of saying that you can put on a condom on other women and not for your wife is right. I can only use a condom on a woman that I do not know, for example somebody I have just met here in Rustenberg. I cannot use a condom on my wife at home … .
> 
> *I*: … So it is difficult for each of you to suggest using a condom.
> 
> *P3*: Yes, a condom makes us not to trust each other. Yes (Rustenberg mineworkers).

In discussions on safe sex, participants also spoke of being able to differentiate between those who are 'safe' and 'unsafe' sexual partners. This perception has been well documented in the literature on the social construction of AIDS that shows how men distinguish between 'clean' and 'unclean' women (Waldby *et al.*, 1993; Wood and Foster, 1995), in which 'unclean' women constitute those who step outside prescribed feminine sexuality ('promiscuous' women, prostitutes), for example:

> *P*: I can say 'Use a condom on a partner you do not trust'. Because there are people that you can just see that they are suspicious. Those are the people on whom one must use a condom (Rustenberg mineworkers).

The sexworker groups in particular demonstrated women's lack of power in negotiating safe-sex practices. There were clear examples of resistance to safe-sex precautions:

> *P*: I am still trying to handle that issue [of safe sex] as we speak. I have a problem with one male client. If I meet with someone else I don't get this … . If I meet with him, I don't know if this comes out with his sperms when he climaxes or [if] there's something wrong with me. I experience some bleeding afterwards. We were busy discussing that now because he is not used to using a condom and he does not want to. So we decided that we should not have sex until such time that all is okay (Standerton sexworkers).

The following extract exemplifies the vulnerability of sexworkers resulting from competition with other sexworkers in respect of condom usage. The language used, such as the statement 'he has forced someone else', certainly suggests coercion and lack of power on the part of the sexworker. Clearly, economic pressure is seen as inhibiting condom usage, and particularly so, given the higher premium on unprotected sex. Also evident here is an emerging discourse on age, where younger women are constructed as less responsible, as willing to work without condoms and as posing a threat generally to older women:

> *P1*: There are many girls in the business. As you see us now, we are not all here. If I insist on a condom, the client leaves me and goes to another girl. When he gets there he meets the one who does not worry about a condom. Then this means I get nothing in return because he has forced someone else who does not care for these condoms. Even if I play hard to get I cannot do that for long. Then what happens you end up meeting someone else who offers you a very small amount of money. They offer you R30.

*P2*: Then they go to the tavern and get what they want. The thing is there's a lot of us. Because we are older (*all laugh*) once they see the young girls who ran away from school, they take them. So there are no chances of playing hard to get for a long time. So now in the morning they count their money and you become envious because you are hungry. We don't eat without sleeping with these men (Standerton sexworkers).

Another reason given for sexworkers' vulnerability to STD infection related to alcohol and drug dependence.

*P1*: Something else that's a problem is that a lot of girls are on drugs … .
*P2*: No girl that is on drugs is going to turn away a client that is offering R40 or R50 more. Ja, substance abusers … they are not going to turn away a client and they get more for it and that's a fact (Western Cape sexworkers).

*P*: … some of us go and wait for men from the shebeen or pubs. This happens because they also want these beers. So now by the time they have sex she's so drunk she does not care if he uses a condom or not. So when you meet the same man and you insist on a condom then he will tell you that he is going to the tavern because he will find others who are … willing to have sex without it (Standerton sexworkers).

The last quote indicates the constraints on sexworkers to adequately negotiate safe sex given the competition of other sexworkers. Although sexworkers' experiences illustrate the particular vulnerability of this group to STD infection, they provide important insights into the sexual experiences, and vulnerabilities, of women in South Africa more broadly.

## Stigmatising discourse in the prevention and cure of STDs

Discussions about help-seeking behaviour for STDs further highlighted stigmatising and negative discourses framing participants' experiences around prevention and treatment. Participants frequently raised the use of alternative methods of intervention – both preventative and curative – to local clinics. The use of such methods of intervention for STDs when not using condoms emerged particularly, but not exclusively, in the sexworker groups. Methods mentioned highlighted the dangers, pain and discomfort involved in alternative 'cures' as well as a discourse of dirt/clean. Having an STD, particularly for the women, was constructed as 'dirty', as involving 'contaminated blood' and therefore needing to be sanitised by as stringent a cleanser as possible. Popular 'cleansers' included 'dip' (apparently those used to disinfect animals from ticks, fleas, etc.), potassium permanganate and Jeyes Fluid (usually used as a toilet cleaner):

*I*: But otherwise if you insist on using condoms they look for someone else?
*P1*: Yes they do. So what we do – we drink '*ama* double buy'.
*I*: What do you drink?
*P1*: Double buy, that's '*uzifo zonke*', and clean ourselves.
*P2*: We also drink dip. This is the dip you mix with water. We drink this in the morning

so as to cleanse ourselves of this contaminated blood and leave it behind in the toilet if possible. You then are okay. You can do this for a week.

*I:* Please tell me more about these 'double buys' ... .

*P3:* Okay, that's potassium permanganate, something like that, that's what they use, and Jeyes Fluid.

*I:* Do you drink it?

*P4:* Yes, yes we do, all.

*I:* What does it do?

*P2:* It cleans you from within and it's also some sort of laxative.

*I:* Whoow ... .

*I2:* (*co-interviewer*) But I believe that the ladies are not aware that this kills.

*P1:* It works – it cleanses us – but it's dangerous (Standerton sexworkers).

Men appeared to use equally painful alternative methods of intervention in attempting to 'drain' the infection, by putting physical pressure on the penis – 'hammering' it, in one case – which also emphasises the construction of the illness as something distasteful and invasive that should be acted upon aggressively:

*I:* Is there anything else you used for treatment before going to the hospital?

*P1:* I asked others and they said you should just put the penis on a hard surface then you hammer it.

*I:* What?

(*background laughter*)

*I:* What did they say?

*P1:* Someone said at the hospital they use the same kind of treatment. They just use a rubber hammer. Instead of going there I tried to do it myself. I did not use the rubber hammer as advised by, I tried to drain it myself. I realised then that it was not working (Butterworth prisoners).

Discussions on intervention through clinics and other medical routes also illuminate the way in which STDs are 'othered' and negatively constructed, even by those apparently well educated about them. Many participants spoke about clinic staff's disrespect, rudeness and judgemental attitudes towards and stigmatisation of their illness:

*P:* Yes it's true, they examine you. What also scares you in hospitals, you might be examined by a nurse old enough to be your mother, so they shout at you like anything. I was once scolded by a nurse there (Butterworth prisoners).

*P1:* On Friday ... last week I was there, and they treated me badly in such a way that I decided to go ... rather than being treated badly. They treat us ... the same way as women, especially when they see that you cannot do anything [and that] you need their help ... .

*I:* Is that just for STDs, or generally?

*P1:* It is also with STD, but includes everything else ... whether you have STD or anything else ... they also treat you bad. But it is worse when you have STD, much worse, and there are some cases that you cannot even bear to think about ... just, it's bad. I will never come here (Standerton volunteer healthworkers).

> *P1*: That's why most people don't go to the clinic. Even our kids when we send them there for contraception won't go. They just turn right round and come home.
> *P2*: Because they humiliate them ….
> *P3*: The nurses are rude, they are so rude.
> *P4*: Even the clerk.
> *P2*: She is worse. She tells you they are knocking off and don't have the time …. These clinic nurses are the reason people don't want to go there. They make you feel like a fool, a piece of rubbish, until you don't even know yourself anymore. You regret why you actually went there …. You'd probably just think of leaving the place, if you think of how humiliated and put down you'll feel when she finds out what disease you have (Katlehong residents group).

Participants also expressed concerns about both the lack of privacy and confidentiality during treatment. Visits to the clinic are often described as alienating experiences in which patients are disparagingly labelled:

> *P1*: The other thing they do if I go there suffering from gonorrhoea, my problem will not end at the clinic. When I am in the community I will hear it, they tell other people who are in the clinic not to sit or go with me because I've got gonorrhoea and everybody will be looking at me for what I've got.
> *P2*: That is why we are having a problem. Clinics are not secretive, that is why we have a problem to go to the clinics … (Standerton volunteer healthworkers).

> *P1*: Sisters are the ones who call the people 'cases'. If you go there and speak with them about your problem, your problem is supposed to be a secret, it's between you and the sister attending you, but when you come back next time another sister who was not there, you will hear them saying, 'Phindi, there comes that case'.
> *P2*: Nurses are the ones who label people, calling them 'cases', it's really them, and they discuss your problem.
> *P1*: Makes you feel bad (Standerton volunteer healthworkers).

Some participants felt that STD patients, especially those with HIV, were alienated by discriminatory and exclusionary practices in clinics:

> *P1*: They are isolated in the clinics.
> *P2*: Ja, they discriminate and isolate them.
> *P3*: Yes, they do isolate, for instance like here …. They do not treat people in the same way, so if you are a patient you can see that you are not welcome and you will end up stopping to come for the treatment because you are not accepted. I think this is lowering their self-esteems and make them to lose hope that they can be cured ….
> *P3*: There at hospital if someone has AIDS they will shout at people around the victim and [tell] … them to stay away from the victim and the nurses will shout at others to double their gloves …. Now the people know that if the nurses say to others, '3 or 4 gloves', they know that the patient is suffering from STDs … (White River church group).

Many participants also felt that they simply did not receive adequate and appropriate diagnoses and treatment, including medication and information, at the clinic, for example:

> P1: The other thing is, [if] they do suspect STD, if you go to the clinic having any pain, they suspect that you've got STD. They do not take you to the consulting room and see what is wrong with you, ja, they do not examine and look what is your problem.
> (*several voices at once*)
> I: They just diagnose?
> P1: Ja, yes, once you tell them about a pain, you are STD positive, even if you've got infection caused by high temperature, or rash, for them you've got STD (Standerton volunteer healthworkers).

Other gender and class differences also emerged as playing a role in the way in which patients were treated, illustrating the differential stigmatisation of illnesses. Some participants felt that men were treated better than women and that status and class in particular played a role in this:

> P1: They treat men differently. They take care of them.
> P2: They don't give us the same treatment.
> P3: They actually laughs, swear and shout at us.
> P1: If your boyfriend takes you there they help you both (Standerton sexworkers).

> P1: And the other thing, the community does not contribute a lot to discriminate women but with hospitals/clinics …. If P [name of participant] as a male has one of these diseases the nurse will say nothing to him, but if I, myself as female goes inside with the same disease they will say a lot. That is why it looks as if females are the ones who spread this disease because they are confronted, shouted and get names that they do not even expect. One would rather stay with it for that matter if it is not sore.
> I: Is the problem in the clinics that they treat male and female differently?
> P2: Even for male, it depends on who you are. They consider your status. If they do not know you, they will play around with you, even if you are male! (Standerton volunteer healthworkers).

Furthermore, the popular notion that women are to blame for STDs was apparently also prevalent among clinic staff, as illustrated in this quote:

> P: I once had it [an STD] and the nurses did explain the treatment to me. I enquired if it was okay to bring my partner and they said I should. I went to fetch her. After examination it was confirmed I had got this from her.
> I: Who confirmed this?
> P: The doctor did (Butterworth prisoners).

Sexworkers spoke about specific forms of discrimination that they had experienced in clinics, with some having been refused any help because of the double stigma attached to their occupation and illness by clinic staff. When they finally did receive help, they spoke of being 'disciplined' and scolded by clinic staff:

> P: … you know they [sexworkers] find it very difficult at some clinics because you know the reception you get there, it's not always nice, especially when they know

you are a sexworker, you know. I am not going to tell everybody the clinic is nice, they are treating me nice …. They treat the sexworkers like shit at … [name of clinic], they look down on sexworkers (Western Cape sexworkers).

P: They [clinic staff] first want to know how you might have gotten the illness. If you tell them that you are a prostitute, then it becomes difficult to get treatment. If you do not tell them then you are given all the treatment you need (Standerton sexworkers).

P1: They say we are bitches.
P2: They even say we are prostitutes for whites.
P1: These are the reasons why I never go to the clinic here in the location. I believe in going to [name of clinic] – they treated me with respect (Standerton sexworkers).

Again here, abusive treatment and lack of confidentiality emerge as strong themes. In the above example, stigmatising discourse is paired with racist talk. By deciding to leave, rather than submitting and staying for the sake of medical treatment, the participant in the above extract resists abusive treatment and stigmatising constructions of her illness and identity, but at the cost of her long-term health. This dilemma of stigma and the ways it proves obstructive to attaining effective treatment appears to lie at the centre of the losing battle that South Africa appears to be waging against STDs:

P: I once went to the clinic here in the location at [name of clinic]. I had small pimples in my vagina which were very itchy … I realised that the pimples were getting worse so I went to the clinic. There I told the sister my problem. They asked us one by one as we were sitting there. One sister shouted in front of people saying that she had heard that we were sleeping with white men without using condoms. She said those white men were going to give us AIDS. She shouted at me in front of people who were there and she never talked to me in private. I was very angry, so I left (Standerton sexworkers).

## ■ Conclusions

The analysis of focus-group material revealed how powerfully entrenched stigmatising discourses of STDs continue to be in sectors of South African society. 'Othering' and distancing discursive strategies proved to be extremely prevalent in focus-group discussions. Pronounced 'asymmetries of blame' were likewise prevalent, with women blamed consistently more than men as the cause of STDs, and with women practising non-monogamous sexuality blamed more than those women categorised as 'in stable relationships' with 'good men'. A sense of 'blameworthiness' was also actively implemented, and enforced through the construction of individuals or practices as 'deviant' or 'loose'. Promiscuity, with its own attendant stigmatising connotations of deviance or amorality, proved to be the most pervasive stereotype associated with STDs. Importantly, however, the notion of promiscuity was undeniably and differentially gendered in the sense that female promiscuity was powerfully problematised and made strongly blameworthy, whereas male promiscuity was less of an issue (and was even rewarded in certain contexts), and constructed as far less responsible for the spreading of disease. One should note, however, that although women were typically more blamed and made far more responsible for the advent of STDs than were men, women did also – within these focus groups, at least – point to the blameworthiness of non-monogamous men in bringing STDs to their stable partners.

An important difference here lies in the fact that when males were blamed for the spread of STDs, this blame was generally diffused through recourse to naturalising levels of explanation. By locating the cause of STDs within the sphere of natural processes, blame becomes less centred at the intrinsic or essential level of the individual man. Similarly, questions of that individual's agency, and of his personal responsibility for the couple's sexual actions, were notably diluted. Whereas the responsibility and blameworthiness of men with STDs was typically diffused in these ways, females with STDs, by contrast, were thoroughly degraded and stigmatised. These gender differences were particularly pronounced in the case of an individual having had sex with multiple partners. In this context, men were relatively blameless, whereas for women, blame was far more essentially or intrinsically tied to qualities of the woman herself. These constructions reflect entrenched asymmetrical patterns of power, where men maintained dominance and relative impunity over disempowered and 'blameworthy' women.

Similarly, such constructions privileged seemingly normative practices and forms of sexuality over ostensibly 'deviant' forms. Rather than facilitating the understanding of safer sexual practices, or facilitating the access to effective treatment, these constructions frequently functioned instead to entrench denial of infection, and to disqualify or marginalise legitimate information about how and under what conditions one might be vulnerable to STDs.

Constructions of female responsibility for the spread of STDs hinged around very specific notions of the female body. Female bodies were consistently constructed as being particularly prone or vulnerable to infections. The vagina, for example, was frequently constructed as a 'compost-like' environment, from which disease was easily bred. The negative, demeaning and misogynistic constructions of female genitalia, and by extension, female bodies and sexuality more generally, were a striking and disturbing feature across focus groups.

Another key difference in the gendered construction of STDs was that, in the case of men, there was always an ambiguity of sorts around the status of having contracted an STD. Though a concern, an STD was emblematic of a positive masculine problem, an affirmation of masculinity, especially given its irrefutable proof of having 'scored' sexually. This was perhaps one of the most dramatic examples of the gendered double standards within predominant constructions of STDs and their effects.

The view of STDs as an invasive force that had to be dealt with aggressively was shared among all groups. This view mirrored the militarist discourse identified in the social construction of HIV/AIDS (cf. Sontag, 1988). Clearly, the examples of the use of hammering and of stringent household cleaners such as Jeyes Fluid to combat STDs reiterated such metaphors of aggression. In this connection, the unsympathetic construction of STDs as repulsive and dirtying threats, as tainting and corrupting of the self, set STDs apart from other 'normal' illnesses. This construction of STDs as a special category of abhorrence and threat, even amongst other diseases, further reproduced the stigmatisation of having contracted an STD, both for men and women.

This study reiterated the importance of engaging with dominant constructions and social understandings of a disease as vital aspects of the effective implementation of intervention and prevention strategies. In obvious terms, current and popular discourses exert a powerful bearing on the given practices of a given community. Thinking about facilitating treatment and prevention hence requires, as a near essential component, a critical engagement with the discourses of the relevant affliction, disorder, pathology or psychopathology. Deconstructing dominant constructions of illness, as it seems this study so strongly shows, can importantly identify those social understandings and prejudices working to block the potential control of the disease in question. As this study has tried to show, misconceptions, stereotyping, blaming and counter-blaming around the spread of STDs are pervasive. These factors will no doubt continue to influence the ways in which people think about STDs. And as such, the attempt to challenge and/or change these attitudes, values, discourses and prejudices must rank highly amongst the imperatives of treating and preventing STDs in South Africa.

Lastly, it soon became evident, in the analysis of focus-group material, that the dominant discourses on HIV/STDs reflected broader discourses and broader social patterns of power, which framed the everyday lived realities of the communities under study. Significantly, such discourses and such asymmetries of power appeared to reflect and to reproduce certain of the most prevalent forms of oppression and marginalisation alive in contemporary South African society, such as racism, gender inequality, the oppression of women and cultural subordination. Such findings throw light on much of the overall construction of pathology. It seems apparent that central to the construction of pathology are the ways in which social constructions emerge out of, and are utilised by, dominant discursive practices in the maintenance of hegemonic power and subordination. It therefore seems evident that any talk about illness and pathology needs to be carefully scrutinised, so that we might explore and explode the powerful linkages between the social construction of illness, on the one hand, and the exclusionary, marginalising and oppressive practices so prevalent in the broader South African social context, on the other.

## ■ Acknowledgements

This research was commissioned by the National Health Department. Thanks go to the other members of the research team, Anna Strebel, Leickness Simbayi, Tanya Wilson, Nokuthula Shabalala, Michelle Andipatin and Cheryl Potgieter.

## ■ References

Abdool Karim, Q., Mathews, C. and Gutmacher, S. (1997). *HIV/AIDS and STDs in South Africa: The National HIV/AIDS and STD Review.* Pretoria: Department of Health.

Abdool Karim, S. S., Abdool Karim, Q., Preston-Whyte, E. and Sankar, N. (1992). Reasons for lack of condom use among high school students. *South African Medical Journal,* 82, 107–10.

Bartky, S. L. (1990). *Femininity and Domination: Studies in the Phenomenology of Oppression.* New York and London: Routledge.

Block, R. and Dehaeck, C. M. C. (1987). Human papillomavirus and the squamous epithelium of the female genital tract. *South African Medical Journal,* 72, 557–8.

Brandt, A. (1988). AIDS and metaphor: Toward the social meaning of epidemic disease. *Social Research,* 55 (3), 413–32.

Buga, G., Amoko, D. and Ncayiyana, D. (1996). Sexual behaviour, contraceptive practice and reproductive health among school adolescents in rural Transkei. *South African Medical Journal*, 86, 523–7.

Buve, A., Laga, M. and Piot, P. (1993). Where are we now? Sexually transmitted diseases. *Health Policy and Planning*, 8, 277–81.

Coward, R. (1984). *Female Desire: Women's Sexuality Today*. London: Paladin Books.

Department of Health, Directorate of HIV/AIDS and STDs (1996). Consensus seminar on the syndromic management of sexually transmitted diseases in South Africa. Johannesburg.

Gilman, S. (1988). *Disease and Representation: Images of Illness from Madness to AIDS*. Ithaca: Cornell University Press.

Gilmore, N. and Somerville, M. A. (1994). Stigmatization, scapegoating and discrimination in sexually transmitted diseases: Overcoming 'them' and 'us'. *Social Science and Medicine*, 39, 1339–58.

Greer, G. (1992). *The Change: Women, Aging, and Menopause*. New York: Alfred Knopf.

Holland, J., Ramazanoglu, C. and Scott, S. (1990). AIDS: From panic stations to power relations: Sociological perspectives and problems. *Sociology*, 25 (3), 499–518.

Holland, J., Ramazanoglu, C., Scott, S., Sharpe, S. and Thomson, R. (1991). *Pressure, Resistance, Empowerment: Young Women and the Negotiation of Safer Sex*. Women Risk and Aids Project (WRAP), paper no. 6. London: Tufnell Press.

Holland, J., Ramazanoglu, C. and Thomson, R. (1996). In the same boat? The gendered (in)experience of first heterosex. In D. Richardson (ed.), *Theorising Heterosexuality*, pp. 143–60. Milton Keynes: Open University Press.

Hollway, W. (1989). *Subjectivity and Method in Psychology: Gender, Meaning and Science*. London: Sage.

Kitzinger, J. and Miller, D. (1991). In black and white: A preliminary report on the role of the media in audience understanding of 'African AIDS'. Medical Sociology Unit, working paper no. 27. Glasgow: Medical Research Unit.

Laga, M., Nzila, N. and Gorman, J. (1991). *The Interrelationship of Sexually Transmitted Diseases and HIV Infection: Implications for the Control of Both Epidemics in Africa*. Antwerp: Collaborating Centre on AIDS, World Health Organisation.

Legion, V. (1992). Breaking the chain: STDs and HIV. *World AIDS*, 22, 18–22.

Leiman, G. (1976). Cervical cancer screening in a Johannesburg family planning centre. *South African Medical Journal*, 52, 611–15.

McNiel, D. (1999). Loose talk about Aids causes more deaths. *Mail and Guardian*, 28 May, 32.

National AIDS Research Programme of the Medical Research Council (1993). *AIDS Bulletin*, 2, 1–24.

National Progressive Primary Health Care Network (NPPHCN) (1995). *Youth Speak out for a Healthy Future: A Study on Youth Sexuality*. Braamfontein: NPPHCN/UNICEF.

Northrup, C. (1995). *Women's Bodies, Women's Wisdom: The Complete Guide to Women's Health and Wellbeing*. London: Judy Piatkus.

Patton, C. (1990). *Inventing AIDS*. New York: Routledge.

Pham-Kanter, G. B. T., Steinberg, M. H. and Ballard, R. C. (1996). Sexually transmitted diseases in South Africa. *Genitourinology Medicine*, 72, 160–71.

Plummer, K. (1988). Organising AIDS. In P. Aggleton and H. Homans (eds), *Social Aspects of AIDS*, pp. 20–51. London: Falmer Press.

Richmond-Abbot, M. (1992). *Masculine and Feminine: Gender Roles over the Life Cycle*. New York: McGraw-Hill.

Sabatier, R. (1988). *Blaming Others: Prejudice, Race and Worldwide AIDS*. London: Panos.

Shefer, T. (1999). *Discourses of Heterosexual Subjectivity and Negotiation*. Unpublished doctoral thesis, University of the Western Cape, Cape Town.

Shefer, T., Potgieter, C. and Strebel, A. (1999). Teaching gender in psychology at a South African university. *Feminism and Psychology*, 9 (2), 127–33.

Sontag, S. (1988). *AIDS and its Metaphors*. Harmondsworth: Penguin.

Strebel, A. (1993). Women and Aids: a study of issues in the prevention of HIV infection. Unpublished doctoral thesis, University of Cape Town, Cape Town.
Tavris, C. (1992). *The Mismeasure of Woman*. New York: Simon and Schuster.
Treichler, P. (1987). AIDS, homophobia and biomedical discourse: An epidemic of signification. *Cultural Studies*, 1 (3), 263–303.
Varga, C. and Makubalo, L. (1996). Sexual non-negotiation. *Agenda*, 28, 31–8.
Waldby, C., Kippax, S. and Crawford, J. (1993). *Cordon Sanitaire*: 'Clean' and 'unclean' women in the AIDS discourse of young heterosexual men. In P. Aggleton, P. Davies and G. Hart (eds), *AIDS: Facing the Second Decade*, pp. 29–39. London: Falmer Press.
Wasserheit, J. N. (1992). Interrelationships between human immunodeficiency virus infection and other sexually transmitted diseases. *Sexually Transmitted Diseases*, 19, 16–77.
Watney, S. (1987). *Policing Desire: Pornography, AIDS and the Media*. Minneapolis: University of Minnesota Press.
Weeks, J. (1989). Aids: The intellectual agenda. In P. Aggleton, G. Hart and P. Davis (eds), *AIDS: Social Representations, Social Practices*, pp. 1–19. London: Falmer Press.
Wellings, K. (1988). Perceptions of risk – media treatment of AIDS. In P. Aggleton and H. Homans (eds), *Social Aspects of AIDS*, pp. 83–105. London: Falmer Press.
Wood, J. T. (1997). *Communication, Gender, and Culture* (2nd edn). California: Wadsworth.
Wood, K. and Foster, D. (1995). 'Being the type of lover ...': Gender-differentiated reasons for non-use of condoms by sexually active heterosexual students. *Psychology in Society*, 20, 13–35.
Wood, K. and Jewkes, R. (1998). *'Love is a Dangerous Thing': Micro-dynamics of Violence in Sexual Relationships of Young People in Umtata*. Tygerberg: Medical Research Council.
Wood, K., Maforah, F. and Jewkes, R. (1996). *Sex, Violence and Constructions of Love among Xhosa Adolescents: Putting Violence on the Sexuality Education Agenda*. Tygerberg: Medical Research Council.

# CHAPTER 11

# Witches and watchers: Witchcraft beliefs and practices in South African rural communities of the Northern Province

*Teboho Lebakeng, Susan Sedumedi & Gillian Eagle*

## ■ Introduction

At the outset of this chapter, it may well be worth posing the question as to why a focus on witchcraft should be included in a text on psychopathology. Despite evidence of witchcraft beliefs and practices across several centuries in many parts of the world, including Africa (Garret, 1977), there has been an uneasy tension between the domain of psychopathology and clinical medicine and the domain of belief in supernatural forces and related practices. It would appear that engaging with the realm of the metaphysical becomes a problem for psychiatry and clinical psychology, since explanatory systems concerning the origin and nature of events become widely divergent and contestable. In addition, in the African and South African contexts, belief in witchcraft is associated with an indigenous cosmology that is seen to lie outside the rational, scientific framework of Western thought (on which scientific mental-health systems are based), extending into what is often somewhat imprecisely referred to as 'cross-cultural' or 'transcultural' psychiatry. However, as was illustrated in Long and Zietkiewicz's chapter in this book (Chapter 8), people who find themselves being treated and evaluated in psychiatric settings cannot always clearly be located as holding Western beliefs, to the exclusion of traditional premises. For example, there have been numerous instances in which patients have been sent for forensic psychiatric observation following the commission of crimes ostensibly under the sway of supernatural forces (including that of witches), leading to often fascinating, if difficult, debates as to the role of such beliefs in relation to the mental status, appreciation of wrongfulness and voluntarism of the patient under observation.

## ■ Witchcraft-related practices as pathology?

Gobodo-Madikizela (1990), in discussing the difficulties inherent in bringing a (white) Western psychiatric lens to bear on mental-health problems among African clients, highlights the phenomenon of witchcraft as illustrating key paradoxes in the interface between two different explanatory systems. Representing as it does the potential for anti-social, paranoid and irrational thinking and behaviour in psychiatric terms, witchcraft as a phenomenon clearly potentially falls within the ambit of the mental-health system. Whereas sociological traditions support the position that witchcraft beliefs and practices (i.e. manifestations of evil believed to stem from a human source) have their origins in social and cultural realities, psychological traditions seek to explain such occurrences as abnormal behaviour stemming from disturbances in the body (as in possession) and disturbances in interpersonal relations (Bootzin and Ancella, 1988). Having located the phenomenon of witchcraft within the realm of the abnormal, then, the discussion in this chapter aims to extend the debates in the field by examining witchcraft within a particular historical and socio-political context. The focus of this chapter, unlike that of Long and Zietkiewicz, is not primarily on witchcraft as a culturally embedded problem, but rather on other tensions and forces associated with witchcraft practices.

In relation to this chapter in particular, the focus on witchcraft also allows for a further examination of what has been referred to as a 'social pathology' in other instances in the book. Such beliefs and practices are social to the extent that they characterise whole communities and groups of people, and result in collective action of a destructive and ostensibly pathological nature. Such phenomena force one to rethink some of the individualising assumptions about the occurrence of psychopathology as a function of personal, either biophysical or intrapsychic (personality), maladaptation. If a significant proportion of a particular population holds to a set of irrational beliefs and acts accordingly, how does this push the explanatory and labelling boundaries of psychopathology? Recent reports of hysterical presentations in entire classes of schoolgirls have been explained as relating to demon possession stemming from bewitchment (*Star*, 2000). Garret's earlier comments on similar cases seem to apply here: 'Anthropologists have long regarded possession as a socio-cultural phenomenon as well as a psychological syndrome whose symptoms may be described as "hysterical". In societies that believe that human witches cause possession, the likeliest remedy will be the punishment or destruction of the alleged culprit' (1977: 467). In the South African case cited above, although there were suspicions of witchcraft, no direct agent/s were identified and the girls were treated through exorcism by spiritual healers or priests, an interesting intersection between Christian and indigenous beliefs that will not be pursued further in this chapter.

What is salient for the purpose of the normality-abnormality debate is that such phenomena provide evidence of susceptibility to 'pathological' behaviour on a group rather than individual basis. However, the primary subject matter of this discussion will be the occurrence of witch-hunts and killings in the Northern Province region of South Africa over the last several years. This case study of witchcraft-related phenomena represents an ideal basis from which to interrogate some of the explanatory assumptions relating to such events and their implications for alternative understandings of the psychopathological. It should also be borne in mind that what is being problematised as pathological is not the belief in witchcraft *per se*, but the consequences of such beliefs when they are enacted in anxiety, suspicion, hostility, witch-hunting, persecution, ostracisation, injury and murder in a community. Therefore, it is the link between the holding of the belief and social disharmony and interpersonal violence that in this instance renders witchcraft a legitimate target of scrutiny as a form of pathology.

## The Northern Province witch persecutions

'During the period 1990–April 1995, 455 witchcraft-related cases were reported to the South African Police Service (SAPS) in the Northern Province' (Minnaar *et al.*,

1997: 25), 55% of these being reported in a one-year period between 1994 and 1995. Therefore, it appears that following the transition to democracy, far from a decrease in such cases, there was in fact an escalation. From January to May 1996, more than 100 witchcraft-related cases were reported to police in the Northern Province of South Africa and 164 people were removed from their places of residence to places of safety for fear of harm related to accusations of practising witchcraft (Minnaar *et al.*, 1997: 25). Statistics presented by the Crime Prevention Unit of the Northern Province over a similar period indicate that for every 10 unnatural deaths dealt with by the police and justice system, one was attributable to the phenomenon of witchcraft. It is also worth noting that in analyses of the pattern of witchcraft-related incidents: 'while all the victims were 50 years or older, the majority of perpetrators varied in age between 16 and 25 years' (Minnaar *et al.*, 1997: 25). As in most societies across the world (Garret, 1977), what was also characteristic was that the vast majority of accusations were directed against women (Straker, 1998). In the Northern Province, the most common feature was that it was usually elderly women who were (and are) accused of witchcraft by young men, who often invoke the assistance of traditional healers such as *inyangas* or *sangomas* to 'sniff out' the culprits. So, not only are levels of witchcraft-related accusations and related crimes extremely high, but the demography of the accusers and the accused also seems to reflect particular kinds of social tensions or characteristic beliefs.

Such demographic indicators have made witchcraft-related crimes a cause of considerable concern in the province, such that the provincial government prioritised initiatives to assist in understanding and combatting the widespread negative impact of witchcraft-related practices. Seth Nthai, the Nothern Province's MEC for Safety and Security, set up a commission of enquiry in 1995, which in 1996 produced a report analysing the phenomenon (Minnaar *et al.*, 1997). In addition, the Northern Province Council of Churches has reacted with alarm to the increase in acts of violence related to allegations or suspicion of witchcraft practices.

Not only do witchcraft-related crimes appear to be largely specific to the Northern Province, but within the province there are more reported cases of witchcraft-related crimes in the Lebowa, Lowveld and Far North areas than in the Bushveld and Central regions. These are the more remote and poverty-stricken sub-regions of the province. The province has come to be called 'the province of witchcraft', and the *Northern Times* and its sister newspaper, the *Northern Review*, as well as other popular media, have consistently commented on the horrors of witchcraft-related violence over recent years (Kgatla, 1995). Therefore, not only is there a real problem, in the sense that statistics provide verification of pervasive violence and disruption to people's lives as a result of allegations of witchcraft practice, but there is also an associated stigmatisation of the province. Witchcraft beliefs and practices are generally associated with the primitive, and people entertaining such beliefs are characterised as superstitious and backward in their beliefs. The fact that such beliefs appear to flourish in the Northern Province lends to the stereotyping of African and rurally based people as having these characteristics. However, before adopting such an explanation unproblematically, it is important to examine the context within which the phenomenon flourishes more carefully.

## The demographic and historical context

The Northern Province has a population of 5 120 600, and is one of the poorest regions in South Africa. It is generally a highly differentiated rural area with an agrarian economy and a significant migrant-labour population, the bulk of whom work in Gauteng. Nevertheless, it has a complex social structure, including rich landowners, peasants, tenants, artisans, traders, farmworkers and labourers. Essentially, most community settlements are populated largely by illiterate and extremely poor African people. The majority of people live below the poverty datum line, i.e. they earn an income insufficient to meet their basic needs of food, water, housing and education. Their grinding poverty within a context of relative economic prosperity for other South African citizens is not because the process of economic prosperity accidentally missed them, but because they were systematically marginalised in the racialised economic and social structure of apartheid. It seems incontrovertible that the underdevelopment in the province is a legacy of more widespread policies and practices related to the operation of racialised capitalism and the particular vagaries of apartheid (Rodney, 1976). Such underdevelopment has not changed substantially under the new ANC government.

Historically, rural communities were traditionally projected as free of, and uncontaminated by, the complexities of modern social pathologies and psychopathologies. In somewhat idealised vein, these communities were perceived as homogenous, cohesive, peaceful and harmonious, guided more by the customs of tradition than the principles of rationality and the civilising (but corrupting) virtues of Western cultures. Such portrayals of rural communal life represent a hankering after a state of being unsullied by 'civilisation', a picture far rosier than the reality discussed above (Nzula, 1979). Traditional beliefs and practices were similarly idealised within such portrayals. Global developments have, however, impacted significantly on the existence of such rural communities. Such developments can be understood either in terms of the diffusion thesis of modernisation theory or in terms of the imperialism thesis of classical Marxism. Diffusion of modernity implied the transfer of technology to developing countries by the advanced West so that the former could ostensibly catch up in the development stage. However, it has been argued that this transfer in actual fact cut across/impeded the normal development path of underdeveloped countries and imposed new dynamics and processes (Rodney, 1976). For instance, in the area of farming, local farming was subordinated to imperialistic tendencies, as colonialists and post-colonialists monopolised the trading and marketing operations of developing countries (Nzula, 1979).

Such developments brought major social changes and contributed to a general deterioration in the material conditions of underdeveloped populations. Deepening poverty became the key feature of these communities, and this in turn bred a range of pathological phenomena. It is the central assertion of this chapter that the prevalence of witchcraft-related accusations and attacks is a phenomenon that can most productively be understood as a consequence of underdevelopment rather than within alternative more individualised, medicalised or even traditionalised or cross-cultural explanatory frameworks. Before exploring the relationship between the witchcraft-related attacks in the Northern Province and underdevelopment in the region, it is important to elucidate some of the existing theoretical frameworks that have been brought to bear on witchcraft-related practices.

## The origins of witchcraft-related accusations and attacks: contesting explanations

As will have been suggested by the discussions thus far, there are multiple explanations for the kind of phenomenon being addressed in this chapter. Witchcraft beliefs and accusations and witchcraft-related attacks and killings may be understood as hysterical phenomena in psychiatric terms, as reflecting location within a traditional epistemological frame of reference in anthropological terms and/or as a form of cultural scapegoating in sociological terms. In relation to the latter, a number of theoretical perspectives have been propounded, including tension theory, projection theory, moral theory, functionalist theory, conflict theory, labelling theory and critical theory. Essentially, what such theoretical positions posit is that witch-hunting is reflective of collective social tensions that result in scapegoating onto specific targets, and that this collective behaviour is justified by alternative means, usually metaphysical or spiritual. In comparing witchcraft beliefs in England and Africa, Thomas viewed these as identifiably a '"social phenomenon", a means for explaining, and also, through counter-magic and persecution, for dealing with the misfortunes of village life' (in Garret, 1977: 462). Thomas argued that the rise of such accusations in England corresponded with 'the Protestant Reformation and the breakdown of the communal interrelationships of village society' (in Garret, 1977: 463). Such broad historical influences could be understood as reflecting the impact of development on traditional social relationships. In addition, Evans-Pritchard noted that when misfortune occurred among the African community of the Azande, 'witchcraft offered a logical, coherent, and self-confirming explanation of illnesses or accidents; since the witch could be dealt with through countermagic or accusation' (in Garret, 1977: 464) and relief could be gained through some form of ensuing action. Witch-hunts are therefore much more likely to occur in contexts of deprivation and misery or when traumatic events have taken place.

It seems then that witchcraft accusations flourish in communities that entertain supernatural cosmologies and gain ascendance at times of socio-historic upheaval and individual and collective adversity. Which sectors of the population become the targets of such accusations and consequent persecution is also not incidental (or supernaturally determined), but reflects additional social tensions and a relative lack of, or possession of, power. In most instances, elderly women have been the target of attack (Garret, 1977; Straker, 1998), although there are, of course, exceptions to this. Among the Azande, for example, accusations 'tended to fall on older women because they were marginal, dependent members of the community and therefore more likely to arouse feelings of both hostility and guilt' (Garret, 1977: 465). Delius, in his research into witchcraft in the Northern Province, notes that in this environment, as in many societies, 'traditionally the powers of witches are believed to be transmitted down the female line'(in Straker, 1998: 17). Citing the response of one activist interviewee about the fact that in the main women were the targets of witchcraft accusations, Delius quotes as follows: 'that is our tradition all the time, linking women to witchcraft, that is how we grew up. Bad things are actually associated with women .... Men don't trust women' (in Straker, 1998: 18). Adding this piece to the puzzle, it seems that witchcraft reflects tensions between dominant (colonial) and traditional (colonised) epistemologies, historical transitions, competition over resources, adverse circumstances, gender stereotypes and politics. It is this complex interlocking of forces that ultimately eventuates in suspicions, accusations, expulsion, harm and even murder. All these factors are primarily social in origin, and seem to point to the fact that what could be construed as a pathological phenomenon in a psychiatric sense (i.e. the delusional belief in the power of witches and anti-social violence enacted against them), cannot be understood outside of this social matrix.

However, in *Culture, Behaviour and Personality*, LeVine argues for a 'psychoanalytic ethnography', claiming that 'Social-structural explanations of witchcraft with individual experience and psychological processes left out ... are incomplete ... and inadequate' (in Garret, 1977: 469). Such psychoanalytically based explanations understand witchcraft beliefs and attacks to stem from projections, which then translate into paranoid behaviour. Although such perspectives have been criticised for individualising a communal phenomenon, it seems that there may be a basis for entertaining a more synthesised social and psychoanalytic causal explanation. As Ann Parsons has shown in her psychoanalytic study, belief in witches and paranoia are both forms of projection, but the former are expressed in 'culturally formulated terms' and are therefore fully comprehensible to other believers in the society. There is what Parsons calls a 'reversible relationship between symbol and situation' (in Garret, 1977: 469), since the putative victim of witchcraft can explain the nature of his/her affliction and name the alleged witch, a real person known to the accuser. As Garret puts it: 'Whereas the symbols used in the language of paranoia are private and personal, those of witchcraft accusations are both cognitive and expressive, and they operate in clearly definable situations of social and psychological tension' (1977: 469). What this fairly lengthy series of quotations re-emphasises is that the same behaviour under different conditions may be viewed as a manifestation of psychiatric disorder or as a socially explicable (even if undesirable) occurrence. As in other cases in the book, it appears that social context and consensual validation create the parameters within which such a distinction is drawn. In the framework of a civilised, developed, modern, industrialised nation, as in the 'new' post-democracy South Africa, even this parameter becomes problematic, since what is consensually validated among specific sectors of the population (belief in witchcraft) may be considered 'crazy' by other sectors of the population.

It seems that the more thoroughly we seek to understand witchcraft beliefs and witch-purging, the more complex the explication becomes. Depending upon which precipitating dimension one seeks to explore, a range of disciplinary frameworks have their place, centrally including anthropology, sociology, gender studies and psychology, but also more indirectly, economics, politics and theology. Returning to the case study at hand, in the context of the Northern Province, most of the arguments presented so far appear to have considerable validity. In the following section we will continue with a discussion of the applicability of these hypothesised precipitants to witchcraft practices that have been observed in the Northern Province. However, as we suggested earlier in the chapter, the final emphasis of this discussion will be on the implications of such practices for understanding underdevelopment as a dimension that both influences, and is influenced by, the phenomenon of witchcraft-related offences.

## The relevance of interdisciplinary understandings for the Northern Province situation

In bringing a multifaceted lens to bear on witch-purging in the Northern Province, it is fascinating to note the relevance of the theoretical understandings presented above, although there are also context-specific aspects.

Research in a variety of contexts unrelated to witchcraft has demonstrated that traditional African belief systems continue to exist in contemporary South Africa. While some aspects of African cosmology have remained relatively unchanged, other dimensions have undergone transformation as the result of social, economic and political changes such as urbanisation and Western acculturation. In some instances, as in Zionist church movements, there appears to have been a fusion of traditional customs with Christian beliefs (Nzimande, 1989). The fact that African traditional beliefs and practices play an important role in the lives of many black South Africans has been recognised in mental-health research and policy development (Freeman, 1989; Korber, 1990). It has also been noted that many African people discriminate between the two healing systems of Western medicine and traditional practitioners, and tend to favour a particular system depending on the nature of their difficulty, particularly in the field of mental-health problems (Swartz, 1987). The positive value of traditional beliefs and practices is taken seriously in mental-health policy, and at this point in South African history the two explanatory systems of Western medicine and traditional healing co-exist as a matter of fact, albeit that tensions exist at the interface.

The belief in witchcraft represents the other face of traditional practices, the notion that supernatural forces can be harnessed for destruction as well as for healing. In African cosmology, there is an emphasis on harmony and disharmony in relation to the supernatural realm, including one's ancestors and the environment as a whole. In addition, mind-body links are viewed as integral, as is the individual's relationship to the communal (Ngubane, 1981). Related to such understandings is the belief that misfortune does not occur by accident, but reflects some kind of potentially identifiable disharmony (Ngubane, 1977). One central hypothesis in such instances is that the causative agent is an unknown member of one's community who has employed the services of a 'witch' (a kind of perverted healer) to bring harm upon one. In this respect, witchcraft can be considered the negative face of prosocial traditional healing or spiritual practices.

There is therefore a close association between spiritual diviners (such as *sangomas* and *inyangas*), who employ their skills for healing, and sorcerers or witches, who employ their powers to harmful ends. Perhaps in part to disassociate themselves from their negative counterparts, traditional healers have often been implicated in the 'diagnosis' of witchcraft at work. Within traditional practice 'a "witch" could only be exposed after consultation with an *inyanga* or *sangoma*, who would then identify or "smell out" the culprit' (Minnaar et al., 1997: 26). Delius describes how in one instance in Ga-Sekhukhune 'a *sangoma* would hang a blank sheet on the wall of her hut and facilitate the process of divining the witch by allowing people to project onto this sheet the identity of the witches in a strange marriage of traditional beliefs with representations reminiscent of modern, western inventions such as the TV and video' (in Straker, 1998: 17).

What is interesting in the case of the Northern Province/Lebowa witch-hunts is that while in part adhering to tradition, the youth involved in such purgings also transgressed recognised practices in such circumstances. For example, in some instances, identification bypassed the employment of diviners. 'In one case (in the village of Makubung near Pietersburg), three women villagers at such a meeting were "pointed out" without any evidence being presented by their accusers. They were rounded up, assaulted and then stoned by a group of villagers before being burnt to death' (Minnaar et al., 1997: 26). Delius (1996) also observes that killings and necklacings of women identified as witches ran counter to conventional practices, since traditional punishment had been less extreme, taking the form of banishment from the community. Such deviation from traditional practices was viewed by those engaging with the problem as reflecting social breakdown, and complicates our understandings of normality and abnormality in this situation even further. Whilst it may be difficult to accept the normality of traditional practices in relation to witchcraft from a modern, scientific, realist epistemology, it appears that the notion of what is normal *within* an African cosmological framework can also not be assumed. Deviation from a norm that is already located within an alternative epistemology represents a more complex form of abnormality, requiring a differentiated analysis of the problem. While it may be acceptable to entertain alternative cultural belief systems, at what point do interventionists decide that digression from the norm within a norm is unacceptable? In this way, tensions inherent in such engagement make interventions in the field more difficult, as we will discuss later.

Having confirmed that the context for the holding of witchcraft-related beliefs exists in South Africa and the Northern Province, what are some of the other parameters that pertain? The context of deprivation and exposure to changing sociohistorical circumstances has already been established at the outset of the paper in describing some of the demographic features of the province. To re-emphasise this, the Northern Province contains some of the poorest and most remote communities in South Africa. The area has been impacted upon by earlier forces of colonialism and more recently by South Africa's transition to a fully fledged democracy. As noted, the escalation in witch attacks corresponded with the post-1994-election period. Indeed, some of the youth justified their actions by 'going around to villages and promising to rid the area of witches so that the freedom in South Africa would be "real freedom which includes being free from super-natural forces"' (Mohola, in Minnaar et al., 1997: 26). Therefore, it seems that social upheaval related to historical transitions can also be implicated in the Northern Province case. In respect of misfortune, it could be argued that widespread unemployment and unmet expectations among the youth constituted a form of affliction in the community. In addition, Minnaar et al. (1997) note that the Northern Province region (including Lebowa) is one of the most lightning-prone places in the world and that witches are commonly held to have the power to control lightning through the 'lightning bird'. Lightning-related deaths, injuries and homestead losses are thus often attributed to purported witches. In these respects, it seems that misfortune occurs to the extent that allegations of witchcraft have fertile ground in which to be engendered.

From the characteristics of documented attacks described earlier, it is also clear that most of the victims of attack are elderly women. The focus on such targets appears to reflect the relative weakness of the marginalised and the strength of gender stereotyping and power relations. A further interesting observation has been made in relation to economics. In the context of high unemployment, it may be that the only tangible source of income for many communities in the Northern Province is in the form of old-age pensions. Therefore, elderly women may be the focus of attack as a result of the combination of their vulnerability and their capacity to evoke envy (Ritchken, 1987). The role of envy in the Northern Province situation is particularly pertinent in relation to issues of advancement and underdevelopment. Having established that the generic contributory factors identified in the literature do pertain in the case of the Northern Province witch-hunts, in the next section we will consider the more specific contextual impact of underdevelopment, the aspect of this case study that the paper seeks to highlight as offering a somewhat unique angle on abnormality and witchcraft-related practices.

## Witchcraft located in relation to underdevelopment

Based primarily on anecdotal evidence and participant observation, it is the contention of the first two of the authors of the paper (located at a university in the 'witchcraft province'), that envy and competition over scarce resources play a pivotal role in witch identification and the heated engagement in witch-purging. Although, as we have argued previously, the majority of witch suspects are marginalised community members and more particularly often elderly women, other individuals are not immune to such accusations. People may be subject to attack not only for being accused of directly practising witchcraft, but in addition for being accused of associating with witches or even for appearing to have employed and benefited from their intervention. In many instances (in accord with earlier arguments) it is community members whose positions or resources invite envy that may become the focus of witch-hunt-related violence. Based on everyday observation, it appears that often those who are targeted tend to be individuals who have managed to achieve some degree of upward mobility or access to wealth. Within the context of high unemployment, even access to employment and the attainment of a job may induce envy and jealousy, emotions that can contribute to witchcraft accusations and consequent actions. A number of companies, businesses and even non-governmental organisations (NGOs) have indicated that employees who gain promotion run the risk of becoming witchcraft-related suspects, as fellow employees tend to accuse them of using strong medicine to gain unfair advantage over them. In addition, political opponents may be discredited and put out of action through making allegations of witchcraft stick. Minnaar *et al.* indicate that Nthai's Commission of Enquiry identified a similar dynamic: 'communal jealousy of a particular individual (because of success in business, farming or sexual exploits), often triggered the attack on and burning of an individual alleged to be a witch' (1997: 29).

The discourse of witchcraft thus becomes the framework within which many poor, struggling and competitive individuals express their frustration, disappointment, anger and disillusionment. In the light of unmet political expectations, community members are particularly likely to experience such feelings and to seek for a means through which to channel them. Given the already established background context for the promotion of witchcraft beliefs and practices discussed earlier, the discursive frame of witchcraft is ripe for exploitation under these circumstances. What we are arguing is essentially that witchcraft-related anti-social practices are a form of displacement derived inextricably from a situation of economic deprivation and underdevelopment. In other similarly poor and unevenly developed communities, such displacement may take another form; however, in the Northern Province, the coalescence of a range of further factors (e.g. the strength of traditional beliefs, rural encapsulation, lightning-proneness, pre-existing gender and transgenerational relations) allows for the specific channelling of frustration into witchcraft allegations. The discourse of witchcraft and its related practices can then be turned to the ends of enactment, scapegoating, revenge and the inducement of fear and anxiety in individuals and the broader community. Rather than this process being understood as an individualised psychoanalytic defence mechanism, displacement in this instance is understood in a broader sense, as a communal phenomenon dependent on cultural and socio-historical forces rather than primarily on intraindividual functioning (much in the same vein as Parsons' and LeVine's theorisation presented earlier). From this perspective, what we are arguing is that the abnormality of witch-purging cannot be appreciated without recourse to a multifacetted lens informed by a multidisciplinary observational stance.

Ironically, it could be argued that what is produced within a context of underdevelopment contributes in turn to further underdevelopment. Again based on personal observations, it is our contention that fear of witchcraft allegations has become pervasive in the Northern Province, such that many community members avoid engaging in activities that may make them stand out or become the focus of envy. Individuals may resist promotion, may quell their industriousness and refuse public office in order to blend in with the background rather than become foregrounded. The possibility of being labelled as a witch contributes to social withdrawal, which also ironically may in turn be construed as a sign of being a witch. People's lives are moulded by rumours and accusations relating to witchcraft, and the employment of the discourse comes to hold an inanimate power over whole communities, whose obsession with 'truth-finding' may consume considerable energy and resources. In this respect, witchcraft beliefs, accusations, stigmatisation and punishment have become critical stumbling-blocks to sustainable social and economic development in the Northern Province, and this is perhaps the aspect of abnormality that most needs recognition.

## ■ The way forward

Various intervention strategies have been suggested to address the problem of witchcraft and its consequences. The most common recommendation is that education is required to alleviate the problem and accelerate development. The emphasis of such education is to change people's mind-set from location within a traditional belief system to a more rational scientific understanding. Interestingly, in the recommendations of the Commission of Inquiry into Witchcraft Violence it was accepted that 'witchcraft beliefs were very real and that their existence should be acknowledged' (in Minnaar *et al.*, 1997: 27), so the commissioners aimed to curb certain practices more modestly, rather than recommending an attempt to radically transform a deeply entrenched belief system. Essentially, the commission seemed to argue pragmatically for a return to earlier more constrained methods for dealing with witchcraft suspicions, i.e. for a return to 'normality' as couched within pre-existing traditional belief systems. Education at school level was, however, recognised as important in the recommendations: 'A comprehensive educational programme should be implemented to "liberate the people from participating in the killing and causing harm" that results from their belief in witchcraft; and that courses be included in the school syllabi in areas where witch-killing and "muti" murders were commonplace in order to explain the traditional methods to deal with witches' (in Minnaar *et al.*, 1997: 29). However, if, as we have argued, it is not so much witchcraft beliefs *per se* that are the problem, but the fact that witchcraft accusations and trials mushroom in times of economic, political, social and ecological stress and distress, then educative intervention cannot be seen as sufficient.

Obviously a more totalising strategy is needed to effectively address the problem of witchcraft. In this case, what is needed is sustainable social and economic development in the region. In other words, intervention strategies should attempt to eliminate the root causes that seem to give rise to this social pathology. It is therefore important to involve communities in the region in problem solving so that they can begin to lay claim to the process of development. In order to achieve this, indigenous knowledge and skills need to be harnessed in prosocial endeavours so as to be more effectively employed in the conceptualisation and implementation of the development process.

## Conclusion

By focusing on a very real South African contemporary pathology, i.e. witchcraft purgings and killings in the Northern Province, we hope that this chapter has provided an opportunity to critically interrogate conventional understandings of normality and abnormality. In summarising the key arguments of the chapter, what we are emphasising is that there are forms of pathology that may involve group rather than individual activity and appear to reflect a kind of collective delusion. Rather than understanding this phenomenon from the perspective of cross-cultural psychology or psychiatry, which has tended to locate such behaviour within the framework of competing epistemologies, what we have argued is that even within an alternative epistemology, the witch-hunts of the Northern Province constitute an aberration, and cannot therefore be understood solely as an indigenous set of practices. Instead, by examining a range of explanatory perspectives that have been brought to bear on witchcraft elsewhere, as well as by investigating the specific characteristics of the environment in which the purgings took place (and continue to take place) and key players involved, we sought to do justice to the complexity of the understanding required. While arguing that underdevelopment (particularly of an economic nature) was the pivotal factor at play in producing displacement of frustration and aggression, we propose that multiple co-existing factors led to enactment in the form it took. We recognise that our analysis is not exhaustive, but hope that what this case examination has illustrated is the importance of a multidisciplinary perspective in seeking to understand non-conventional 'abnormalities' in the social fabric and that intervention strategies in turn need to be informed by such multidisciplinary understanding.

# References

Bootzin, R. R. and Ancella, J. R. (1988). *Abnormal Psychology: Current Perspectives*. New York: McGraw-Hill.
Buhrmann, M. V. (1987). The feminine in witchcraft, Part II. *Journal of Analytic Psychology*, 32, 257–77.
Delius, P. (1996). *A Lion Amongst the Cattle: Reconstruction and Resistance in the Northern Transvaal*. Johannesburg: Ravan Press.
Freeman, M. (1989). Mental health crisis in South Africa. Paper no. 16, Centre for the Study of Health Policy, University of the Witwatersrand, Johannesburg.
Garret, C. (1977). Women and witches: Patterns of analysis. *Signs: Journal of Women in Culture and Society*, 3 (2), 461–70.
Gobodo-Madikizela, P. (1990). Notions about culture in understanding black psychotherapy: Are we trying to raise the dead? *South African Journal of Psychology*, 20 (2), 93–8.
Junod, H. A. (1927). *The Life of an African Tribe*, Vol. 2. London: Macmillan.
Kgatla, S. T. (1995). Beliefs about witchcraft in the Northern Region. *Theologia Viatorum*, 22, December, 53–79.
Korber, I. (1990). Indigenous healers in a future mental health system: A case for co-operation. *Psychology in Society*, 14, 47–62.
Krige, E. and Krige, J. D. (1943). Witchcraft and sorcery. In *The Realm of a Rain-queen: A Study of the Pattern of Lovedu Society*, pp. 250–70. London: Oxford University Press for the International African Institute.
Laubscher, B. J. F. (1975). *The Pagan Soul*. Cape Town: Timmins Hammond Tooke.
LeVine, R. (1977). Properties of culture: An ethnographic view. In R. Shweder and R. LeVine (eds), *Essays on Mind, Self and Emotion*, pp. 67–87. Cambridge: Cambridge University Press.
Magesa, L. (1997). *African Religion: The Moral Traditional Abundant Life*. New York: Orbis Books.
Middleton, J. (1967). *Magic, Witchcraft and Curing*. Austin: University of Texas Press.
Minnaar, A., Wentzel, M. and Payze, C. (1997). Witch-purging in the Northern Province. *Focus Forum*, 4 (5), 25–9.
Ngubane, H. (1977). *Body and Mind in Zulu Medicine*. London: Academic Press.
Ngubane, H. (1981). Aspects of clinical practice and traditional organization of indigenous healers in South Africa. *Social Science and Medicine*, 15, 361–5.
Nindi, B. C. (1998). Why the poor stay poor. *Sowetan*, 14 May.
Nzimande, B. (1989). African life and the 'Hidden abode of mental life'. In *Proceedings of the Third National Conference of the Organisation for Appropriate Social Services in South Africa*, pp. 76–85. Durban: University of Natal, Durban.
Nzula, A. J. (1979). *Forced Labour in Colonial Africa*. London: Zed Books.
Ritchken, E. (1987). Burning the herbs. *Work in Progress*, 48, 17–22.
Rodney, W. (1972). *How Europe Underdeveloped Africa*. Dar es Salaam: Tanzania Publishing House.
Sow, I. (1980). *Anthropological Structures of Madness in Black Africa*. New York: International Universities Press.

Straker, G. (1998). When is a woman a woman? Multiple identities and coalition politics. *International Review of Women and Leadership*, 4 (2), 15–23.

*Star* (2000). Johannesburg, 16 November.

Swartz, L. (1987). Transcultural psychiatry in South Africa, Part II. *Transcultural Psychiatric Research Review*, 23, 273–303.

# SECTION 4

# PHILOSOPHIES OF PATHOLOGY

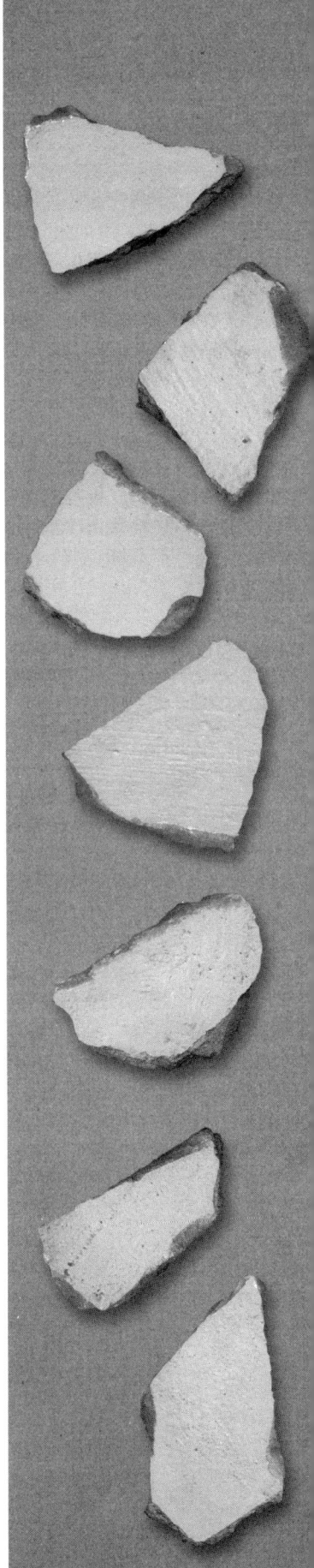

# CHAPTER 12

# Memory, madness and the market

*Erica Burman*

The nourishing fruit of the historically understood contains time like a precious, but tasteless, seed (Benjamin, 1955/1973: 254).

Unfortunately, when subject to excessive external influence, both collective and individual narrated memories may resemble less art than kitsch (Lambek, 1996: 252, fn. 15).

## ■ Introduction

These opening statements appropriately frame my perambulations here, inspired as they were by a footnote to more general discussions of memorial practices and their relations to cultural-historical trajectories. My objective in this chapter is to juxtapose the current media preoccupation with narratives of traumatic remembering and forgetting alongside an equivalent proliferation of representations of madness. While it may be banal to talk of discourses of pathology as shifting to accommodate a postmodern or consumer acceptance/celebration of the psychopathology of everyday life, my particular focus here is on how these intersect with available forms of individuality and sociality. That is, my concern lies with the political subjectivities facilitated/instigated by this discursive explosion. After all, Freud's (1902/1962) *Psychopathology of Everyday Life* not only asserts that our madness is shared, in the sense that we are all equally subject to it, but also that the forms our madness takes are structured according to each unique and idiosyncratic history (as a function of contingency, as well as trauma and overdetermination). Within the psychological and psychoanalytic culture of late modernity (Parker, 1997), then, the question arises of the extent to which these common interpretive resources become a means for shared action and reflection.

At this point, I should admit that there is something Lacanian in the process of the construction of this chapter – it was inspired by an advertising image (aptly titled 'You Can Forget') that I have been unable since to trace, despite much searching (but which I discuss later). However, as is the way with an elusive object of desire, the journey has uncovered all kinds of interesting avenues on the way. Firstly, I should briefly indicate that most of the popular cultural and advertising material I will comment upon here appeared in Britain within the latter quarter of 1999, and is hence relatively recent. Given the effects of globalisation, the British origin of much of this material should not prove an obstacle for the majority of readers living outside Britain. (In fact the similarity, across national boundaries, of many of the advertising images/slogans to be discussed here is itself indicative of the importance of the generality and popularity of the discursive themes to be discussed *internationally*.) Given the various problems and difficulties of reproducing these adverts visually (i.e. as original images), I will instead try – insofar as is possible within a written text – to refer to these slogans and advertising images in a written form, in the body of this text, as I go along.

The conviction driving my narrative here is that there is a current socialisation of psychopathology that, alongside a dynamic of normalisation, has also given rise to further forms of individualisation. Notwithstanding how these discussions may promote greater tolerance for these forms of madness, I will be suggesting that these in fact ward off socially located explanations in ways that *repathologise* the individual at the expense of maintaining the normality of the social. I will attempt to intimate some of the manifold political consequences of this movement through reference to cultural examples as well as 'real-life' events. For as a symptom of psychoanalytic culture (Parker, 1997), the forms of subjectivity cultivated within these cultural-political arenas can be read as much from the crafted images and slogans emerging in popular magazines and advertising campaigns as from the more explicitly therapeutic projects of self-construction and destabilisation of clinical consulting rooms. Hence, as Goffman (1979) pointed out some time ago, advertisements are interesting precisely because their crafted/idealised status offers sedimented cultural types for analysis.

Therefore, this chapter is framed under the mantle – so to speak – of Michel Foucault. However, precisely within the terms of his analyses (cf. Foucault, 1977, 1986, 1988), it is necessary to elaborate these in relation to further shifts and drifts of cultural-subjective forms. The analyses I want to develop here take as their starting point the inter-relations between, and mutually constitutive character of, normality and pathology, as reviewed by Foucault principally in *Discipline and Punish* (1977) but also elsewhere (Foucault, 1980, 1986, 1988), i.e.:

1) that the definition of the limit-cases of pathology (whether educational, sexual, legal or otherwise mental) produces their disciplining norms;
2) that the talk about the vilified or abnormal, far from repressing or silencing these, itself constitutes them. Thus, such discourses betray a structural interest in what they disavow (playing here on Foucault's own ambivalence/agnosticism about psychoanalysis); and
3) that disciplinary practices are moral (rather than 'scientific' or 'natural' in character), and thereby inevitably culturally situated.

In particular, I want to attend to this moral-political character of disciplines, to explore how contemporary discussions of memory relate to representations of subjectivity, including those of madness. For if we are all now allowed (or even mandated) to be mad in some ways, within the contemporary and globalising psychological and psychoanalytic cultures (of therapy, talk shows, agony-aunt newspaper columns, etc.), we are also subject to powerful injunctions to remember (some things) and to forget (others). Therefore, memorial practices, within the various everyday and professional contexts that I will go on to discuss, take their place alongside other more familiar disciplinary apparatuses (of sexuality, pedagogy, the clinic, etc.).

Far from being a private space of contemplative reminiscence, memories have, at the beginning of the 21st century, become the site of dramatic struggle, which has wrenched their forms and processes into the public sphere. Taking up contemporary discussions of memory as symbolic practice rather than personal possession (Lambek, 1996), we can see such discussion and debate on representations of memory as a key arena for the articulation of forms of individual and collective subjectivities. Therefore, the apparent increasing 'disorder' of (individual and social) memory can perhaps intimate something of the ordering processes that correspondingly attempt to 'fix' it in place. Just as (traumatic) kinds of life events occupy a key place in current debates on madness, so too do (increasingly medicalised) disorders associated with memory (of, for example, post-traumatic stress disorder (PTSD) and multiple personality disorder) now seem to hold the key to secret or subjugated subjectivities.

Meanwhile, the fact that the contest seems to consist of determining which memories are true or false threatens to obscure the more general institutionalisation of a model of memory as an entity that is (more or less well) stored or retrieved within a singular individual, internal and private mind. However, if we move away from this traditional and widely circulating psychological conception of memory as a commodity or product to focus instead on remembering as an *activity performed within relationships*, then we arrive at a characterisation of memory as moral by virtue of its role as a 'culturally mediated expression of the temporal dimension of experience, in particular, of social commitments and identifications' (Lambek, 1996: 248).

Lest it appear that I am trying to press together too-divergent themes, let me highlight how models of memory can be seen as significant repositories of representations of subjectivity: indeed, awareness of one's own spatial and temporal existence has been put forward as constituting memory itself (Lambek, 1996: 241). Moreover, within modern industrialised societies (but beyond these through various forms of globalisation that themselves produce dislocations of memory and identity) and their corresponding subjectivities, notions of memory and identity reinforce each other. The fact that my notion of 'who I am' depends on that of 'who I was' means that models of memory and subjectivity are mutually constitutive – through the shared commitment to some notion of experiential continuity. A key political question, then, is firstly how cultural narratives of madness connect with forms of subjectivity, and secondly how these forms of subjectivity correspondingly link up with representations of memory.

## ■ Disciplining memories

We seem to be living in a post-Foucauldian parody, a context that exaggerates those certain political (i.e. power) forms identified by Foucault (1977, 1980, 1986, 1988). Biopolitics, for example, flourishes in multiple forms, e.g. the 'body fascism' of fashion aesthetics; the revival of evolutionary psychology; the rise and rise of biological psychiatry (and the corresponding popularity of biochemical/genetic explanations for mental illness); the proliferation of the medicalisation of educational difficulties (such as dyslexia, autism and attention-deficit hyperactivity disorder), with corresponding focus on drug treatments, rather than the provision of material resources and interpersonal support.

Such strange distortions of chronology and location produced by new disciplinary knowledges of (individual) minds and bodies occlude social agency and turn contingent effect (i.e. the outcome of such processes) into cause. So, discourses of the body have now shifted temporally and spatially to include 'risk' as situated within the body, portrayed as an inherent vulnerability rather than as environmentally produced or even triggered. We are beyond psychological notions of personality, 'life-style' or even 'life events' here, and into the far reaches of biogenetics. A specific and worrying development of this discourse bolsters the already existing moral panic around personality disorder (with the usual sensationalism around – the very few – violent offences committed by people with diagnoses of mental illness). Indeed, new draft legislation in Britain threatens to lock up anyone considered to meet the (very loose) diagnostic characteristics *before* they commit any crime. The creation of such collective processes in the name of public protection therefore implies a greater intensification of disciplinary practices of individualisation.

Trajectories of madness are therefore not only being foreshortened in causal/temporal perspective, but also the time and timeliness of memory are currently sites of intense scrutiny. Contests over memory, or memory wars, form a current focus of legal-juridical practices, with the stakes for individuals (as victims, accusers, 'recanters') ever increasing. Haaken (1998) points out the significance of these debates as not only bolstering the backlash to the small successes of feminism in the US, but also as displacing generational conflicts between women, including feminists, who are focused on different strategies and orientations towards institutional access to power. In terms of motley political allegiances – and if it is hard to avoid taking positions in this vexed debate, it is even harder to elaborate one (Burman, 1996/1997) – we might note how fundamentalism (the commitment to a natural, unmediated model of memory) lives happily alongside constructionism. So, paradoxically, it is not that False Memory advocates are constructionists opposing the evil (or, alternatively, gullible) fundamentalist survivors/therapists (depending on your model), who in turn claim the integrity and veracity of memory. The problem is that False Memory supporters are *in*sufficiently constructionist, for they want to freeze the moment of construction at the point of alleged manipulation by therapists, rather than admit the continuous memory work of construction and reconstruction – including through their own practices (Burman, 1999). Further, despite their polarisations (but perhaps by virtue of its legal construction as such), both sides of this dispute converge in focusing on the individual body as the site of work, feeling and memory.

This representation of individual memory so beloved of psychologists (and lawyers) is of course a powerful reflection of the modern Western model of possessive individualism. This model extends beyond representations of individual subjectivities to their collections, resulting in national identities constructed along lines of models of individual ones. This is a point I will return to later. Kirmayer (1996) takes up this disjunction between individual and collective thresholds for memory in his discussion of different forms of traumatic response. He points to the documented contrast between narratives of victims of child sexual abuse and Holocaust survivors, and offers a socio-cultural explanation for the prevalence of dissociative disorders in the former and PTSD in the latter. (He omits to discuss compensation claims as a key factor driving the creation of the diagnostic category PTSD.) He discusses the gaps of narrative that characterise 'dissociation' as a reflection of the difficulty of telling (and – I would add – getting a hearing for) the private non-sanctioned story that disrupts conventional images of the past. For apart from New Right historical revisionists (whose influence should not be underestimated, cf. the British court case against David Irving in 2000), unlike victims of child sexual abuse, the events experienced are not themselves in doubt for Holocaust survivors. Thus, the pathology of individual memory *arises as an effect of the disorder of social memory* that will not admit the violence and abuse of normal families. Kirmayer develops his conclusions in the following way:

> The moral function of memory is to compel us to confront what we – and all around us – wish to leave behind. It might seem that for memories to be true they must be unfettered. Yet the evidence is that memories are most fully and vividly accessed and developed when they fit cultural templates and have a receptive audience. Societies then must provide cultural forms and occasions for remembering. It is a paradox of freedom that the moral function of memory depends on the constraints of social and cultural worlds to provide a limited range of narrative forms with which to construct the coherent stories of our selves (1996: 103).

Developing these ideas, I want to move on now to explore collective representations of memory, especially as they connect with those of madness, in relation to the 'stories of our selves' they afford. Clearly, these stories require specific cultural-historical situating, and some may indeed be very specific to Britain or the Anglo-US 'chattering classes'. However, the preoccupation around individual and collective discourses of responsibility, and memory as a moral form, seem to form part of the cultural fabric of South Africa too, as indicated by the recent explicit harnessing of public memory-making within the Truth and Reconciliation Commission as a tool of healing and nation-building.

## ■ Madness and the market

I want to suggest that the contemporary context of an increasingly 'mad' (incomprehensible/insecure) world produces a proliferation of further forms of madness that are tolerated – even celebrated – within the discursive realm of the norm. So let us go window-shopping for some banal (but not thereby uninteresting!) examples. There is a longstanding discourse of madness as a marketing strategy, which portrays selling at bargain rates as a disregard for or unawareness of exchange value: slogans of 'crazy cuts' and 'mad deals' are sometimes supplemented by the tired old cultural slip between mad and bad with notions of price 'slashes'. Just in case this is so well worn as to have escaped our notice, let me highlight that the norm for sanity implied here is one of making money, i.e. the normalisation of capitalism.

Within this, there is a current nuance within youth culture of madness as chic. This commutes discourses of madness and badness to 'naughty', and murder as merely transgression (cf. how the slogan '94.7% good' on a free card for 'Vodka Sour' accompanies the image of two smiling bikini-clad women on water beds in a swimming pool with their tray of drinks balanced on the body of a drowned man). Madness is seemingly portrayed as relational rather than purely individual (as in 'Are you still mad at me?' in Per Grankvist card promotions). Moreover, there are consumer 'treatments' available for some of the corollaries of madness, such as the stigma of difference. So the designation 'freak' can be taken up as an advertising slogan to highlight how this label is remediable by the purchase of a product (in a particular case, a skin-improvement product from the promotional card for Lutsia Laboratoires Dermatologiques, with the statement: 'Only 25% of people never suffer from problem skin. Problem skin is normal skin. Lutsia can help you control it'). Indeed, purchasing in general was recommended as 'Retail therapy' in the July 1999 issue of the British young women's magazine *Sugar*.

Hence, there is an increasing normalisation of pathology, with more pathology assimilated into the realm of the 'normal' as a by-product of maintaining these as individual attributes. There are clear illustrations of political investments in such individualised representations. During the Gulf War of the early 1990s, and again during the recent Balkan War, documentaries were screened in Britain investigating the personality profiles of Saddam Hussein and Slobodan Milosovic. Equally, we see an exoneration of moral lapses through a medicalisation of discourses of madness/abuse as illness – as in Hillary Clinton's recent likening of 'her husband's infidelity to an addiction such as drinking or gambling', and the citing of the 'childhood abuse which may have caused him to philander and experience "bimbo eruptions" in later life' (*Guardian*, 2 August 1999: 2).

## Individual and social

The proliferation of discourses of badness as madness and the everyday permeation of representations of madness also facilitate a playing with distributions between individual and social attribution, which I want to move on to explore. Returning to the market, the successful perfume/body-fragrance industries offer a socio-cultural legitimation of the 'sins' of envy and obsession (as they are titled by Calvin Klein). Interestingly, these more-recent titles address something more stable, internal and psychological than the earlier varieties (such as 'poison' – which still implies the incorporation of an external agent), with an explicit celebration of class mobility recently imported by the fragrance 'Bourjois'.

If there is a socialisation of cardinal sins into consumer items on the one hand, then on the other there is increasing discussion of *rage*. In some sense, anger thereby becomes public, yet it remains expressed by individuals. As Harre (1999) points out, within Western societies, anger was only recently thought of as an individual, internal state. Rage would seem currently to occupy an intermediary position between the social and the individual. Those actions glorified with the title 'rage' – road rage, air rage, supermarket rage – all indicate behaviour that is somehow both incomprehensible and unacceptable, but also potentially within the scope of identification.

The film *Falling Down* (1992) is the story of a man who within one day graduates from intolerance of urban traffic jams to making a racist attack on an Asian shopkeeper, and then to seemingly arbitrary terrorism and murderous rampaging – all in the course of his frustrations in trying to fulfil the everyday 'normal' tasks of the North American male, white, middle-class breadwinner, i.e. of getting to work, buying a drink and a hamburger, making a phone call and getting home for his daughter's birthday party. The only thing is, he's out of work, misses breakfast at the diner, can't find a call-box that works, gets caught up in Latino gang territory and mixed up with white supremacists, *and* is estranged from the wife and daughter he wants to return to. In short, he is the unanchored, de-roled white man, whose briefcase is literally empty.

The film can be described as a fascinating movie on urban life, with a protaganist who is both hero and villain (cf. Walker, 1997). Furthermore, it can be seen 'as a vigilante film, an attempt to claim a position for White Anglo-Saxon Protestants as among the victims of modern society, or a satire on over-reaction to city living' (Walker, 1997: 247). Walker also noted: 'It's hard to decide whether it's a fascist movie made by a liberal or a liberal film made by a fascist' (1997: 247). Is this how the emotionally and financially bankrupt white man becomes a terrorist? Like *Falling Down*, other forms of designated rage have something of the individual bearing the brunt of social conditions about him/her. Indeed, the very label seems to treat *as* the pathology the incursion of an intolerable social situation on the vulnerable individual. This is unlike the 19th-century discourse of the crowd, which constructs the persons therein as de-individualised and merged with others – and thereby deprived of moral/reflective capacities (cf. Le Bon, 1896). For the identity that joins those so subject to these 'rages' remains individual, as well as shared. The discussion of supermarket rage in the British popular press in December 1998 concerned men's dislike of accompanying their female partners on (Christmas) shopping expeditions. 'Rage' therefore offers an external vindicator for internal and uncontrollable emotion, and not least a collective legitimation for (what are thereby allocated as) pre-social and natural gender roles.

Significantly, although in its current discursive constructions it seems to be more frequently attributed to men, 'rage' was something that second-wave feminists sought to reclaim as a primitive revival of self-assertion and response to injustice that all the trappings of patriarchy could not eradicate. And there remains something of the underdog and of the oppressed in rage stories. Indeed, as far as 'air rage' goes, for all the hype and headlines, what emerged on TV news screens in the British case reported in early 1999 was a group of working-class people of Irish descent who had started their celebrations for their foreign holidays so early they weren't even allowed to land and start the actual vacation. A more recent case reported in *Skyport* (the Heathrow Airport newspaper) on 13 August 1999 was of a man becoming abusive and violent (with the aid of alcohol) to cabin crew on a flight from London to New York. Significantly, not only was this man Colombian and resident in Italy (and therefore constituted as an infiltrator into Europe), but he was also a travel agent, and therefore hardly uninformed as to airline codes and practices.

Moreover, the rapid take-up of discourses of rage *as metaphor* indicates a media/cultural-friendly and quasi-constructed character. Hence 'road rage' was also used to refer to car drivers' concerns and interests (in the absence of any proper plan for the development of public transport) being taken up as an electoral issue in Britain (*Guardian*, 12 July 1999). Indeed, the first court case claiming to be about road rage in Britain turned out to be (a nearly successful) hoax by a woman to distract investigations away from her murder of her male companion, whom she later claimed had been oppressing/abusing her.

It would seem that 'rage' is regarded as something that lies within us all, but is only expressed under conditions of extreme duress – a popular psychoanalytic discourse if ever there were one. If rage – that supposedly most primitive and unsocial emotion – has entered the social sphere, does this rearrange thresholds of tolerance for other forms of social dysfunction/indiscipline? But the partial admission of the social within the individual (or is it the individual within the social?) still leaves lots of room for the evaluation of unacceptable/incomprehensible actions as outside humanity. The recent cases in the US and Britain of gun-crazed attacks on schools and of explicitly fascist attacks by white supremacists on black communities, gay bars and Jewish synagogues were not designated as rage, for 'rage' is regarded as somehow deeply justified. While these attacks were apparently perpetrated by individual men rather than organisations, they were certainly steeped in racist, sexist and homophobic cultures that explicitly incited such actions. But somehow, being able to situate these within the domain of the incomprehensible, overwhelming discourse of the mad (individual) allows us to ward off exploration of such actions as expressing more collective desires or implicating wider politico-economic explanations.

## ■ 'Forget the pain'

If 'rage' elaborates a traditional psychological arena that maintains an individual psyche floating amid a social swirl, contemporary discussions of *memory* focus on pain as social and correspondingly amenable to manipulation. 'Forget the pain' was the slogan for the latest sequence of painkiller ads, with the statement 'No wonder Anadin is Britain's most popular brand of pain killer' invoking the statistical discourse of population alongside various different images appearing each week – images of intimate abandon, sometimes domestic, often recreational (in such magazines as *Take a Break* and *New Woman*). The invitation to 'forget' does not allow for an implicit 'IF' before 'you can forget'. Rather (with the magic pill) the headache, your pain, *will* disappear and you *will* enjoy yourself – in what seems like an exemplary Lacanian exegesis of the covert injunction to enjoy what is overtly forbidden (Zizek, 1989). The direct address (to 'you') alongside a statistical discourse of generality ('Britain's most popular brand') situates 'you' as a particular who is also like others. Similarly, marketing strategies for other products seem to be coalescing around themes of forgetting. That the paradigm for these (including the first Anadin one that alerted me to this theme) concerns specifically feminine (menstrual) pain must give pause for thought (the exhortation 'Discover how comfortable New Brevia pantyliners are. Then forget them' appeared twice in one issue of *New Woman,* August 1999, as well as 'Now Nurofen Longlasting can give period pain the push for up to 12 hours'). In some cases, the narrative of freedom (from pain, for activity) is not even disguised as meaning sexual availability (as in 'Forget the lemsip [a cold-cure drink], have sex', which appeared in *New Woman* (August 1999: 172)).

The producers of other products use forms of memorial agency that are also saturated with psychoanalytic themes. The massively successful British National Lottery, launched by the Conservative Party in 1996, maintained by New Labour at present in power, justifies itself in a current promotional leaflet (available wherever lottery tickets are sold) as a charity that provides 'Fun for you. Funds for projects like these' (alongside images of rural/ecological preservation and children trampolining). The initial publicity for the scratch cards launched a year later, which can be bought at any British newsagent or corner shop, reads 'Forget it all for an instant' – an invitation that explicitly transgressed (perhaps precisely because of) the then-dominant discourses of economic recession, with corresponding moral injunctions to look to the future (now fulfilled by your purchase of the card that supports future-oriented causes).

'Forget it all for an instant' has always enraged me (so to speak), not least because 'instants' seemed to be the total time for enjoyment accorded poor people, and because 'an instant' is so meagre a claim to life's pleasures and political utopias. There are perhaps shades here of Walter Benjamin's notion of the 'weak Messianic power' (1955/1973: 246) with which we are all endowed, a power '[that] cannot be settled cheaply' and moreover that, because 'our image of happiness is thoroughly coloured by the time to which the course of our existence has assigned us' (1955/1973: 245), is also a redemptive image of the future 'to which the past has a claim' (1955/1973: 246).

There are contrasting images of forgetting here: a wish for escape versus a fantasy that forgetting/oblivion leaves no trace of what it erases. Perhaps that is why we are only invited to 'Forget it all' for an *instant*. Forgetting it for longer (for forever perhaps?) would somehow be morally reprehensible. Or perhaps there is a fear fuelling the injunction to forget (like Benjamin's storm of progress blowing from Paradise). For what might happen if, instead of forgetting, we *remembered* what 'it all' is really like? How elliptical is this way of referring to the totality of the (putatively) miserable conditions of one's life: such small relief to circumscribe such large issues by the most minimal words of the English language ('it all'). Moreover (to again invite a Lacanian twist), the acknowledgement of the pain of 'it all' only arises within the invitation to forget 'it'.

## ▪ Changing images

By contrast, the current (1999 onwards) National Lottery slogan runs 'maybe, just maybe'. It thus wobbles between offering transportation from an oppressive present to a liberation from a traumatic past. Like 'Forget it all ...', the absence of person markers facilitates a shift of subjective identity as well as condition. 'Maybe, just maybe' you can be a different person, as well as live in different circumstances. But in a shift away from such gloriously unspecified fantasy slogans, the current version of Instants now announce themselves with a slightly menacing 'It could be you'. This is combined with the symbol of the crossed fingers – which signifies not only luck, but also has resonances of British HIV awareness campaigns of the 1980s, and before that family-planning poster campaigns (which went something like 'There are lots of ways of making sure you don't get pregnant. This isn't one of them'). As Darien Leader (1996) points out, the National Lottery's 'It could be you' incites a desire that installs guilt as the condition for enjoyment. It thereby elaborates a more *reflexive* relation between images of oneself (as one is versus as one would like to be), unlike the previous football-pools campaigns that worked *comparatively*, inciting envy with images of 'people like you' enjoying themselves with their winnings.

If a secularised but originally religious discourse of guilty/repudiated pleasure is implicit in the National Lottery campaigns, it becomes more explicit – because parodied – in a soft-drink promotion in 1999 for Diet Tango, with its slogan: 'You need it because you're weak'. Here 'need' is explicitly ironised as a social/personal construction. It is 'weak' to want junk food – of which Diet Tango is simply a slightly less-fattening version (adding to the layers of meaning and interpellation within a moral/religious discourse of confession). But this weak, private need, 'yours' but now public (playing on the ambiguity of 'you need' as shameful description or injunction), has acquired cultural celebrity status (a bit like the do-nut and diet coke syndrome?). Like 'Forget it all' of the National Lottery, the desire is accorded public expression and permission at the same moment of its prohibition. Tango campaigns specialise in violent, surprising stunts (hence the slogan 'You've been Tango'd'), which in this case both attest to gluttonous desires (the slogan accompanies close-up lurid images of old greasy takeaway chips or boxes of instant noodles) and therefore produce the 'need' to impose 'Diet Tango makeovers' on 'winning' 'greasy spoon' caffs (cf. the 'promotion': 'Grease is the word: You need it because you're weak', in *Loaded,* August 1999). The modern ritual of the 'makeover' recalls the public spectacle of catharsis in religious and legal practices of confession, with corresponding dynamics of humiliation and victimisation – but also identification – between viewers and subjects. However, instead of punishment, here – as in talk shows – the transformation is contingent on the exposure of the *pre-transformed* state (the vilified state to be repudiated), which is yet another example of the social construction of *nachtraglichkeit* (the retroactive installation of a traumatic event).

## ▪ Nationality and social memory

So far, I have been dealing largely with banalised practices of socially engineered memory-making – the kitsch end of the very commercial Western line, so to speak. Yet even these – even in their emphatic reiteration of the singular subject who wields and wears memories like the fragrances she/he buys in the shops, or constructs in the Lottery – are thereby of unstable identity. Lambek (1996) points out the parallelism between discussions of imagined communities and the imaginary character of individual histories, by both of which we live accordingly (Anderson, 1991). For it is precisely because as individuals we cannot remember – either our childhoods or each moment of our histories – that we subscribe to cultural narratives that allow for the creation of subjective continuity. Moreover, Lambek (1996) argues, these discourses of selfhood, like discourses of collective identity, are poetic or rhetorical, rather than foundational. Both personal memory and historical accounts are therefore far less fixed than they would seem: 'The critical distinction is one of fluidity, the degree to which any particular narrative is open to continuous reformulation, any event or document to reinterpretation, and how such changes are legitimated' (Lambek, 1996: 43).

Issues of legitimation are – of course – what are crucially at issue in struggles over individual and collective memory, i.e. issues of the construction of tradition and of experience, and of what is to be remembered and what passed over and forgotten. It would seem that there are, firstly, some experiences that cannot be remembered precisely because they so structure the reflexive subject that they elude being the object of reflection. Secondly, there are others that are constituted as outside the threshold of tolerance for remembering, i.e. supposedly traumatic forgetting of material that – so the theory goes – can only break through to consciousness in fragments or under certain conditions. It is this second kind of remembering that exercises us the most. Just as marketers manipulate individual and collective memorial practices, so also political events acquire different memorial classifications. Clearly, the South African Truth and Reconciliation Commission represents one very explicit means of attempting to manage this as a social process.

In Britain, discussions of racism have recently been focused on the case of Stephen Lawrence, a young black man who was murdered by a gang of white youths in April 1993. The police response to and investigation of this murder was handled so incompetently and offhandedly that public pressure generated a very damning independent inquiry (the *Macpherson Report*), after two previous police inquiries failed to discipline culpable police officers who had failed to take appropriate action and allowed the case to remain without a conviction. Not only did the events and the inquiry highlight endemic institutional racism, they also foregrounded the dangers for black men on British streets. Shifting the analytic territory from social-structural to personal-individual, the report of the final inquiry (released in March 1999) talked of 'unconscious racism' fuelling the catalogue of mishaps and misunderstandings in the official process. By such means, a psychoanalytic rendering of racism as pathology comes to be applied to organisational and political processes, and collective memory becomes constructed as analogous to that of a traumatised and traumatising individual. The longer-term political nuances of this rendering of institutional racism remain to be seen, but the cultural framework of individualisation of such forms of interpretation gives grounds for concern.

## ■ Limiting dilemmas

In this chapter, I have been focusing largely on popular cultural and public examples, on the crass 'excessive external influence' (Lambek, 1996: 252, fn. 15) upon memorial constructions and their corresponding subjectivities. In drawing to a close, I want to try to strike a slightly different note. For all my attention to the malign character of manipulations of individual and collective histories, this does at least highlight the flexibility of such representations – even within societies apparently committed to a fixed and rational unitary subject. Moreover, a whole range of possibilities flow from this for elaborating a different range of culturally sanctioned relations to being in history, not all of which depict the subject as wielding the past as a picture book – a book that may be either open or closed, but that is always linear and successive.

The psychoanalytic account that has come to dominate Western conceptions of memory both subverts, and in some ways leaves intact, the individualist and 'storebox' theories of psychology and neurology. Nevertheless, as Hacking (1996) argues, it has become the modern secular forum in which broader questions about the soul and society are posed. If we can come to see this account as the narrative it is (rather than truth), then perhaps we can begin to identify other cultural-political trajectories made possible by unfixing dominant relations to time and history. While anthropologists look to non-Western – often African – cultures for intimations of alternative accounts of subjective being and directionality in history (e.g. Bloch, 1996), I am suggesting these narratives already abound even in the market centres of late modernity, with their shifting sands of madness and civilisation. This is not merely to indulge in a post-modern celebration of flexible identities produced through consumption, although my account here clearly could be read in such a way. Rather, my aim has been to return the gaze from the multiple 'others' of capitalism's centres, to look again, perhaps a little awry (Zizek, 1991), at how European and US subjectivities partake of that which they repudiate, and then seek elsewhere – in this case, a diversity of relationships to lived time and sociality. Questions of who remembers and what is remembered are very much on the agenda in the elaboration of post-colonial positions – both on the part of the (historical) colonisers and the (historically) colonised. The fact that global capitalism and its penetration through cultural imperialism represents another colonising force should not obscure the ways popular culture can also intimate (and shape) forms of subjectivity that at least jar against each other, and against the dominant received notions of Western subjectivity.

Acknowledgement of the unfinished, incomplete character of the past, of a 'past imperfect' (Lambek, 1996) that is always changing through engagement with the present, is central to the elaboration of the conditions for Kristeva's (1981) politically radical 'future conditional' conception of (women's) time. She critiques the genre of *ecriture feminine* (women's writing) as essentialising and rendering static and homogeneous the radical possibilities of women's political activity, including writing, and advocates forms of subjectivity (as elaborated through writing) that do not presume fixed gendered positions, but rather envisage the temporal-historical possibilities of how the current conditions could be different. Similarly, we must not foreclose radical possibilities by overstating the fixity of current subjective forms, with their attendant follies and foibles. Nevertheless, highlighting the constructive character of both individual and social memory institutes responsibilities towards the politics of subjectivity, responsibilities that marketers and politicians clearly take too lightly. Such are the dilemmas and political responsibilities fashioned through institutional memorial construction, i.e. to create subjects capable not only of remembering and forgetting, but, in doing so, also of changing:

> Central to Freud's understanding of the genesis of the person is the idea that we must have a history that we get wrong. Similarly, two commentators on nationalism, Anderson (1991) and Hobsbawm (1992), draw on Renan's remarks of 1882: *'Or, l'essence d'une nation est que tous les individues aient beaucoup de choses en commun et aussi que tous oublie bien des choses'* [For the essence of a nation is that all the individuals have many things in common and also that they forget many things (my translation)], recognising that the ethical quandaries of the historian and psychoanalyst are similar. In telling the stories of their subjects, must both remember the very things those subjects are determined to forget? Is their responsibility to support current identity politics or to break through the defences in order to reposition the subject for new self-interpretations or radical change? (Lambek, 1996: 249–50).

## References

Anderson, B. (1991). *Imagined Communities*. London: Verso.

Benjamin, W. (1955/1973). *Illuminations*. London: Jonathan Cape.

Bloch, M. (1996). Internal and external memory: Different ways of being in history. In P. Antze and M. Lambek (eds), *Tense Past: Cultural Essays in Trauma and Memory*, pp. 215–34. New York: Routledge.

Burman, E. (1996/1997). False memories, true hopes: Revenge of the postmodern on therapy. *New Formations*, 30, 122–34.

Burman, E. (1999). Feminist approaches to false memory controversies. Paper presented to the Annual General Meeting of the North West Division of the Royal College of Psychiatrists, June.

*Falling Down* (1992). Dir. J. Schumacher, dis. Warner.

Foucault, M. (1977). *Discipline and Punish: The Birth of the Prison*. Harmondsworth: Penguin.

Foucault, M. (1980). *The History of Sexuality: An Introduction*, Vol. 1. New York: Vintage Books.

Foucault, M. (1986). *The History of Sexuality: The Use of Pleasure*, Vol. 2. New York: Vintage Books.

Foucault, M. (1988). *The History of Sexuality: The Care of the Self*, Vol. 3. New York: Vintage Books.

Freud, S. (1902/1962). *The Psychopathology of Everyday Life*, Vol. 6. London: Hogarth Press.

Goffman, E. (1979). *Gender Advertisements*. London: Macmillan.

Haaken, J. (1998). *Pillar of Salt: Gender, Meaning and the Perils of Looking Back*. London: Free Associations Books.

Hacking, I. (1996). Memory sciences, memory politics. In P. Antze and M. Lambek (eds), *Tense Past: Cultural Essays in Trauma and Memory*, pp. 67–88. New York: Routledge.

Harre, R. (1999). The social construction of emotions. Paper presented at the Qualitative Methods Conference, Sheffield Hallam University, 12–15 July.

Kirmayer, L. (1996). Landscapes of memory: Trauma, narrative and dissociation. In P. Antze and M. Lambek (eds), *Tense Past: Cultural Essays in Trauma and Memory*, pp. 173–98. New York: Routledge.

Kristeva, J. (1981). Women's time. *Signs: Journal of Women in Culture and Society*, 7 (1), 13–35.

Lambek, M. (1996). The past imperfect: Remembering as a moral practice. In P. Antze and M. Lambek (eds), *Tense Past: Cultural Essays in Trauma and Memory*, pp. 235–54. New York: Routledge.

Leader, D. (1996). *Why do Women Write More Letters than they Post?* London: Faber and Faber.

Le Bon, G. (1896). *The Crowd*. London: Ernest Benn.

Macpherson, Sir W. (1999). *The Stephen Lawrence Inquiry: Report of an Inquiry by Sir William Macpherson*. London: Stationery Office.

Parker, I. (1997). *Psychoanalytic Culture*. London: Sage.

Walker, J. (1997). *Halliwell's Film and Video Guide*. London: Harper Collins.

Zizek, S. (1989). *For They Know Not What They Do: Enjoyment as a Political Factor*. London: Verso.

Zizek, S. (1991). *Looking Awry*. London: October Books/MIT Press.

# CHAPTER 13

# Rethinking normality through post-disciplinary practices

*Mark Smith*

## ■ Introduction

What we think of as 'the normal' is always bound up with our culturally specific preconceptions of the pathological, signifying not merely what is different between individuals or groups, but, through the operation of power, the construction of 'otherness'. To engage in the pathologisation of a specific social category implicitly invokes the process of normalisation, which in turn involves classificatory practices. The choice of the word 'category' here is especially significant, for it signifies the imaginary constitution and classification of groups and communities in a specific location, while at the same time acknowledging that the identities fixed through racial classificatory practices have a real impact. For example, we can see how the attribution of specific qualities to racial categories (such as intelligence or athletic ability) can be used to reinforce cultural stereotypes. What part does social science play in this?

There has been a fixation on the excluded and marginalised as objects of moral concern as much as objects of analysis throughout the history of the social sciences from the 18th century onwards. Quite late in this process, Emile Durkheim rationalised the development of social-scientific disciplines as a direct response to the need to explain discrete objects of analysis (such as the mind, the economy, the polity and so on). Moreover, the possession of a discrete object was the entry ticket to disciplinarity within the academy. This was, in Durkheim's case, motivated by the desire to ring-fence 'society' as the sole preserve of the disciplinary project of sociology and to establish markers of competence and expertise in relation to psychology and philosophy. In his *The Rules of Sociological Method* (1895), a project for dealing with facts as things and for establishing the appropriate procedures for knowing, Durkheim explicitly tied sociological method to the distinction between normality and pathology in identifying the character and function of what can be known. We can see this in the analogies and metaphors developed in his sociological narratives:

> The word 'sickness' always signifies something which tends to be the total or partial destruction of the organism. If there is not destruction, there is cure, but never stability, such as exists in several abnormalities ... [T]he abnormal is also, in the average case, a threat to the living creature. It is true that this is not always so, but the dangers that sickness entails likewise exist in average circumstances. As for the absence of stability allegedly distinctive of the morbid, this leaves out of account chronic illnesses and is to divide the study of monstrosities from that of the pathological. The monstrosities are permanent (Durkheim, 1895: 105).

Within the terms of reference of the social as an organism, we can find a complex account of sickness, morbidity, pathology, abnormality and monstrosity tied to their degree of permanency (one which is open to criticism on a number of fronts: see Smith, 2002b). This classificatory system conceals a sophisticated treatment of normality/pathology as interconnected, mutually essential (for all social orders presuppose both) and subject to variability across time and cultures. Significantly, criminality is viewed as the exemplification of a universally pathologised predisposition (hence the selection of criminology later in this chapter):

> The Criminal no longer appears as an utterly unsociable creature, a sort of parasitic element, a foreign, unassimilable body introduced into the bosom of society. He plays a normal role in social life .... The principle purpose of any science of life, whether individual or social, is in the end to define and explain the normal state and distinguish it from the abnormal .... For sociology really to be a science of things, the generality of phenomena must be taken as the criterion of their normality (Durkheim, 1895: 102–4).

For Durkheim, criminality is evidence of how the pathological is an extension of the normal. This valuable point of the dynamic and historical specificity of the normality/pathology distinction is obscured by the preference for nomothesis (i.e. general explanations) and for detachment of the knowing subject from the object of analysis (i.e. characterising objects as referents independent of the discursive conditions of their constitution).

Working through similar problems in reconstructing the normality/pathology distinction in the history of medicine, Georges Canguilhem also sought to historicise knowledge (in so doing, indicating that progress was an inadequate descriptive term for characterising the changing definitions of concepts or the evolution of social institutions). Unlike Durkheim, he challenged the separation between orders of thought and referent, providing a framework for recognising how scientific knowledge of the world was in the same breath situated in the institutional practices that it putatively explained. However, Canguilhem retains the idea of a separation of scientific from pre-scientific thought in order to demonstrate the normativity of science in the face of error (i.e. the regulation of the production of knowledge through the distinction between truth and falsity), so retaining a commitment to a fallibilistic conception of knowledge. This is something that has been repeatedly challenged in the sociology of scientific knowledge, and for good reason. Recent ethnographic research on the level of laboratory practice demonstrates how conventions evolve (so science is itself a shifting terrain), while at any given time and place indicating resistance to the implications of anomalies or disconfirming evidence (Canguilhem, 1991; Rose, 1998). It is better to distinguish between the normativity of science in general (a rhetorical device that can be rearticulated in different ways) from the precise conditions in which it is (re-)articulated. Knowledge is always produced within the institutional practices, rules of conduct and textual references that give an academic discipline its coherence and plausibility.

Unlike theories that surface as a way of stringing together concepts after the event, Canguilhem suggested that concepts have lives of their own. Concepts are manufactured through rational thought; moreover, they create objects as well as generate hypothesis and experimentation. So, we can talk of a plurality of rationalities with specific versions tied to specific historically specific conditions. Rather than viewing pathological and abnormal characteristics as statistical generalities (on the margins of a normal distribution of behaviour types), Canguilhem argues that the normal and pathological symbolise deeply embedded values in a given social order: 'Every preference for a possible order is accompanied, most often implicitly, by the aversion for the opposite possible order. That which diverges from the preferable in a given area of evaluation is not the indifferent but the repulsive or more exactly, the repulsed, the detestable' (Canguilhem 1991: 240).

Nevertheless, the pathological should be seen as a type of normal. That is, rather than viewing the pathological as *against the normal*, one might view it as *another normality*. Michel Foucault developed this insight into a series of accounts of the institutional locations (the asylum, the clinic, the prison, the school and so on) within which the process of normalisation has a crucial role in capturing the body. In *Discipline and Punish* (1977), for example, his concern is with the operation of power to maximise the usefulness of a population (with the body as a productive element of a social order). In this context, norms are the means by which the 'analysable body' and 'manipulable body' are conjoined through observations, measurement, comparison, averaging and (if necessary) reform; in short, the means through which active bodies become docile in order to be 'subjected, used, transformed, and improved' (Foucault, 1977: 136). The story of normality and pathology is one involved in the management of human populations, in which normalisation becomes the evolution of procedures for judgement (in setting the standard of the distinction ranks) that assesses and distributes bodies within a complex social order:

> The practice of placing individuals under observation is a natural extension of a justice imbued with disciplinary methods and examination procedures. Is it surprising that the cellular prison, with its regular chronologies, forced labour, its authorities of surveillance and registration, its experts in normality, who continue and multiply the functions of the judge, should have become the modern instrument of penalty? Is it surprising that prisons resemble factories, schools, barracks, hospitals, which all resemble prisons? (Foucault, 1977: 227–8).

This has been acknowledged in both clinical and social-scientific practice in a number of ways. Within clinical practice, the role of diagnostics in pinpointing 'disorders' and 'abnormalities' as if they were neutral denotations for clusters of symptoms ignores the social significance of such categories, as well as the classificatory systems in which they have a place. These classificatory systems are in part the evolved systems of thought through which the meaning of scientific knowledge is produced. Social scientists operate as the custodians of established procedures for classifying people, but, in drawing upon clinical experience, they maintain the relevance of established analytic frameworks, hence legitimating the pathologisation of specific groups within social relations of inclusion and exclusion. The use of language that carries negative connotations encodes the words with messages about the way the world is organised. So it is not so much the words themselves that are important as their meanings, their relationship to how we understand and organise the social world and the concrete effects such categories have on people's lives. To think through the meaning of normality, we have to rethink the relation between normality and pathology.

Judgements about cultural differences and the associated values involve the operationalisation of complex classification procedures that are to some extent shared, and serve as the tacit basis for producing meanings. These approaches are, in their different ways, very effective in exploring the rules of conduct that permit particular kinds of offensive talk and indiscretions. For example, the categorisations of groups according to 'race' are manufactured through the constant repetition and reformulation of narratives and stories constructed in everyday life. The close relationship between ethnocentric bias in psychopathological and psychiatric research and their role in defining culturally specific behaviour as abnormal, and hence in need of treatment and/or detainment, has been identified in a number of studies (for recent examples see Fernando *et al.*, 1997; Littlewood and Lipsedge, 1997). These studies attempt to understand the unacknowledged conditions of racist values within situated conversations and texts (as well as in psychological knowledges).

In this way, the plausibility of disciplinary narratives was achieved through the operationalisation of the distinction between the normal and the pathological. As a result, social-scientific practices have been tied to power relations by translating cultural values into authoritative knowledge. We have experienced two centuries of disciplinarity, where the study of the social has presumed that 'objects of analysis' are concrete things with a definite structure, or alternatively that they are constituted by a set of components accessible to some procedure of knowing. All disciplinary projects need a guiding purpose, whether this involves some generalised commitment to progress or more specific ends such as public safety. The normalising and pathologising tendencies of social-scientific practices are now in question, and with them the present institutional basis of academic governance.

## Disciplinarity and complexity

Objects of analysis are not what they used to be. Once, so the history of social science tells us, they were secure and fixed, a matter of definition and not in question. Now they are in doubt, problematic, under erasure and without foundation. This does not signify a fundamental change in the social structure. Both the natural and social worlds have always been complex and discursively constituted. Despite enormous argumentation and considerable dispute about the 'proper' focus and character of social inquiry, there have been strong continuities in academic practices over time and across fields of knowledge. The emergence of disciplinary fields of knowledge is also tied to the emergence of particular forms of governmentality in the institutions of the academy. Yet each has been destabilised over the last two decades. In contemporary social science, objects of analysis are increasingly seen as complex, uncertain and contested spaces. Debates on difference and otherness have played a significant role in this. To understand this process, this chapter explores the changes in classificatory practices and judgements involved in contemporary social-scientific practices. We have been very effective at convincing ourselves that the world is simple, atomistic, a collection of empirical regularities and subject to the whims of phenomenalists and nominalists (who have argued that what we see is what we get and that the names we devise for things are accurate reflections of what they are). As I will argue later, it is the adoption of a closed-system analysis of the social that has served to shore up the social-science disciplines (see the table below).

## Closed and open systems in the social sciences

|   |   | Closed systems | Open systems |
|---|---|---|---|
| 1 | **Simplicity and complexity** | A limited number of measurable variables is used to increase the possibility of identifying and predicting clear relationships. | A state of complexity is acknowledged as the condition of one's objects of analysis and the relations between them. |
| 2 | **External boundary** | Exclusion clauses ensure that the confusing mass of possible influences are screened out (such as the *ceteris paribus* clause that, holding all other things constant, *x* will lead to *y*). | No external boundary is assumed to exist, so that each object can be part of multiple causal relations and one cannot predict an outcome with any degree of certainty. |
| 3 | **Intrinsic properties** | All objects of analysis are taken at face value, so that the intrinsic properties of an object are not considered. | It is recognised that all objects have intrinsic properties and structures that affect their performance in different conditions. |

Source: Smith, 1998b: 45

By examining the implication of closed-system analysis in the study of people within social relationships and institutions, it is possible to establish how the disciplines of sociology, psychology and economics were able to consolidate their professional academic status. Emulating the successful natural sciences through a series of analogies and metaphors offered a fast track to building up trust in the knowledge produced. Science is a very powerful and evocative word or idea in Western culture. It conveys legitimacy and authenticity upon the people, ideas and institutions with which it is associated. A claim to authenticity means that a statement is 'true to life', the real thing, rather than an imitation. To be effective, disciplinary projects had to (have to) engage with a variety of audiences (within the academy, within policy communities and in the public sphere). Disciplinary projects had to (have to) establish some degree of plausibility with these audiences, so that they come to be seen as authentic accounts of the social world or, at least, a discrete portion of it. In Durkheimian fashion, each discipline sought to (seeks to) construct its own distinctive object of analysis and establish its respective claim to be able to speak authoritatively upon it.

The idea of closure has been an important part of all disciplines that have sought to establish objective knowledge. The assumption that closure can be achieved, whereby extraneous variables can be excluded in order to achieve an 'interference-free' zone for identifying clear-cut relations (i.e. conjunctions between empirical variables) remains extremely popular as a technique.

The application of this model of inquiry in different social-scientific disciplines is closely related to the way the object of analysis is constructed in each case. For instance, in the development of political science, the specification of 'the state' and political institutions was also tied to the adoption of behaviourist assumptions about observable concrete decisions and the operation of power. Political science sought to explain the dynamic process of political choices and the exercise of power with the supposed precision of a natural science. Dahl and Polsby explicitly adopted the scientific approach towards social research when constructing the pluralist model of the state and politics. Dahl presents a useful definition of this method as the 'examination of the political relationships of men [sic] ... with the object of formulating and testing hypotheses concerning uniformities of behaviour' (Dahl, 1961: 764). The concept of power is treated as an empirical regularity whereby the behaviour of one agent causes the behaviour of another, so that the latter does things that it would not otherwise do. For Dahl, 'A has the power over B to the extent that he can get B to do something that B would not otherwise do' (Dahl, 1957: 203–4).

This approach limits research on power to actual decision-making behaviour by groups of individuals within situations where observable conflicts of interests exist. These interests are defined as 'expressed policy preferences' (such as demands for change or supports for the status quo), which are, in turn, revealed through political participation. This means that we should take what political actors say and what they do to be a direct expression of their interests. By focusing upon the specific outcomes of observable behaviour, the pluralist approach is able to gather 'reliable evidence' (which has been subject to further tests and which produces the same or similar results). This usually takes the form of quantitative data in order to facilitate correlations between variables (i.e. statistical comparisons). Pluralists used statistical controls to simulate a closed system involving a limited number of simple variables (cf. Blalock, 1964). In effect, in order to establish a plausible scientific approach, the disciplinary project had to construct a 'political subject' that fitted the bill regardless of the complexities of political decision-making and, as Dahl came to accept, the need to understand the wider cultural conditions of political relations and processes.

This example draws our attention to the relationship between *what* is known and *how* we know; between our various ontological assumptions and presuppositions about the social world and the epistemological procedures for knowing the social. In the search for plausibility, social scientists have assumed that their simplifications of social processes are a mimetic (reflectionist) account of the way the world operates. In such a context, it is important to establish what complexity means. In research work on social-scientific practice (Smith, 1998b), I identified a number of kinds of complexity.

- **Practical complexity:** This involves recognising that simple relations are artificial human inventions, for other factors always have a part to play when we are reconstructing social existence (i.e. that the empirical world is always much more complex than we expect).
- **Imaginative complexity:** Rather than seeing thoughts as a reflection of the things we study, it is important to recognise the way imaginative thinking organises our perceptions, sensations and impressions (i.e. that we simplify empirical complexity through imaginative thought).
- **Situated complexity:** All forms of knowledge, including scientific knowledge, are the complex product of the practices established in historical and social locations where they were produced. As such, they carry the cultural values upon which they were grounded, although they may be received in other locations in quite different ways.
- **Representational complexity:** The production of meaning is itself a complex process, composed of linguistic, symbolic, discursive and cultural elements, all of which can have dramatic affects on how social scientists construct evidence and communicate arguments to others.
- **Structural or deep complexity:** In order to see science as an intelligible activity, the things we study must have real internal properties (i.e. real powers and liabilities), but our only way of expressing these things is through representation.

Each kind of complexity involves a further step away from the conventional view of what it means to be scientific. If we accept that studying people involves acknowledging these aspects of social complexity, then we must also acknowledge that the adoption of a closed-system approach is inappropriate. However, there is no agreement on which of these we should take seriously, and you may find some kinds of complexity more convincing than others, depending on how you assess the alternatives to the closed-system approach.

How can we address these transformations in knowledge construction? To start with, we have to have a clear idea of what disciplinarity means as a conceptual tool. Two closely connected dimensions stand out:

1. The *discursive dimension* highlights the unifying characteristic of a discipline – its capacity for self-reference and self-regulation (autopoiesis). Disciplinary discourses are effective to the extent that they provide a framework within which meanings can be regulated. They attempt to shut down the possibility of alternative interpretations by drawing upon the stock of common-sense knowledge that has come to be accepted. Discourses regulate the production of meaning with reference to an established set of textual sources (often canonised) and within the institutional practices through which we classify people. One way in which this is achieved is through directly tapping into tacit prejudices, values and taken-forgranted assumptions about cultural differences. For a disciplinary discourse to work, the use of language has to make sense through good storytelling (McCloskey, 1983), enabling its deployment within the inclusionary and exclusionary relations of everyday life. This is achieved through the construction of subject positions. However, this kind of strategy for fixing meaning is never fully

successful, for audiences can produce meanings in unanticipated ways and people resist classification (Laclau and Mouffe, 1985).

2. **The *contextual dimension*** indicates the important role played by social scientists as cultural agents. Since we can never be separate from the things we study (i.e. the system of language and specific cultural values, the rules of conduct and the established social practices, the institutional and textual conditions of knowledge production and so on), then the best position we can maintain is to acknowledge this condition and try to be aware of the way we draw upon and articulate classificatory systems in order to engage in classificatory practices (i.e. the location of things in categories). In a discussion of the role of categories such as high, low, mass, elite and popular in relation to culture, Pierre Bourdieu (1986) argues that 'taste classifies the classifier'. In social science, the attachment to markers of authenticity like validity, reliability, rationality, truth, progress and so on raises similar issues. Cultural hierarchies enable us to make a judgement about what is good or poor art. So too, social science has its carefully maintained stable reference points through which we can spot an 'authoritative' piece of work that speaks in the appropriate voice. Many of these markers work through style and terminology, a rhetorical formula instantly recognisable through the subtext – which whispers, 'I am true; believe me'. The distinctions that are at work within knowledge construction serve as a measure of all that is considered to be worthwhile. Social-scientific practices that embody received wisdom and cultural knowledge mimic the 'authoritative voice', and embody the cultural heritage of a specific time and place for a specific audience. In this sense, the processes of communications through which social science has come to be established involve a kind of performance that conveys meaning to an audience, who themselves possess at least some of the skills to decode the messages, ritual and symbolism involved.

This means that social-scientific research is (and always has been) a dialogue between readers and writers. It involves a cultural politics of knowledge construction, a politics based on the contradictory principles of trust and contestation (cf. the contradictory logics of equivalence and difference in Laclau and Mouffe, 1985). In addition, this 'political' dimension indicates how power relations are an inherent part of the way social-scientific practice is conducted, i.e. that the kinds of knowledge produced through social science operate through the normalising and pathologising of different kinds of behaviour and identities. If power is defined in terms of its consequences (even if we just concentrate on gender and ethnicity), then social-scientific knowledge has a lot to answer for. The presence of social prejudice in social research is well documented, but perhaps more significant is the way social-scientific practice can be tacitly androcentric or ethnocentric. We can now start by thinking about how cultural meanings are part of the processes involved in classification. (For a discussion of how this can be understood in environmental studies, see Smith, 1998a, 1999, 2002a, 2002c.) The plausibility of disciplinary narratives is achieved through the operationalisation of the distinction between the normal and the pathological. As a result, social-scientific practices have been tied to power relations by translating cultural values into authoritative knowledge. The normalising and pathologising tendencies of social-scientific practices are also now in question. To see how the normal and pathological operate, we will consider one area of social research that provides a useful meeting point for disciplinary interventions, i.e. the study of crime.

The gradual merging of critical-realist with discursive concerns in this area offers one model for moving away from disciplinarity. Parker *et al.* (1995) focused attention on the need to deconstruct psychopathology as a situated practice, directly challenging the role of experts in mental-health practice, whether they be therapists, psychiatrists or psychologists. This is achieved through careful consideration of oppositional distinctions at work in the diagnosis of specific conditions (reason/unreason, lay/professional, individual/social, form/content, categories/messy real life and, last but not least, normality/pathology). Along similar lines, Burman *et al.* (1996) have offered a detailed exploration of the role of therapeutic practices in the construction of subject positions. However, as critical psychologists, they want to make a difference. Therefore, they also point to the ways in which therapeutic practices (from educational psychology to gender-identity therapists) open up opportunities for resistance by patients to the pathologising tendencies of professional experts. The discourses of psychiatry and psychology attempt to regulate the production of meaning, yet they are always open to destabilisation and subversion, and can even facilitate empowerment. In the case study at the heart of the next section, we will concentrate on the disciplinary field in which psychopathology and psychiatry play a performing role, the discipline of criminology.

## ■ Constructing criminal subjects

The study of crime provides us with a useful terrain to consider the role of disciplinary discourses. Firstly, unlike some areas of inquiry, it provides a terrain where all the social sciences have contributed. Indeed, some of the most important contributions to the study of crime have been one-off interventions by social theorists and researchers from other areas of work. Secondly, there is a central core of social research, the discipline of criminology, that attempts to generate a disciplinary project around the task of identifying the causes of criminality. The hard core of this disciplinary project draws heavily on psychology, but has come into contact with writers from sociology, politics and economics, each leaving its own legacy. This project has attempted to establish firm foundations for a particular subject position, the 'criminal subject'. Hall offers the following outline, which captures the meaning of subject positions in discourse theory:

> The 'subject' is *produced within discourse*. This subject *of* discourse cannot be outside discourse, because it must be *subjected to* discourse. It must submit to its rules and conventions, to its dispositions of power/knowledge. The subject can become the bearer of the kind of knowledge which discourse produces. It can become the object through which power is relayed. But it cannot stand outside power/knowledge as its source and author ... [The] 'subject' seems to be produced through discourse in *two* different senses or places. First, the discourse itself produces 'subjects' – figures who personify the particular forms of knowledge which the discourse produces. These subjects have the attributes we would expect as these are defined by the discourse: the

madman, the hysterical woman, the homosexual, the individualized criminal, and so on. These figures are specific to specific discursive regimes and historical periods. But the discourse also produces a *place for the subject* (i.e. the reader or viewer, who is also 'subjected to' discourse) from which its particular knowledge and meaning most makes sense. It is not inevitable that all individuals in a particular period will become the subjects of a particular discourse in this sense, and thus the bearers of its power/knowledge. But for them – us – to do so, they – we – must locate themselves/ourselves in the *position* from which the discourse makes most sense, and thus become its 'subjects' by 'subjecting' ourselves to its meanings, power and regulation. All discourses, then, construct *subject-positions*, from which alone they make sense (1997: 56).

A short and truncated overview of the succession of criminal subjects is useful for our purposes here. The so-called classical school of criminology came into existence through the work of Cesare de Beccaria (1764/1963), who drew on Enlightenment liberal social-contract theory. Beccaria argued for the severity of punishment to match the crime rather than the personage and standing of the offender (the retributive principle). This was stimulated by the excesses that followed the emergence of police forces and the growth of penal regimes throughout Europe in the 18th century. In particular, he was scathing of the police in Paris for their intervention in response to moral and political opinion as well as in crime. His publications (at first anonymously) challenged the use of arbitrary power and urged consistency in the application of legal codes. Nevertheless, the humanitarian aspect of his work is overstated, for he accepted the need for corporal punishment and judicial torture (Newman and Marongui, 1990). In Britain, Jeremy Bentham (1748–1832) also outlined how the felicific calculus could be used to deter the hedonistic tendencies of individuals. Both approaches were aiming to deter, yet the characterisation of the criminal subject by Beccaria is one where the motives are automatic and completely bound by a web of determination, for he wrote of 'recalcitrant objects who must be angled, steered and forced into law abiding behaviour' (in Beirne, 1991: 812). This approach secured legitimacy for the criminalisation of the emerging urban populations throughout Western Europe.

The development of positivist criminology in the 1870s led to a shift in the characterisation of the criminal subject. It also led to the attribution of the label of the classical school to this criminology. For Cesare Lombroso, the causal basis for establishing criminality could be established through the physiological characteristics of the prison population. This account combined phrenology (the study of skull shapes) with other anatomical stigmata (physiological features that supposedly differed from the norm), such as webbed feet, large jaws, large ears, skin colour, thick hair, the inability to blush, the possession of an extra nipple and diminished sensitivity to pain. His attribution of criminality and moral degeneracy to epilepsy ensured that this particular disability became the object of intense interventions by eugenicists. Lombroso used evidence from the crania of 383 dead and 3 839 living criminals to construct a model for predicting the criminal tendencies of the population as a whole (Lombroso, 1876/1911). Underlying the construction of the criminal subject was the assumption that criminals were throwbacks to an earlier stage of evolution, so dehumanising as well as pathologising those concerned. Similarly, he attributed female prostitution to the possession of a big toe somewhat separated from the other toes (Lombroso and Ferrero, 1895/1915). The focus on exterior signs of an underlying constitutional disorder would, he argued, deliver a capacity for distinguishing the chronic recidivists from those amenable to reform.

As the search for biological determinants came under question in the early 20th century, criminological theories were supplemented by social determinations. Cyril Burt, better known for his work and fraudulent research on intelligence, made his name in British criminology, specifically in juvenile delinquency. Indeed, in discussing crime, he was probably the first to attribute a causal basis for media effects in this area. His affable descriptions and storytelling mode yielded a large audience among those working in the British penal system. The publication of *The Young Delinquent* (1925) had an enormous impact on the treatment of young offenders throughout much of the 20th century in Britain. Burt's account of criminal inheritance is worth a little further scrutiny. Using genotype analysis, he pinpointed the patterns of pathologies that existed in the families of his case studies, and argued that inherent propensities to criminality were potentially controllable if spotted in the very young. Needless to say, if we applied such categories to our own families, then few of us would be beyond suspicion!

In the systematic research work of the team led by W. H. Sheldon, this explanation achieved a new level of sophistication. Using evidence relating to the social and physical characteristics of young men who had opted for military service rather than prison, Sheldon explores the relationship between physique and propensity for crime. In this case, he uses the military identification photograph to classify bodies as physical types and matches this with social-service, medical and psychiatric documents in order to identify patterns of behaviour. He discovered that a series of agencies had conducted investigations to monitor the social background of those examined in the study. Everyone, it seems, had a say, except, of course, the young men in question. Look more closely and you find a wealth of subjective judgements masquerading as factual indicators of pathology. One subject is described as having a 'highly energised, extroverted, dramatic sociability', he is a 'shrewd successful thief' probably destined for 'big time crime' who 'picks up Freudian and Christian profanity like a sponge' (Sheldon, 1949: 200). Another is remarkable for his gnarled physique, loudness, hair-trigger temper and his love of nudity. In each case, family background is considered for its difference from the norm. Each subject is classified through a complex set of factors organised within the terms of reference of the opposition of the normal and the pathological. Whether the causes of criminality are seen as biogenic, the product of anomie or the consequence of status deprivation, subcultural norms or the subject's ecological location, each 'criminal subject' has been pathologised.

In each of the previous cases, the 'criminal subject' is constructed in a manner that matches the system of representation at work in the criminological discourses concerned, so that the people convicted of illegal actions are punished within the rules of conduct, established texts and institutions that make sense of the world through these discourses. Recent criminology appears to be broadly consistent with these attempts to establish patterns of pathological behaviour, but differs in one important way. In contemporary accounts of pathologies, the focus on clinical assessment of the individual has given way to the 'language of probabilistic calculations' and investigation into the statistical propensity of population groups towards criminality. This new criminology is concerned more with managing sub-populations and maintaining public safety. The language of these discourses draws from systems analysis and social utility. In the United Kingdom, proposals to detain 'seriously disturbed individuals' (without an offence being committed) have been justified by the Blair administration in terms of the balance of probabilities, risk and public safety. This actually reinforces the function of clinical judgement in identifying potentially dangerous forms of behaviour and personality traits. In relation to penal policy, one figure that has featured in the construction of criminal subjects to date – the individualised 'chronic recidivist' – has begun to disappear from penal discourses. According to Feeley and Simon, 'Instead of social norms like the elimination of crime, reintegration into the community, or public safety, institutions begin to measure their own outputs as indicators of performance. Thus courts may look at docket flow. Similarly, parole agencies may shift evaluations to, say, the time elapsed between arrests and due process hearings' (1992: 456).

So the processing of people in an efficient manner (something the processors can control) becomes the measure of performance, just as educational performance is increasingly measured by conducting standardised tests rather than the outputs of certain levels of literacy and numeracy. If reoffending became a measure of performance, then those involved would be unlikely to achieve any targets. Feeley and Simon suggest new forms of custodial control, such as electronic tagging and curfews for persistent offenders, instead of rehabilitation (1992: 457). As a consequence, the discourses on criminality and penology are now in transformation. Whether they will be consolidated into a new, unified disciplinary project or become part of a wider managerialist discourse concerned with public policy is uncertain. What we can conclude is that we should not ignore the complex relationship between discourses and institutional practices.

Foucault was concerned with exploring the disciplinary processes through which people are turned into 'docile bodies'. In short, individuals regulate themselves in the way that the institution norms would anticipate. Similarly, he argues that the same practices of surveillance combined with the careful use of punishment can be seen in all institutions in modern societies, whether this is the school, the hospital, the housing estate, the shopping centre, the football terraces or elsewhere. It is for this that Foucault's intervention has been described as the 'best account of the dark side of the social sciences' (Rorty, 1994: 58). This means that the carceral practices of the prison system are part of a move towards a 'disciplinary' or 'panoptic' society (where surveillance is maximised). At the heart of this account of the history of punishment is the emergence of a new system of power, control and surveillance apparent in all aspects of the institutional life of modern societies. In Foucault's words:

> The carceral texture of society assures both the real capture of the body and its perpetual observation; it is, by its very nature, the apparatus of punishment that conforms

most completely to the new economy of power and the instrument of the formation of knowledge that this economy needs. Its panoptic functioning enables it to play this double role. By virtue of its methods of fixing, dividing, recording, it has been one of the simplest ... most indispensable conditions for the development of this immense activity of examination that has objectified human behaviour .... I am not saying that the human sciences emerged from the prison ... [but] it is because they have been conveyed by a specific and new modality of power ... [and] a certain way of rendering the group of men docile and useful. This policy required the involvement of definite relations of knowledge in relations of power; it called for the technique of overlapping subjection and objectification; it brought with it new procedures of individualization. The carceral network constituted one of the armatures of this power-knowledge that has made the human sciences historically possible. Knowable man (soul, individuality, consciousness, conduct, whatever it is called) is the object effect of this analytical investment, of this domination-observation (1977: 304–5).

However, there is also a message of hope in this account. While Foucault demonstrates how the links between power and knowledge are very effective, discourses only work as systems of domination through the rules of conduct, texts and institutional practices where meaning is produced. Power always generates its own forms of resistance, and if meanings are produced, they can also be subverted and changed. Any attempt to destabilise the emergent discourses of crime also has to address the way they organise knowledge and how they are connected to more general discourses constructing social problems. Discourses tell us what is worth knowing and, to greater or lesser extent, regulate what can be said in a meaningful way in a particular time and place. Discourses shape, and become institutionalised in, social policies and the organisations through which they are carried out. This also means that we need to pay attention to the little things, e.g. the informal arrangements by which practices operate and the tacit assumptions that help institutions adapt. They also produce the 'norms' against which deviation or abnormality is marked (the norm of 'not being criminal', for example). If we look at Clarke and Cochrane's consideration of the institutionalisation of discourses in relation to poverty, we can see how state institutions and agencies monitor and intervene to encourage individuals to invest in particular kinds of subject positions (such as the 'deserving poor'):

- *Poor people have to prove they are poor.* The systems of doing something about poverty ... have always involved various sorts of tests that poor people have to pass to prove their need .... There have also been morality tests – mainly directed at women – which examine whether they have been cohabiting ....
- *Poor people must present themselves as poor.* They are claimants – an inferior and dependent social status, asking for something from society ... [and are] subjects of the discourse [of poverty] ....
- *Poor people have things done to them.* Being poor is to be placed in a position where other people have rights over you. Society's institutional arrangements have sometimes been focussed on *segregating* the poor – putting them in workhouses, for instance – to keep them away from the rest of 'us'. Sometimes they have been concerned to *normalize* the poor – giving lessons in budgetary management, good

housekeeping, or parenting – with the aim of making 'them' more like 'us'. At other times the emphasis has been on maintaining surveillance on the poor – monitoring their behaviour to ensure they behave 'properly' (1998: 35–6).

In these practical examples, we can see how Foucault's account of the carceral character of the social order provides a vocabulary for analysis. In a variety of fields, we should focus on the 'authorities of surveillance and registration' and the 'experts in normality', and in so doing identify how judgements operate, but not without due consideration of the classificatory practices involved. In this way, the resemblances between factories, schools, barracks, prisons, hospitals and so on will become more visible as forms of governance.

## Towards a conclusion

Despite enormous argumentation and considerable dispute about the 'proper' focus and character of social inquiry, there have been strong continuities in academic practices over time and across fields of knowledge. These continuities were acquired through the adoption of closed-system analysis to study the social world, although this was achieved in slightly different ways (see Smith, 1998b, Chs. 1–3). There they carried a price tag, i.e. the loss of an awareness of complexity and diversity in social identities. The emergence of disciplinary fields of knowledge was also tied to the emergence of particular forms of governmentality in the institutions of the academy. Through disciplinary discourses and the emergence of organised academic communities (such as professional associations and the development of a compartmentalised departmental institutional structure), the production of meaning in academic work became intensely regulated. The work on disciplinarity in the academy has barely begun. Three areas of work can be highlighted: firstly, mapping the shifting identities of organised academic knowledges (specifically, in relation to this chapter, the social sciences); secondly, research on the regulation of meaning and the institutional practices within which disciplines have emerged; and thirdly, identifying the impact of academic governance on audiences in historically and socially specific cultures. For practical reasons, such a project must be a post-disciplinary one.

Yet we must also bear in mind that disciplinary discourses have been destabilised over the last two decades. In contemporary social science, objects of analysis are increasingly seen as complex, uncertain and contested spaces. What we may be witnessing is the emergence of the first post-disciplinary academic discourses. As with disciplinary discourses, we should distinguish two dimensions:

1. The *discursive dimension* of a post-disciplinary approach highlights capacity for self-reference and self-regulation (autopoiesis), but also acknowledges the ways within which meanings are produced by audiences as well as social scientists. Practitioners will attempt to open up the possibility of alternative interpretations and recognise that their work is plausible within the terms of the stock of common-sense knowledge of different audiences. They will not see textual sources as unquestionable points of reference, and the institutional practices through which they classify people will be conducted in a more sensitive way, so that they do not shore up the inclusionary and exclusionary relations of everyday life that

lead to injustice. This will also be achieved through the construction of subject positions in which an investment of identity will not lead to disempowerment.
2. **The *contextual dimension*** of a post-disciplinary approach will acknowledge the system of language and specific cultural values, the rules of conduct and the established social practices, as well the institutional and textual conditions of knowledge production. In short, practitioners must define objects of analysis as complex and uncertain, drawing upon concepts, arguments and evidence in a way that avoids partial and one-sided accounts. Of particular importance is their being aware of the way in which they draw upon and articulate classificatory systems in order to engage in social-research practices. It is not only the way they locate people in categories that must be challenged, but practitioners should also destabilise the classificatory systems responsible for pathologies, so that such systems are negotiated and not fixed inventories.

To summarise the discussion:
- The institutionalisation of **disciplinary knowledge** is the key problem in social science, for it generates a narrow focus on one ring-fenced area of concern, often producing one-sided accounts of the social. In particular, it ignores important lessons that have been learned in other fields of knowledge. The existence of disciplines presumes clearly defined objects of analysis amenable to closed-system analysis (see the table above).
- **Interdisciplinary knowledge** is credited with leading to the generation of interesting new questions, posing problems in new ways and shaking up complacency, but tends to produce a retreat back into disciplinary research in order to answer these new questions. Multidisciplinary research often attempts to draw together the work of different fields of knowledge, but tends to bolt the work together in an unintegrated way. On the positive side, objects of analysis are seen as complex and multidimensional, but there is still a tendency to view objects as definite objective entities, neglecting the representational and symbolic aspects of knowledge production.
- **Post-disciplinary knowledge** assumes that it is possible to establish connections between the ways these questions are addressed across the social sciences, and to develop social research that regards the boundaries established by disciplinary and interdisciplinary social science as permeable. A post-disciplinary approach acknowledges objects of analysis as complex contested spaces.

This chapter has considered discursive approaches at length. Other approaches to knowledge construction exist – the critical-realist approaches – that have also acknowledged the problems of closed systems in studying both natural and social objects. I have discussed this at length elsewhere (Smith, 1998b, Ch. 7; 1999, 2000a). Some critical realists have begun to develop a post-disciplinary account of the social (Sayer, 1999). Broadly speaking, critical realism has a contradictory position in discussing the normality/pathology distinction. On the one hand, in the transformational model of social action (Bhaskar, 1979), it offers an account of how knowledge can emancipate the pathologised from unwanted determinations. Yet the reluctance to address the symbolic and classificatory systems at work in social science is a major problem for this approach. More cogently here, critical realism is concerned with identifying unobservable social relations, and uses 'disorders', 'breakdowns' and 'dysfunctionality' in order to specify the normal. Certainly we need better theoretical accounts of the processes of normalisation to match the growing work on specific context-bound pathologies, but I am not convinced that reproducing the language of disorder and abnormality in such a direct way is the best way to approach them.

# References

Beccaria, C. de (1764/1963). *Dei Delitti e Delle Pene (On Crime and Punishments)*. New York: Bobbs-Merrill.
Beirne, P. (1991). Inventing criminology: The 'science of man' in Cesare Beccaria's *Dei Delitti e Delle Pene*. *Criminology*, 29 (4), 777–820.
Bhaskar, R. (1979). *The Possibility of Naturalism*. Brighton: Harvester Wheatsheaf.
Blalock, H. (1964). *Causal Inferences in Non-experimental Research*. Chapel Hill: University of North Carolina Press.
Bordieu, P. (1986). *Distinction: A Social Critique of the Judgment of Taste*. London: Routledge.
Burman, E., Aitken, G., Alldred, P., Allwood, R., Billington, T., Goldberg, B., Gordo-Lopez, A. J., Heenan, C., Marks, D. and Warner, S. (1996). *Psychology Discourse Practice: From Regulation to Resistance*. London: Taylor and Francis.
Burt, C. (1925/1961). *The Young Delinquent* (4th edn). London: University of London Press.
Canguilhem, G. (1991). *The Normal and the Pathological*. New York: Zone Books.
Clarke, J. and Cochrane, A. (1998). The social construction of social problems. In E. Saraga (ed.), *Embodying the Social: Constructions of Difference*, pp. 3–42. London: Sage.
Dahl, R. A. (1957). The concept of power. *Behavioural Science*, 2, 201–5.
Dahl, R. A. (1961). The behavioural approach in political science: Epitaph for a monument to a succesful protest. *American Political Science Review*, 55 (4), 763–72.
Durkheim, E. (1895). *The Rules of Sociological Method and Selected Texts on Sociology and its Method*. Basingtoke: Macmillan.
Feeley, M. M. and Simon, J. (1992). The new penology: Notes on the emerging strategy of corrections and its implications. *Criminology*, 30 (4), 449–74.
Fernando, S., Ndegwa, D. and Wilson, M. (1997). *Forensic Psychiatry, Race and Culture*. London: Routledge.
Foucault, M. (1977). *Discipline and Punish: The Birth of the Prison*. Harmondsworth: Penguin.
Garland, D. (1988). British criminology before 1935. *British Journal of Criminology*, 28 (2), 1–17.
Hall, S. (ed.) (1997). *Representation: Cultural Representations and Signifying Practices*. London: Sage.
Laclau, E. and Mouffe, C. (1985). *Hegemony and Socialist Strategy*. London: Verso.
Littlewood, R. and Lipsedge, M. (1997). *Aliens and Alienists: Ethnic Minorities and Psychiatry* (3rd ed.). London: Routledge.
Lombroso, C. (1876/1911). *L'Uomo Delinquente (The Criminal Man)*. Harmondsworth: Penguin.
Lombroso, C. and Ferrero, W. (1895/1915). *The Female Offender*. New York: Appleton.
McCloskey, D. (1983). The rhetoric of economics. *Journal of Economic Literature*, XXI, 481–571.
Newman, G. and Marongui, P. (1990). Penological reform and the myth of Beccaria. *Criminology*, 28 (2), 325–46.
Parker, I., Georgaca, E., Harper, D., McLaughlin, T. and Stowell-Smith, M. (1995). *Deconstructing Psychopathology*. London: Sage.
Rorty, R. (1994). Method, social science and social hope. In S. Seidman (ed.), *The Postmodern Turn*, pp. 46–64. New York: Cambridge University Press.

Rose, N. (1998). Life, reason and history: Reading Georges Canguilhem today. *Economy and Society*, 27 (2–3), 154–70.
Sayer, A. (2000). For postdisciplinary studies: Sociology and the curse of disciplinary parochialism and imperialism. In J. Eldridge, J. MacInnes, S. Scott, C. Warhurst and A. Witz (eds), *For Sociology: Legacies and Prospects*, pp. 83–91. Durham: Sociologypress.
Sheldon, W. H. (1949). *Varieties of Delinquent Youth*. New York: Harper and Brothers.
Smith, M. J. (1998a). *Ecologism: Towards Ecological Citizenship*. Buckingham: Open University Press and Minneapolis: University of Minnesota Press.
Smith, M. J. (1998b). *Social Science in Question: Towards a Postdisciplinary Framework*. London: Sage.
Smith, M. J. (ed.) (1999). *Thinking Through the Environment*. London: Routledge.
Smith, M. J. (2000a). *Culture: Reinventing the Social Sciences*. Buckingham: Open University Press.
Smith, M. J. (2000b). *Rethinking State Theory*. London: Routledge.
Smith, M. J. (2002a). *An Invitation to Ecological Thinking*. London: Sage.
Smith, M. J. (2002b; forthcoming). Deconstructing sickness, pathology, abnormality and monstrosity: The soft underbelly of the formation of social problems.
Smith, M. J. (2002c; forthcoming). Understanding environmental discourses: Contested ethics and social scientific practice.
Sparks, R. (1996). Prisons, punishment and penalty. In E. McLaughlin and J. Muncie (eds), *Controlling Crime*, pp. 197–247. London: Sage.

# Norms, normativity and normalisation: Between the vital and the social

*Ulrike Kistner*

## ■ Introduction

The works of Georges Canguilhem and Michel Foucault have always been closely associated with one another. Through their mutual celebrations and defences of each other's work, a perception of a convergence of their respective projects has been conjured up. What emerges is a picture of an unproblematic inter-relation between Foucault and Canguilhem; of a cross-fertilisation of their respective work; and of a strong mutual influence of their thinking. This picture, however, as I will attempt to show, is misleading. Moreover, it goes against both Foucault's and Canguilhem's attempts to place the history of science and philosophy on a new footing. Contrary to received scholarly wisdom, their procedures and goals in doing so diverge in important aspects, making them into each other's most radical critics. Foucault's writings on the clinic and on the history of sexuality have coined a notion of 'normalisation' that has become near-canonical to his readers. To prevent the normalisation of the concepts of the normal and normalisation, I believe it is important to reopen the elided controversy between Canguilhem and Foucault. To unearth this elided controversy and to restate and reinstate the terms of the debate *within theories of pathology and psychopathology* is the principal aim of this chapter.

## ■ Canguilhem on norms, normativity and pathology

### Monstrosity and pathology

Canguilhem provides a positive critique of the traditional historiography of science by reference to Bachelard's notion of the epistemological obstacle. Canguilhem locates such an obstacle – error, monstrosity, anomaly, elements resisting the order of knowledge – within the logic of science itself, rather than considering it as an external constraint or as an impediment to the advance of the sciences at any particular point. On the basis of these ruptures, Canguilhem attempts to establish a constantly renewable relationship between the superseded and the officially recognised elements within the history of science (Canguilhem, 1979). It is with this in mind that Canguilhem revisits the history of the relationship between the normal and the pathological within the order of knowledge in modernity.[1]

The notion that the pathological opens singular pathways to discover the functionality of the normal has a long history that shares some of its presuppositions with pre-scientific teratology. However, it attained scientific interest only once it had ceased to be viewed as a spectacular singularity and once it was inserted into a spectrum of variability (Canguilhem, 1979). With the foundation of a scientifically based, methodologically elaborated teratology at the turn of the 18th and 19th centuries, the functional equivalence of the results of both normal and anomalous developmental processes was acknowledged. Normal phenomena were explained by reference to pathological ones. In the process of the formulation of these insights, the distinction between physiology and pathology was effaced (Lepenies, 1976). Canguilhem (1979) acknowledges his debts to teratology, and retains teratology as the discursive limit of pathological physiology.

## The normal and the pathological in 19th-century physiology

The question of the delimitation of the normal and the pathological became *the* exemplar of the inter-relation of medicine (and of physiology in particular) and the newly arrived social sciences in the 19th century. August Comte (1798–1857), one of the most vociferous advocates of this idea, saw biology as a necessary condition of sociology: his 'sociology' was elaborated in strict analogy with physiology. Based on the notion that organisation was the normative property of organisms, Comte developed a theory of the biological organism that he applied to psychic and social organisation. Through the postulated link between physiology and sociology, the problem of the delimitation of the normal and the pathological was imported into the emerging social sciences and psychology.

It was in physiology that the doctrine of the identity-in-functions between the healthy and diseased body took hold. The figure who lent his name to this principle was François-Joseph-Victor Broussais (1772–1838). Broussais was not prepared to grant illness its own ontological status. On the contrary, he viewed illness as nothing more than a functional disturbance in the organism, varying from healthy bodily processes only by quantitative determinations. Celebrating 'fellow citizen Monsieur Broussais'' genius, Comte provided an exposition of Broussais' 'principle' (which was termed a 'principle' not by Broussais, but by Comte) in his *Philosophie première: cours de philosophie positive* (1838). Comte maintained, with Broussais, that the pathological state is not radically distinct from the normal (physiological) one. In fact, says Comte, the pathological state was nothing else than 'excess or deficiency of stimulation ... either rising above or below the degree which constitutes the normal condition' (in Gane, 1998: 302) – in other words, a simple extension or prolongation of either the upper or lower limits of variation, which characterises every normal organism. Comte hailed this insight as opening the way to a pathology concerned with 'intensity in the action of stimulants indispensable for maintaining health' (in Gane, 1998: 302). Comte was to accord pathology the privileged position that afforded unique possibilities to the sciences of man – i.e. those of spontaneous experimentation, which would, in turn, allow for a comparison between the normal and the pathological states of an organism.

Both Auguste Comte and Claude Bernard (1813–1878; Bernard was called the 'philosophical physiologist' by Canguilhem (1994: 261)) relied heavily on the insights of Broussais. Bernard, in turn, was a careful reader of Comte. He adopted the principle of the fundamental identity between the normal and the pathological from Broussais. Health and illness were, for Bernard, determined by the same laws: 'Common sense shows that if we are thoroughly acquainted with a physiological phenomenon, we should be in a position to account for all the disturbances to which it is susceptible in the pathological state: Physiology and pathology are intermingled and are essentially one and the same thing' (in Canguilhem, 1991: 67).

Like those of Broussais and Comte, however, Bernard's variations on the theme of the normal and the pathological – which describe the pathological in terms of disturbance, disproportion and discordance – reveal a lack of distinction between quantitative and qualitative concepts in the definition of pathological phenomena (Canguilhem, 1991). The test for Broussais' principle, which it was ostensibly not to survive, came with the outbreak of the cholera epidemic in London, Calais and Paris in 1832. The same challenge awaited Claude Bernard. While for Bernard the pathological did not constitute a functional innovation, the findings of the bacteriologists posed the question as to what normal state would correspond to smallpox, measles, scarlet fever, etc. The theory initially popularised as 'germ theory' by Pasteur was to bring about the demise of 19th-century medical theories.

### Canguilhem's monstrous history of the life sciences

Nevertheless, Canguilhem returns to physiology and teratology in uncovering a hitherto hidden history of these concepts – which for Canguilhem becomes imperative for dismantling the current conception of 'the normal' and 'the pathological', ever since their unproblematic transposition into the psychological and social fields. Canguilhem's retrospective history, which revolutionises the value-laden delimitation of the normal and the pathological, takes him firstly to teratology, in which signs of 'abnormality' were prototypically described. Nevertheless, the interest aroused by monstrosity is based on the scientific curiosity about the pathological as opening the way to discover the functionality of the normal. Firstly, error and monstrosity henceforth are treated not as falsity or deviation to be eliminated in the course of the advance of science, but as that which arouses theoretical interest in the normal.

Secondly, teratology offers him the notion of the functional equivalence of normal and anomalous developmental processes. In 19th-century physiology, illness was de-ontologised, and health and illness were seen to be determined by the same laws, producing an identity of functions, albeit with quantitative variations. Canguilhem needed to rediscover these tenets in order to bring about his own reversal in thinking about the normal, norms and normativity. In medical training, from the second half of the 19th century up to the time of Canguilhem's writings, disease or malfunction was understood as the deviation from a fixed, static norm. Returning the patient to health consequently meant re-establishing the norm from which she/he had strayed in her/his pathology (Rabinow in Canguilhem, 1994; Rabinow, 1998).

### Canguilhem on the normal and the pathological

Canguilhem's *The Normal and the Pathological*, in contrast, opens the path for a new nomenclature of disease, 'referring disease not to the individual considered in its totality but to its morphological and functional constituents …' (Canguilhem, 1988: 140). Thus, the science of living things, in the genealogy provided by Canguilhem (1988), far from having eliminated the contrast between normal and abnormal, has 'grounded that contrast in the structure of the living things themselves' (Canguilhem, 1988: 141). For Canguilhem, placing the relationship between the normal and the pathological on a scientific footing means the elimination of all qualitative judgement and criteria. It was Michel Leriche and the neuropsychiatrist Kurt Goldstein who, in Canguilhem's view, came closest to formulating an alternative. It is from them that Canguilhem learns that 'diseases are new ways of life' (Canguilhem, 1991: 100): 'That which produces disease in us touches life's ordinary resiliences so subtly that their responses are less that of a physiology gone wrong than that of a new physiology where many things, tuned in a new key, have unusual resonance' (Leriche, in Canguilhem, 1991: 97).

This is the notion of the normal that Canguilhem makes his own, and thereby finally overturns traditional renderings of 'the normal':

> In biology the normal is not so much the old as the new form, if it finds conditions of existence in which it will appear normative .... There is no fact which is normal or pathological in itself. An anomaly or a mutation is not in itself pathological. These two express other possible norms of life ... [N]ormality [comes] from ... normativity. The pathological is not the absence of a biological norm: it is another norm but one which is, comparatively speaking, pushed aside by life' (Canguilhem, 1991: 144).

Therefore, the pathological can never be abnormal in an absolute sense. While it signifies the reduction of the norms of life, it calls for new norms of life, for which it paves the way. The pathological, indeed, is one kind of normal. However, it is not identical with the previously normal. The norms that it attempts to establish are new in the sense that they do not arise from the (previous) state of the normal (Canguilhem, 1991).

## Foucault on biopower and biopolitics

In contrast to Canguilhem's insistence on the irreducibility of the vital and the social, Foucault makes the normal the object of normalisation processes in the clinic and in the social arena at large. In Foucault's account of processes of normalisation, 'the living has ceased to be the subject of normativity in order to become no more than the point of application ...' (Macherey, 1998: 111). In linking norms to normalisation, epistemology and ontology are shown to be historically and politically inflected. This is exemplified, among other things, in the medical gaze that became pivotal for 19th-century anatomo-clinical medicine, i.e. the creation of a distinct place for the homogenisation, stabilisation, observation and supervision of, and intervention in, the relationship between the individual and pathology, this place being the hospital and the social network that supports it by tightening its grip on individuals. The consequent medicalisation of society meant that medicine became a task for the nation that was linked to the state, with the task of doctors becoming increasingly politicised (Foucault, 1976). In his historical/archaeological accounts of the clinic and the penal institution, and in his discourses of sexuality, Foucault extends the field of the functioning of norms from the vital to the social. From the end of the 18th century onwards, according to Foucault, the crystallisation of positive notions of health is linked to normality and normalisation:

> Medicine must no longer be confined to a body of techniques for curing ills and of the knowledge that they require; it will also embrace a knowledge of the healthy man, that is, a study of the non-sick man and a definition of the model man. In the ordering of human existence it assumes a normative posture, which authorizes it not only to distribute advice as to healthy life, but also to dictate the standards for physical and moral relations of the individual and of the society in which he lives. It takes place in that borderline, but for modern man paramount, area where a certain organic, unruffled, sensory happiness communicates by right with the order of a nation, the rigor of its armies, the fertility of its people, and the patient advance of its labours (Foucault, 1976: 34–5).

For Foucault, the establishment of norms, the normal and normativity is based on a prior homogenisation, on quantification, on statistics and on the establishment of equivalences and averages. Normalisation, he contends, is a process based on the disciplining of the body in medical, psychiatric, penal, military, industrial and educational practices and institutions at a particular historical moment, i.e. it is integral to a range of discursive practices that have sprung up around these practices and institutions.

What Foucault has retained from Canguilhem's elaborations on the normal and the pathological is a limited notion of the perception in the 19th century whereby the norms of life and health became positive as life came to be defined by death, and health by pathology, with death founding the truth of disease and of life (Foucault, 1976). Following the normalisation processes based on the disciplines of the body (which occurred from the end of the 18th through the 19th century), there came a politicisation of health that moved from individualisation to the constitution of masses and from individualisation to the species, i.e. from the individual body to the population, contributing to the medicalisation of society. This second move is what Foucault termed 'biopolitics' (see Foucault, 1992). The disciplines of the body (anatomo-politics) and the regulations of the population (biopolitics) 'constituted the two poles around which the organization of power over life was deployed' (Foucault, 1990: 139).

### Foucault on norms: the circumvention of law

Foucault therefore transposes norms from the juridical sphere of the law to the social sphere of regulation. Law emanating from the principle of sovereign power is related to the power over life and death. According to Foucault, with the process by which sovereign power is drawn into the field of the social, external power and law are being translated into processes of regulation, correction and normalisation of life through immanently functioning norms: 'the law operates more and more as a norm, and … the judicial institution is increasingly incorporated into a continuum of apparatuses (medical, administrative, and so on) whose functions are for the most part regulatory' (Foucault, 1990: 144). Transforming sovereignty, with its power of law and power over death, from the principle instituting society into the instituted of society, simultaneously transforms the power over death into a matter of regulating life.

What is elided in the outline of this transformation in Foucault's work is a factor that would make for a strong distinction between the vital and the social. This elision concerns the principle of sovereignty in Foucault's genealogical writings on modern power. The fate of sovereign power in modernity is treated simply in terms of a 'juridical regression'. In Foucault's genealogical writings, hand in hand with a short-circuiting of the problem of the place of the instituting principle in modern society goes a disavowal of the category of 'bare life' or *zoe*, i.e. the simple fact of living common to all animate beings – or, in the terms of a modern episteme, biological life. This has been shown to be intimately tied up with the original nucleus of sovereign power, to the extent that 'it can even be said that the production of a biopolitical body is the original activity of sovereign power' (Agamben, 1998: 6). Sovereign power, which effects the inclusion of bare life in the state, presupposes itself as the state of nature outside of the social contract (Agamben, 1998: 107). Foucault, however, remains largely blind to the modalities of sovereign power in relation to the politicisation of bare life. By unproblematically transposing norms from the vital to the social, Foucault produces a slippage between the vital and the social. What largely eludes him in the process is the fact that it remains 'bare life', i.e. the object of biopolitics. Foucault's lack of attention to the distinction between *zoe* and *bios*, between the vital and the social, as a condition for accounting for the politicisation of bare life, with biological life and sexuality as its avatars, becomes an indictment. As Agamben points out, 'Foucault never brought his insights to bear on what could well have appeared to be the exemplary place of modern biopolitics: the politics of the great totalitarian states of the twentieth century. The inquiry that began with a reconstruction of the *grand enfermement* in hospitals and prisons did not end with an analysis of the concentration camp' (Agamben, 1998: 119).

If Foucault's inquiry had ended with an analysis of the concentration camp, Agamben implies, it would have hit against its own limitations, and this might have caused Foucault to question his conflation of the vital and the social; for 'once modern politics enters into an intimate symbiosis with bare life, it loses the intelligibility that still seems ... to characterize the juridico-political foundation of classical politics' (Agamben, 1998: 120). Yet it is precisely the reference to the original political space of the West – with its primary distinction between *zoe* and *bios* and its secondary localisation of bare life in relation to sovereign power – that can serve as the locus of critique. This is the locus that Canguilhem seems to want to guard. It is this locus that he accords primacy over empirical and sociological descriptions of modern power.

While Canguilhem recognises Foucault's self-styled pose as a 'denouncer of the normality of anonymous norms', he sees in Foucault's work something that Foucault himself was to disavow, i.e. a notion of secular networks of power that have become unmoored from the law, from sovereignty and from any transcendental localisation of power, truth and knowledge, but that cannot, for all that, negate their transcendental origins. Foucault's refusal to recognise in a retrospective history an important lever of critique is all the more puzzling, as he recognises precisely this move as the moment of psychoanalysis' resistance to fascism:

> It is to the political credit of psychoanalysis – or at least, of what was most coherent in it – that it regarded with suspicion (and this from its inception, that is, from the

moment it broke away from the neuropsychiatry of degenerescence) the irrevocably proliferating aspects which might be contained in these power mechanisms aimed at controlling and administering the everyday life of sexuality: whence the Freudian endeavour (out of reaction no doubt to the great surge of racism that was contemporary with it) to ground sexuality in the law – the law of alliance, tabooed consanguinity, and the Sovereign-Father, in short, to surround desire with all the trappings of the old order of power. It was owing to this that psychoanalysis was – in the main, with a few exceptions – in theoretical and practical opposition to fascism (Foucault, 1990: 150).

In assessing the critical stance of psychoanalysis, Foucault ultimately returns to a damning verdict. He labels the critical position of psychoanalysis a 'retro-version' with limited legitimacy – a legitimacy that arises from and declines with the contingencies of the specific historical conjuncture. In opposition to this 'retro-versive' perspective, Foucault argues, 'we must conceptualize the deployment of sexuality on the basis of the techniques of power that are contemporary with it' (Foucault, 1990: 150).

This stance amounts to a demotion of philosophy. In calling for an approach '[that] is more empirical, more directly related to our present situation, and [that] implies more relations between theory and practice' (Foucault, 1982: 780), Foucault's genealogy is rendered internal to the techniques of power that it describes. It runs the risk of subordinating philosophy to the analysis of discourse and power, making it complicit with the latter.

## Biopolitics according to Canguilhem

Possibly motivated by his cautiously enthusiastic reception of Foucault's *Histoire de la folie* in 1960 and his insider's preview of the publication of *Naissance de la clinique* in 1963, Canguilhem revisited his 1943 doctoral thesis on *The Normal and the Pathological* exactly twenty years later, inserting a new section as Section II entitled 'New Reflections on the Normal and the Pathological', which was included in the 1966 and 1991 versions of the book. In his own words, 'twenty years later I wanted to measure myself against the same difficulties by other means' (Canguilhem, 1991: 233). These 'other means' were partly provided by the new developments in the life sciences, particularly those in the fields of neurophysiology and in genetics following the discovery of the structure of DNA in 1954 (developed further in 1965), facilitating new types of diagnoses of genetically determined pathologies and biochemical anomalies.

One of the additional considerations mounted in his 'New Reflections on the Normal and the Pathological' concerns the new history of science and medicine in as much as it contributed to what Foucault had termed 'biopower' and 'biopolitics'. Canguilhem entertains the notion of a possible inter-relation between the vital and the social as far as the normal, normativity and normalisation are concerned. Canguilhem here seems to be echoing Foucault's notion that 'for the first time in history ... biological existence was reflected in political existence' (Foucault, 1990: 142). In his outline of the emergence of biopower and biopolitics, Canguilhem follows closely on the heels of Foucault. However, the notion of a conceptual convergence of Canguilhem and Foucault on the inter-relation between the vital and the social is misleading. For Canguilhem, this inter-relation is a highly specified, qualified, circumscribed and conditional one. Acknowledging that the term 'normal' has passed into popular language and has been naturalised, Canguilhem (1991) traces the history of 'the normal' as a category of popular judgement. He emphasises the differences between the structure of an organism and the structure of a social organisation. Unlike the biological organism, a social organisation can put into place new 'organs' and new functionaries. Regulation and integration, while imperative, can only be effected from outside and from above society by religion and/or philosophy, which provide the organs and the norms of their exercise. Social needs and social norms are not internal to the society conceived of as organism. The rules governing members of social collectivities are external to what they regulate. Such rules must be represented, learned, remembered and applied (Canguilhem, 1994). By contrast, in the biological organism, the rules whereby the functions and elements are related and adjusted to each other are inherent in the living organism itself. In the biological organism, there is no externality of particular parts in relation to others; each of its elements co-exists in an immediate present. It is to Claude Bernard that Canguilhem attributes the notion of the internal environment of the organism that becomes crucial in the distinction between the vital and the social. The peculiarities in the functions of the living organism modify the analogy between biological and social organism/organisation.

### Canguilhem's philosophical analysis of life

In delimiting the field of the normal, Canguilhem returns to the physiological model of the individual as the only possible domain of application of 'the normal'. There is a possibility of therapy/cure – i.e. the establishment of a normal state – for the individual organism, while this cannot be said to be a possibility in the case of 'social ills' (Canguilhem, 1991). His descriptive outline of biopower and biopolitics notwithstanding, Canguilhem's earlier insistence on the vital norms of the individual organism as the only legitimate application of the concept of 'norm', 'normality' and 'normativity' remains. As he explains, 'Today, then, as twenty years ago, I am still running the risk of trying to establish the fundamental meaning of the normal by means of a philosophical analysis of life understood as activity of opposition to inertia and indifference. Life tries to win against death in all the senses of the verb to win, foremost in the sense of winning in gambling. Life gambles against growing entropy' (Canguilhem, 1991: 236).

This formulation reveals Canguilhem's indebtedness to Claude Bernard's 'physical vitalism', to the second law of thermodynamics and to the psychoanalytic concept of the death drive. In these references of Canguilhem's writings – i.e. Cuvier, Bernard and Freud – we recognise Canguilhem's insistence on the vital as incommensurable with the social.

Canguilhem's analytical priorities remain clear. In looking at the concepts of norm and normal in the social sciences (sociology, ethnology and economics, with research on social types, criteria of maladjustment to the group, consumer needs and behaviours, and preference systems), he claims that he only wanted to 'clarify *the specific meaning of vital norms* by comparing them with social norms' (Canguilhem, 1991: 235; my emphasis). Canguilhem insists that it is only '*with the organism in view*' that he allows himself some forays into society (Canguilhem, 1991: 235; my emphasis), as when he looks at civilisation in its function to increase entropy, or at the workings of the death drive in fomenting 'aggressive behavior that makes collective life impossible' (Canguilhem, 1998: 324, 325).

## Canguilhem's non-sociological vitalism

Canguilhem criticises the extension and expansion of the notions of 'health', 'normality' and 'pathology' to the social body or the 'body politic' in the strongest terms. These predications are based on qualitative judgements, i.e. on judgements based on value (Canguilhem, 1991). An organism is not a society, and the model of the organism is no longer bound up with a social model (Canguilhem, 1994). Canguilhem wants to restrict the predication of 'pathology' to the deviation from the physiological norm *in the individual body* (Canguilhem, 1989). In dealing with biological norms generally, Canguilhem (1991) insists, one must always refer to the individual. This caution should be more particularly heeded as it is only in and for the individual that the borderline between the normal and the pathological can be precise (whereas for several individuals considered simultaneously, it remains imprecise): 'It is the individual who is the judge of [the transformation from the normal to the pathological] because it is he who suffers from it from the very moment he feels inferior to the tasks which the new situation imposes on him' (Canguilhem, 1991: 181).

A further limiting condition of a generalised predication of 'the normal' lies in the fact that it can only be established experimentally under laboratory conditions. The extension of the predication of 'the normal' to the living being's functional activity considered outside the laboratory remains questionable if not inadmissible (Canguilhem, 1991). This partly explains Canguilhem's critique of the extension of the expressions 'the normal' and 'the pathological' to the sphere of mental illness. Pathology as the laboratory for spontaneous experimentation simply finds no equivalent in mental illness: 'nothing is less well known than the conditions in which nature establishes these experiences, these mental illnesses: the beginning of a psychosis most often escapes the notice of the doctor, the patient, and those surrounding him; its physiopathology, its pathological anatomy are obscure' (Lagache, in Canguilhem, 1991: 116).

This limiting condition provides one of the prongs of Canguilhem's critique of psychology, which he labels as 'a mixture of philosophy without rigour, ethics without obligation and medicine without control' (Canguilhem, 1980: 37). Psychology offers the newly qualified initiate leaving the Sorbonne a choice between two routes – either up the hill to the Pantheon (of philosophy), 'which is the resting place of a few great men', or downhill to the Préfecture of Police (Canguilhem, 1980: 49).

Having mounted all these cautions and critiques, Canguilhem returns to physiology as the only discursive site that would allow for the scientific legitimation of 'the normal' as an original normativity of life. Norms are produced by the very movement of life – not from the outside, but in a completely immanent way (Macherey, 1998: 110).

## Foucault's critique of Canguilhem; Canguilhem's critique of Foucault

Returning to his obliquely critical rejoinder to Foucault, then, Canguilhem arrives at a position that gives him the last laugh. He takes up Foucault's analysis of normalisation in its toughest aspects. The most radical aspect of the analysis of normalisation is reached in Foucault's outline of the convergence of biopower (the disciplining of the body) and biopolitics (the regulations of populations), in which Foucault locates a double normalisation, i.e. the normalisation of the behaviour of the individual, followed historically by the normalisation of the life process of the species itself through 'the modern technologies of power that take life as their objective' (Foucault, 1990: 152). This is the toughest challenge thrown out to Canguilhem and his scholars, whose position is identified and apparently pre-empted by Foucault. Foucault outlines the positions of and disarmingly responds to his potential critics of Canguilhem's ilk as follows:

> People are going to say that I am dealing in a historicism which is more careless than radical; that I am evading the biologically established existence of sexual functions for the benefit of phenomena that are variable, perhaps, but fragile, secondary, and ultimately superficial; and that I speak of sexuality as if sex did not exist ... [T]he purpose of the ... study [of the history of sexuality] is ... to show how deployments of power are directly connected to the body – to bodies, physiological processes, sensations, and pleasures; far from the body having to be effaced, what is needed is to make it visible through an analysis in which the biological and the historical are not consecutive to one another ... but are bound together in an increasingly complex fashion in accordance with the development of the modern technologies of power that take life as their objective. Hence I ... envisage ... a 'history of bodies' and the manner in which what is most material and most vital in them has been invested (Foucault, 1990: 150–2).

Foucault's response is designed to make short shrift of his potential critics. Following his response, he returns to the question of sex as disputed object of (a history of) sexuality. He formulates a stance that could be described as a constructionist one: 'Is "sex" really the anchorage point that supports the manifestations of sexuality, or is it not rather a complex idea that was formed inside the deployment of sexuality? ... [O]ne could show how this idea of sex took form in the different strategies of power and the different role it played therein' (Foucault, 1990: 152).

Canguilhem sees in Foucault's 'effort to track down every surreptitious enterprise of normalisation under the appearance of the sole "authority" of knowledge' (Canguilhem, 1995: 286) a sign of a profound refusal to offer himself as a model, which for Foucault would be tantamount to tyranny. At the source of this refusal, Canguilhem infers, lies an anxiety. This is the point where Canguilhem can reassert his ground for an oblique critique of Foucault's particular version of a constructionist notion of the biological. That ground lies at the heart of Canguilhem's critical enterprise. In this particular case, it is linked to a physiological explanation of anxiety. In response to a physiologically based anxiety, Canguilhem can say, 'it was normal, in the proper axiological sense, that Foucault would undertake the elaboration of an ethics. In the face of normalization and against it, *Le Souci de soi*' (Canguilhem, 1995: 286).

In restating Foucault's 'care of the self' on vitalist grounds, Canguilhem accords to a particular *bios* a *zoe*, instead of the reverse move, which is the biopolitical one, i.e. the politicisation of 'bare life'.

The irreducibility that Canguilhem simultaneously decries and upholds with absolute conviction marks his work as that of a philosophical historian of science, and of a critic of the conflations between the social and the vital that have marked both fascist/genocidal and so-called 'progressive' social-medicine programmes in the 19th and 20th centuries.

## Conclusion

It is Foucault's merit to have painted the scenario of biopower and biopolitics in modernity. Modernity has politicised biological life to such an extent that biological existence becomes reflected in political existence. Human rights, humanitarianism and bioethics are no less part of this politicisation of life than massacres, genocides and human experiments. The capture of *zoe* by *bios* has produced the greatest risk of all times: it has given the life of the species over to its own political strategies. In this context, Foucault acknowledges Aristotle as providing a counterpoint to modern biopower and biopolitics: 'For millennia, man remained what he was for Aristotle: a living animal with the additional capacity for a political existence; modern man is an animal whose politics places his existence as a living being in question' (Foucault, 1990: 143).

Called Foucault's teacher, his influence and his godfather, Canguilhem has reversed the order of intellectual parentage. Before and during his interactions with Foucault, Canguilhem has restated a position that does not fit into transpositions and equations of power/knowledge, vital/social and biopower/biopolitics. Instead, he has provided a space of critique for philosophy, science, psychoanalysis and medicine, inasmuch as they have embarked on staking out a field that has as yet only been outlined by way of a postulate and a set of conditions:

> This biopolitical body that is bare life must itself ... be transformed into the site for the constitution and installation of a form of life that is wholly exhausted in bare life and a bios that is only its own zoe .... If we give the name form-of-life to this being that is only its own bare existence, and to this life that, being its own form, remains inseparable from it, we will witness the emergence of a field of research beyond the terrain defined by the intersection of politics and philosophy, medico-biological sciences and jurisprudence (Agamben, 1998: 188).

## Endnote

1 Canguilhem distinguishes the anomaly from the pathological state, in the terms of the difference between a biological variety and negative vital value, respectively (Canguilhem, 1991). 'Anomaly' is not reducible to 'abnormality'; it is, rather, a statistical deviation; i.e. it is a purely empirical or descriptive concept. 'Anomaly' is derived from the Greek 'an-homalos', meaning 'uneven', 'rough', 'irregular'; 'anomaly' points to a fact, and is a descriptive term, while 'abnormal' implies reference to a value and is an evaluative, normative term (Canguilhem, 1991).

# References

Agamben, G. (1998). *Homo Sacer: Sovereign Power and Bare Life*. Stanford: Stanford University Press.

Canguilhem, G. (1979), *Wissenschaftsgeschichte und Epistemologie: Gesammelte Aufsätze*. Frankfurt: Suhrkamp.

Canguilhem, G. (1980). What is psychology? *Ideology and Consciousness: Technologies of the Human Sciences*, 7, Autumn, 37–50.

Canguilhem, G. (1988). *Ideology and Rationality in the History of the Life Sciences*. Cambridge, Mass.: MIT Press.

Canguilhem, G. (1989). *Grenzen Medizinischer Rationalität: Historisch-epistemologische Untersuchungen*. Tübingen: Edition Diskord.

Canguilhem, G. (1991). *The Normal and the Pathological*. New York: Zone Books.

Canguilhem, G. (1994). *A Vital Rationalist: Selected Writings from Georges Canguilhem*. New York: Zone Books.

Canguilhem, G. (1995). On *Histoire de la folie* as an event. *Critical Inquiry*, 21 (2), 282–6.

Canguilhem, G. (1998). The decline of the idea of progress. *Economy and Society*, 27 (2–3), 313–29.

Comte, A. (1838/1974). *The Positive Philosophy*. New York: AMS Press.

Foucault, M. (1976). *The Birth of the Clinic: An Archaeology of Medical Perception*. London: Tavistock.

Foucault, M. (1982). The subject and power. *Critical Inquiry*, 8 (4), 777–85.

Foucault, M. (1990). *The History of Sexuality: An Introduction*, Vol. 1. Harmondsworth: Penguin.

Foucault, M. (1992). *Leben Machen und Sterben Lassen: Die Geburt des Rassismus*. Duisburg: Duisburger Institut für Sprach- und Sozialforschung.

Gane, M. (1998). Canguilhem and the problem of pathology. *Economy and Society*, 27 (2–3), 298–312.

Lepenies, W. (1976). *Das Ende der Naturgeschichte: Wandel Kultureller Selbstverständlichkeiten in den Wissenschaften des 18. und 19. Jahrhunderts.* München: Carl Hanser.

Macherey, P. (1998). *In a Materialist Way: Selected Essays by Pierre Macherey*. London: Verso.

Rabinow, P. (1998). French enlightenment: Truth and life. *Economy and Society*, 27 (2–3), 193–201.

# Index

abnormal, the 254–5
  constituted by talk about 223
  construed as a threat 235
  contrast between normal and, and structure 254–5
  qualitative judgement/criteria 255
  see also normal, the
abnormal behaviour 25, 207
abnormality, signs of 254 (see also normality)
abuse
  aggression as normal response to 84
  child sexual: narratives of 225, 226
  family 95
  incestuous 83
  interrogative 227
  perpetrated by police 86
  sexual 83, 113, 225, 226
acetylcholine treatment 60
activism in research 100
activist agenda 87 (see also anti-apartheid; anti-racialism)
acute stress disorder 75, 77
advertisements, subjectivity cultivated by 223
aetiological ideas 64, 66
affective disorders 68
African Renaissance agenda, and xenophobia 177, 179
agency of patient(s) 35, 49, 113–18 passim
aggressive behaviour
  death drive and 260
  normal response to battery 84
  in women 23
  xenophobia and 171
  see also anger
AIDS, see HIV/AIDS
alcohol abuse 129, 133, 198
alienation
  between nationalities 182
  of diseased 81, 190
'aliens' (foreigners), see foreigners
Alzheimer's disease 64
amafufunyana 155
American Psychiatric Association 56
amines, deranged 61
analysis 30, 238, 239, 240, 241
analytical investment 247
anatomical stigmata and criminality 244
ancestor possession 157
ancestors and aetiology: case study 161
androcentricity in social research 242
anger 23, 131, 133 (see also aggressive behaviour)
Angolan immigrants 181
anomaly 252, 255
anorexia nervosa 110–23
  active agency of patients 113–18
  collaboration of patient and clinician/researcher 116–18

as control, focused on body 115–16
disempowerment 114, 115
gendered nature of 114–15
as passive resistance/political problem 117, 118–19
role of food 114–15
as strategy against social (dis)order 110–13, 116
victim role 110, 115
anti-apartheid movements 98, 103 (see also activist agenda; anti-racism)
anti-biopsychiatry 67–71 (see also new anti-biopsychiatry)
anti-psychiatry 69, 70, 71
anti-psychotics 59, 60
anti-racialism 146–7 (see also activist agenda; anti-apartheid)
anti-science mode 121
anti-social behaviour and witchcraft 207
anxiety 131, 133
  bio-chemical treatment 60
  in gays 131
  physiological explanation 261
  in psychological phobias 178
  in post-traumatic stress 75
apartheid
  culture of violence a legacy of 180
  isolation and xenophobia consequence of 172–3
appetite, denial of 114–15
Aristotle 262
autonomy
  of experts and therapy of damage 26
  women's socialisation away from 23
auto-therapeutic narrative 35
avoidance manifestations in traumatic stress disorder 78

bacteriology and germ theory 254
barbiturate-induced coma 60
bare life: politicisation of 257, 262
battery: aggression as normal response to 84
battle fatigue 92
Beccaria, Cesare de 244
behaviour(s)
  aberrant: regulated by clinicians 27
  abnormal 25, 207
behaviourism 68
beliefs, breakdown of 133
benevolent assistance and intense repression: strategy 97
Bentham, Jeremy 244
Bernard, Claude 254
biochemical anomalies 258
biochemical concomitants: and affective disorders 68
biochemistry and mental illnesses 224
biocultural hypothesis of xenophobia 173

bioethics 262
biogenetics 225
  and criminality 245
biological diversity: 'race' used to classify 142
biological life/bare life 257
biological/psychological dualism 70
biological psychiatrists 69
biological psychiatry 55–74 (see also biopsychiatry; new biological psychiatry)
biologism, the new 55–8, 69
biology: constructionist notion 261
biomedical discourse: power of: case study 163
biomedical/indigenous taxonomies compared 153, 163–6
biopolitics 224, 255, 256–7, 258–9, 261, 262
biopower 255, 258, 261, 262
biopsychiatric research 62
biopsychiatry 55–74 passim
  anti-biopsychiatry alternatives to 69
  new, see new biological psychiatry
  psychosocial psychiatry reconciled with 68–70
  reconciled with psychodynamics 68
bio-psychosocial model 69
bipolar disorder: genetic-linkage studies 61
body
  image in anorexia nervosa 112, 114–16
  institutional control over 120
  as site of patient's contestation/control 116, 117, 120
borderline personality disorder 26–7, 129
boundaries in social sciences systems 239, 249
boundary maintenance: and xenophobia 172–3
brain
  biology 67
  disease 64
  mind-brain debate 69
  neurochemistry of the 56
'brain psychiatry' vs psychodynamics trends 70
Broussais-principle 253, 254
bulimia 115
  incidence in homosexuals 129
Burt, Cyril 245

Canguilhem, Georges 236–7
  biopolitics according to 258–60
  critique of Foucault 261–2
  Foucault's critique of 261–2
  on norms, normativity and pathology 252–5
carbamazepine 61
carbon dioxide treatment 60
catecholaminergic hypothesis of depression 61

categorical vs dimensional view 155
categorisation: and social identity 139
central authority validated by view of humanity 141, 142
cerebral syphilis 64
characterological changes: chronic stress and 132
chauvinism
  and xenophobia 179
  in-group: and self-identity/social identity 139, 141, 142
  nationalist 144
  racial 145
child sexual abuse victims: narratives of 225, 226
children
  effects of war on 94
  in townships: support organisations 87
chlorpromazine 59, 60, 62
choice of patient 117
  in anorexia nervosa 113, 115, 117
chronic traumatic stress 132
circumcision conflict: case study 161–4
civil rights legislation 143
class inequalities/discrimination 139, 201
  lack of concern with 223
  racialisation of 145
class struggle 145
classical school of criminology 244
classification systems 70
  historical shifting of 155
classificatory practices 238
  and normality 235
clinical detachment: and role-induction 43
clinical involvement: pathology induced or detected 20
clinical practices 237
  political neutrality 86
clinics
  abusiveness of staff to AIDS/STDs 199–202
  diagnosis and treatment inadequate 200
  and functioning of norms 255
  gender and class discrimination in 201
closure in knowledge systems 240
co-construction of meanings of trauma 96, 99–100
coercive instrument: psychotherapy as 25
collaborative approach to trauma 100–5, 116–22 passim
collective action for change 102
collective life: death drive and aggression and 260
colour-blindness notion 143, 144, 146
colour-consciousness 146–8
'combat exhaustion' 92
commensurability of diverse theories 70
communal envy/jealousy: and witch persecution 215–16
communal power relations 146
communicating/sharing experiences 101–2

community(ies)
  collaboration 116–22 passim
  meaning-making with 100
  participation 93, 96, 98
  rebuilding 101
  relations between, and communal/social identities 141
  terror's forces affect 104
community-based treatment and care 71, 158
compensation claims: and PTSD 226
competence, issues of, in anorexia therapy 118
competition theory 139–40, 141
complexity and disciplinarity 238–42
compressed air treatment 60
Comte, August 253
concentration camps 93, 257
concepts 236–7
conditioned stimuli and depression 68
condom use 195–8
confessional, therapeutic situation as 31–2, 121
confinement 63
conflict
  sense of, in absence of conflict 141
  women kept from exploring and resolving 23
conformance: power and non-conformance 159
Congolese immigrants 173, 181
conscience, externalising 32
consciousness raising 76
conservatives, elitist 144
constituents of the individual and pathology 254
constructing (psychopathological) ailments 38, 44–6
constructivist theories 93, 261
consumer culture
  and anorexia 110, 114
  and madness 227
contamination-discourse: and xenophobia 176, 178
contempt, issues of: in anorexic 118
contextual dimensions of disciplinarity 242–3
contextual stress experiences of gays 131
contingency factor 222, 225
control
  body as focus of, in anorexia therapy 116
  community-based treatment as device for 71
  discourse of: not conducive to cure 118
  loss of, in trauma 79
  pathologies problems of 182
  regime of: psychotherapy corresponds to 29
  see also political contol; political control; social control
corporal punishment 244
creation of anomalies, systematic 29
creative deviance: and antibiopsychiatry 69
creative resources 102
criminal inheritance 245

criminal subject(s)
  characterisation of 244
  constructing 243–8
criminalisation of criminal subject 244
criminality
  inherent propensities to 245
  as pathologised disposition 236
  physiological characteristics as causal basis 244–5
  social determinations 245
criminology 243–50
crisis-intervention 76
  organisations 77
cross-cultural psychiatry 207
Crossroads 80
crowd action: psychological defence downplays role of police 85
cultural conflict: case study 161–4
cultural differences: judgements about 238
cultural identities 104
cultural institutions, disruption of 95, 98
cultural meanings in social classification 242
cultural stereotyping 235
cultural values translated to authoritative knowledge 242
cultural victimisation of gays 131
culture
  and mental health 16
  terror's threat to 104
cumulative effects of stress 132
curfews for persistent offenders 246
custodial control, new forms of 246

data, gathering of 96 (see also research)
death: life and 256, 259
death drive 259
  and aggressive behaviour 260
deconstructive approaches 166–7, 243
definition: disciplining norms produced by 223
dehumanising criminal subjects 245
deinstitutionalisation 62, 63
de Kok, Eugene 87
delayed onset disorder 75
delinquency: proliferation of 29
demon possession, alleged 208
demonological era 64
demoralisation 133
dependency in women: effect of therapy 23
depression 133
  biochemical treatment of 56, 59
  catecholaminergenic hypothesis of 61
  prevalence of diagnoses of 27
  recurrent 68
depressive episode, major 68
deprivation and xenophobia 171
desire and power 258
DESNOS 75
  in homosexual people 132–3, 135
detainees 86
  support 76, 87
detention of 'seriously distyrbed individuals' 246
developmental stress 130

deviants:
    AIDS and other STDs associated with 186, 188
    normalisation of: as political object 26
    pathologised by psychotherapy 23, 24, 25
    separated from rest of society 159
deviation from the norm
    contested boundaries 158
    pathology as 254
    see also social deviance
diagnosis
    affected by gender and racial factors 27
    ideological bias 88, 89
    power; subjectivity; bias of 26–7
    practical device: can be changed 156
dialogue 99
disability and social identity 139
'disadvantaged' 145
disciplinarity
    and complexity 238–42
    as a conceptual tool 241–3
    moving away from 243
disciplinary knowledge 249
disciplinary narratives
    distinction between normal and pathological 242
    plausibility of 238
disciplinary power: and construction of madness 159
disciplinary practices: cultural/moral-political 223
disciplinary processes 246
disciplinary projects: plausibility 239
disciplinary society 246
disciplining of the body 256
discordance: pathology described in terms of 254
discourse(s)
    disciplinary 243
    empowerment can be facilitated by 243
    generation/production of pathology 20–54
    of health profession 122; anorexic's ridicule of 111
    ideological: damaging effect 25
    indigenous: incorporation and participation 153
    institutionalised in social policies 247
    interchange between clinician and patient 118
    multiple: collaborative exploration by 103
    open to destabilisation and subversion 243
    power of 26
    prescriptiveness 50
    as regime of control/self-sustaining system 29
    role in representing views and interests of groups 141
    of social regulation: deconstruction of 120
    stuctural interest in what they avow 223
    subject produced within and subjected to 243–4
    subject-positions constructed by 244
    subjectivity and 21, 49, 100, 104, 162
    and taxonomies of madness 153
    traditional institutional 120
discourse theory: meaning of subject positions in 243–4
discrimination
    against gays 131
    legislation 143
    see also class discrimination; gender discrimination; racial discrimination
discursive dimension of disciplinarity 241–2
disease(s)
    abnormal behaviour as 25
    bewitchment and 192
    as new ways of life 255
    see also illness; pathology; sickness
diseased
    alienation of 190
    labelling of 188
disempowerment 249
    in anorexia nervosa 112, 114, 115, 118
    of women: effect of therapy 23
disinhibition as mitigating defence 85
displaced people: traumatic stress symptoms in 87
displacement as communal phenomenon 216
disproportion: pathology in terms of 254
dissociative disorder 70, 225, 226
distress: pathologising 22
disturbance: pathology descibed in terms of 254
divine inspiration: madness regarded as 154
doctors: politicisation of the task of 253
doctrines: imposition of 159
documentation of experiences 102
dominant cultures as invisible norm 147
domination
    agency of 121
    male: anorexia and 110, 116
domination-observation 247
dopaminergic hypothesis of schizophrenia 61
drinking problems: see alcohol abuse
drug addiction/abuse 133, 198
drug dependence in sexworkers 198
drug-takers
    AIDS and stigmatisation of 186
    labelled and stigmatised 25
drug treatments 55, 224
    clinical evaluation 60
    harmful and useful 60
drug-induced disorders 70
Durkheim, Emile 235

eating disorders 114, 115, 133
    issue of control 117
    see also anorexia; bulimia
economic deprivation: lack of concern with 22
economic structures: and psychotherapies of damage 25
educational difficulties: medicalisation 224
egocentrism: outcome of therapy 34, 49
El Salvador 98
electroconvulsive treatment 59, 62, 64
electronic tagging 246
elitist conservatives 144
emotion(s)
    interpellation/construction of 40–2, 48, 50
    in jurisdiction of therapists 50
emotional sounding board: therapist as 31, 37
entropy: civilisation's function 260
environmental factors: inherent vulnerability vs 225
epilepsy: criminality attributed to 244
epistemology: and norms and normalisation 2554
erectile dysfunction 70
error within the order of knowledge 252
established order: psychotherapy as support for 23
ethical problems 25, 52
ethical self-inspection/-evaluation: and madness 159–60
ethnicised conflicts: and social identity 139, 141
ethnicity and ethnic categories
    authentication of national identities 142
    legislation against discrimination based on 143
    and psychopathology of social identity 139–49
    racialised 142–7
ethnocentric bias 238, 242
ethnopsychosis 156
event-related potentials 68
event-related stress 130, 131
evolutionary psychology 224
evolutionary theories of criminality 245
examination procedures as disciplinary methods 237
externalising the problem 119–20

false-memory-syndrome 83
faith, breakdown of 133
family abuse 95
family background as indicator of pathology 245
fascism 257, 258, 262
fat phobia 112, 115
fear
    culture of 97
    in gays 131
    silencing population through 97
    and traumatic stress 79
felicific calculus 244
female physiology viewed as pathological 188, 192, 203
female sexuality viewed as pathological 188

femaleness: anorexia as defence
    against 114
femininity: idealised images of 192
feminist perspectives/agendas 23, 77,
    99, 119
  on rage 229
  in rape counselling 76
fight-flight responses in traumatic
    stress 81
focal infection 60
food
  role in anorexia 114–16
  source of anxiety for women
    114–15
foreign identity
  element of transience 181
  impact of xenophobia on 180–4
  see also immigrants; xenophobia
foreigners (black Africans)/'aliens'
    169–76 passim
  abusive interrogation of 86
  African Renaissance and 179
  AIDS seen as originating among
    186
  attitudes to South Africans 181–2
  communities 181
  coping strategies 182
  criminalisation 176
  police attitude to/treatment of 86,
    170
  responses to xenophobia 181–3
  social networks/support stuctures
    181
  see also immigrants; xenophobia
foreignness 173–4
forgetting 229–30
  historian and psycho-analyst and
    233
  as marketing commodity 229–30
  traumatic 232
Foucault, Michel 223, 237
  on biopower and biopolitics 255–8
  Canguilham's critique of 261–2
  critique of Canguilham 261–2
  on disciplinary/surveillance
    processes 246–8
free will and anti-biopsychiatry 69
freedom: regulation of 159
Freud, Sigmund 222
Freudianism 258
frustration-scapegoat 171
functional\structural dualism 70
functional constituent of individual
    and pathology 254
functionality of the normal:
    pathology and 254
future generations: affected by terror
    104

Galen 64
game theory and social identity
    140–1
gay identity, see homosexual/gay
    identity
gay lifestyle 126, 127–8
gayness, see homosexuality,
    male/gayness
gender
  diagnosis affected by 27
  discrimination 22, 23, 76, 139, 201

meaning systems 126
oppression 23, 76, 157
politics: rape counselling and 76
relations: and STD 195–8; and
    witchcraft 216
role prescriptions 23
socialisation 76
stereotyping, and witchcraft
    accusations 215
  and terror 96–8
  and witchcraft persecutions 212
general paralysis of the insane 64
generational conflicts 225
genetic factors/explanations 61, 66–7,
    224
genetics 66, 225, 258
genius: construction of madness as
    voice of 154
genocide: terror as partial 97
genotype analysis 245
global knowledge, vs 'local'
    collaboration 120
gonorrhoea 191
gravity: pathologising 31, 49, 52
grounded-theory method of analysis
    30
group-related factors of madness 157
group resources: dimensions of social
    identity as 140
Guatemala 93, 96–8, 100–3
guilt feelings reframed 76

healer: ancestor-possession signifies
    calling 157
healing process: dimensions of terror
    and 104
health
  defined by pathology 256
  discourses ridiculed by anorexic
    111
  politicising of 256
hedonistic tendencies 244
helplessness, feeling of: in traumatic
    stress 79, 133
Hippocrates 64
historical revisionism 226
historiography and theoretical
    diversity 70
history/historiography of psychiatry
    55–67
  Commission for Historical
    Clarification 101
  Committee on the Recuperation
    of Historical Memory 101
HIV/AIDS 176, 186–7
hlonipha, system of 157
Holocaust 95
  narratives of survivors 225, 226
homogenisation: establishment of
    norms and 256
homo-negativity 133
homophobia: fuelled by AIDS 186
homosexual behaviour/experimenta-
    tion: in non-homosexuals 126
homosexual/gay identity 125
homosexual(s)(ity),
    male/gay(s)(ness) 124–38
  AIDS and pathologisation of 186
  diagnosis 134

drive for equal treatment and
    privileges 125
gayness as discourse 126–8
human rights discourse 125
inherent nature/genetic
    inevitability of 125
labelling and stigmatising 25, 157
legal problems 134
liberative discourses 126–7
oppressive discourses 127–8
removed from list of mental
    disorders 27
repathologisation: avoiding
    implicit 124–38
stressors 128–35
hopelessness, feelings of 133
horror, feeling of 79
hospital(s) 255, 257
human rights 88, 89, 262
humanitarianism 262
humiliation: anorexia and 114
hydrotherapy 63
hyper-arousal in post-traumatic stress
    78, 81
hysteria
  chemical treatment 60
  group: and witchcraft notion 208

iatrogenic psychopathology see under
    psychopathology
'ideal' concept of self: promotion of
    24
identity(ies)
  African/South African 177
  categorisation and 139
  cultural 104
  disability and 139
  ethnic, and xenophobia 139
  flexible 233
  homosexual 125
  individual 104
  national 225
  psychopathology and 139–49
  religion and 139
  sexuality and 157
  see also social identity(ies)
ideological imperatives 89
illiteracy 96
illness
  chronic: stability of 235
  experience as interpretive
    enterprise 154
  as functional disturbance in the
    organism 253
images of self in advertising 230–31
Imipramine 59, 62
immigrants, black African 170
  criminalization 176–83 passim
  illegal 173–4, 175, 176
  see also foreigners; xenophobia
incestuous abuse 83
indigenous/biomedical taxonomies
    compared 164
indigenous healing 152, 157–8
indigenous/religious discourses: and
    madness 153
indigenous/religious taxonomies of
    madness 152, 164–7
  incorporated as discourses 153

individual, the
  domain of application of 'the normal' 259
  health and 256
  repathologisation 223
  state control of, and psychotherapy 23–5
individualisation, psychotherapeutic 23
'inequality'/'diversity' discourse: social identity and 139
inertia: life as activity of opposition to 259
insanity, see madness
insomnia 131
institutional discourse: and anorexia 120, 121
institutional power 28
institutional practices: discourses and 246
institutions
  and constructions of madness 153, 154, 158–9, 165
  resemblance to prisons 237
insulin-coma treatment 60, 63
insulin therapy 60
interdisciplinary knowledge 249
interest groups 158
intergroup conflict 157
interiorising of problem 22, 49
International Symposium of Children and War 92
interpellations of meaning: and emotion 40–2, 43, 44–6
interpersonal anxiety 133
interpersonal relations: disturbances of, witchcraft and 208
interpersonal sensitivity 133
interpersonal stressors, chronic 132
intervention 75
interventionist power of mental-health experts 29
interview responses: ambiguous and ambivalent 27
intrapsychic causation of problems 22, 208
intrusion manifestations in traumatic stress disorder 78
inyangas 209, 213
iproniazid 59
Ireland, Northern: children in 94
irrational beliefs and actions: and witchcraft 207, 208
isolation 131, 172–3

judicial torture 244
juvenile delinquency 245

Khulumani 103
kin selection: and social identity 139–40, 141
knowledge(s)
  construction: transformations in 241–3
  organising of: and production of pathology 21, 29
  subjugated: distinguished from common sense 121

labelling
  euphemistic/distorting 189
  potential of psychotherapy 25–6, 27
  role of ordinary language 157
  of STD sufferers 188
language
  creative power: and constructions of madness 157
  and xenophobia 170, 173–4
law: circumvention of 256
legal codes, application of 244
Lesotho 174
liberatory perspective of trauma 98–9
librium 59
life: Canguilhem's philosophical analysis of 259
life hassles, cumulative, as cause of distress 131
lightning linked to witch persecutions 215
lineage, 'race' as 142
listening, therapeutic 30–31
  disclosures elicited by 31, 43
lithium treatment for mania 59, 61, 62
lobola 195
'local' collaboration/knowledge 120
Lombroso, Cesare 244

madness: 152–68
  as active process 164
  allowed in some ways 223
  badness as 227
  contingency factor of 222
  diagnosis 157: adaptive qualities 157
  fluidity of boundaries 155, 158
  government: discourse as tool of 162
  individual and social attribution 227–9
  labels, agency wielding 157
  as marketing strategy 226–7
  medicalised as illness 227
  and memory 223, 224
  overdetermination factor of 222
  political power and 161
  post-structuralist account 153–4
  post-structuralist analysis of 164–7
  power-relations in 153, 154, 159–60
  relational portrayal of 227
  representations of 222
  as resistance to the social 157
  shared subjection to 222
  social attribution of 227–8
  social constructions 156, 157
  social responses evoked by 158
  subjectivity and 223, 224
  transcultural validity 154
  trauma: factor of 222
  ukuthwasa and role-change opportunities 157
Malawians 174
male domination: anorexia and 110, 116
male homosexuality, see homosexuality, male
male sexuality: perceptions of 188, 190–91
maleness: exnomination of 145

mania 59, 133
  lithium for 59, 61
manic-depressive psychoses 66
marginalised groups problematised 23 (see also homosexual males)
marginalised persons: minority stressors 134
massacres 92
Maya people, see Guatemala
meanings
  amplification of 42
  interpellation/reflexion of 40–2, 43, 44–6
  negative change in systems or 133
  production, subversion and changing of 243, 247
  ruptures to 79
media effects
  causal basis for 245
  representations of Africa and foreigners 175–6
  representations of madness 222
  representations of xenophobia 178
  role in anorexia 115
  see also advertisements
medical gaze 255
medical profession: anorexia and categorisations of 112
medicalisation of society 255, 256
medicine: and the social sciences: inter-relation 253
memorial agencies, marketing of 229–30
memorial practices 222
  as disciplinary aparatuses 223
  external influences 232
  market manipulation of 232
  of political events 232
memories
  ordering/disciplining processes 224
  storing and retrieval: efficiency of 224
  traumatic 222
  truth or falsity 224
memory
  access to 226
  awareness and 224
  collective representations of 226
  collective threshold of 225
  constructionism of 225
  contests over 225
  continuous work of 225
  cultural templates, provision of 226
  disciplining 224–6
  disorders associated with 224
  feminism and contests over 226
  individual 225
  madness: memory and 223
  making: socially engineered 231–2
  moral role/function of 224, 226
  pathology of 226
  sharing and establishing 101–3
  social: nationality and 231
  and subjectivity 223, 224, 225, 232, 233
  time and timelessness of 225
  tool of healing 229
men: role in cause of STDs 194
menopause: construed as disease 192

menstrual cycles in anorexia nervosa 112
menstrual pain 229
mental health, socio-cultural factors 152–3
mental-health professionals/experts
  challenging the role of 243
  in conflict zones 92, 93
  progressive political agenda 76
mental illness
  as artifact of society/biology 69
  brain chemistry and 56
  community-based treatment 71
  confinement of sufferers, threat of 225
  cultural interactive effect on 152
  damaging effects of psychotherapies 25–6
  neurological basis of 64
  pathology terminology applied to 260
  proliferation of types and sub-types 27
mental retardation 27
metabolites, excess of: mania and 59
migrants 181 (*see also* foreigners; immigrants)
millenarian overtones of New Biological Psychiatry 58, 65
mimesis/mimicry/mockery as strategy in anorexia 110–13
mind-body dualism implied in word 'organic' 70
mind-body duality/split superseded 70
mind-brain debate 69
mineworkers: 'at risk' to AIDS/STDs 187
minorities co-opted into majorities 145
minority groups problematised 23
minority stressors
  cumulative impact 131
  gay-related 130–1, 134
  and trauma symptoms 131
misfits: power relations and 159
monoamine oxidase inhibitors 59
monologue, therapeutic 34
monstrosity(ies) 235
  and pathology 252–3
mood disorders 66
Moprobamate 59
moral codes: imposition of 159
moral degeneracy attributed to epilepsy 244
moral insanity 65
moral responsibility: patient made locus of 22
moral value-judgements implicit in treatments 26
morality
  and anti-biopsychiatry 69
  and permissive sex and AIDS/STDs 188
morbidity 236
morphological constituents of individual and pathology 254
motives, criminal 244
Mozambican immigrants 174, 175, 181
multiculturalism 140, 144
multidisciplinary research 249

Multiple Personality Disorder: memory and 224
mutation 255
narration of self 166
narrative, psychotherapeutic 34–6
  accenting and emphasising statements 42
  auto-therapeutic 35
  co-construction of 39–40, 42, 44, 48
  corrections/amendments 36
  echoing/reflecting sentiments expressed 37, 42
  focusing by therapist 42
  group interactions 120
  interpellations of meaning and emotion 40–2, 44
  prompting, redirecting 36
  psychopathology reconstructed out of 39, 50
  'rhetorical tricks' 38, 42
narrative therapy 120–2
nation-building: foreigners/xenophobia and 176–7, 179
nation-state, creation of: and violence 182
national chauvinism 142
national identity(ies)
  actions and interactions at border of 181
  'race' used to authenticate 142
National Security violations of human rights 92
nationalism: and xenophobia 175, 176, 177, 179, 180, 182
nationalists, chauvinist 144
nationality dimension of social identity 139
natural disaster 93
negative self-concept 131
neo-Darwinian project 139
neoromantic/psychoanalytic interregnum 63, 64
neurobiology 66
neurochemical findings in schizophrenia 61
neurochemical mechanisms 67
neurochemistry of the brain 56, 61
neuroimaging: post-traumatic stress and 79
neurological deficits 68
neurology 64, 65, 68
neuropathological trend 64
neurophysiological processes: traumatic stress and 79
neurophysiology 258
neuroscience(s) 66, 67, 68
  imbued with psycho-analytic meaning 68
  terms of, as codes for mental concepts 70
neurosis: chemotherapy 60
new anti-biopsychiatry 69–70, 71
new biological psychiatry
  combined with psychosocial intervention 68
  distinctive features 58
  logical approach 58–9
  the social construction of a 55–74
new-nation discourse 169

New South Africa and xenophobia 177, 179, 180
Nigerian immigrants 173, 181
non-conformance/power/constructions of madness 159
non-governmental organisations for intervention 77
norm(s) 24, 49, 237, 241
  anorexia as strategy against 111, 113
  consolidation of, in therapy 33
  damage to 98
  definitions 223
  disciplinary power of 159
  generation and policing of 25
  and normalisation: linking of 255
  normativity and: and normalisation 252–63
  pathology as deviation from 254, 255
  patients' voluntary self-evaluation 32, 49
  positive aspect of 256
  unspoken, implicit in listening 31–3
  vital and social 259–60
normal, the
  established under laboratory conditions 260
  in 19th century physiology 253–4
  as object of mormalisation processes 255
  sociological application criticised 260
'normal' self: maintenance and cultivation of 24
normalisation 261
  based on disciplining of the body 256
  dynamic of 223
  norms, normativity and 252–63
  political: damaging effects 25–6
  as procedures of judgement 237
normalising approach: to anorexia 118
normality
  changing definitions 236
  and pathology: inter-ralatedness of 223, 236, 237, 238, 253–4
  prototypically described 254
  rethinking, through post-disciplinary practices 235–51
  *see also* abnormality
normative(ity)
  consolidation/displacement of 33
  the living as subject of 255
  in medicine 256
  norms and, and normalisation 252–63
  prescription of 26, 49, 50
  of science 236
nuclear family
  permissive discourses threat to 187

OASSSA 76, 77, 88
objectification; subjection and 241
observation: placing individuals under 237
  perpetual 246
ontology: and norms and normalisation 255

oppression
  and DESNOS 132
  and STDs 204
  and traumatic stress disorder 78
  see also under gender
oppressive discourse 23
  complicity of medical science in 23
organic aetiologies and treatments 66
organic mental disorders (term) 70
Organisation for Appropriate Social Services in South Africa 76, 77, 88
ostracism
  of and by foreigners 182
  Western-traditional approach 155
'outsider'-perspective
  on AIDS 186
  and reflexivity 99

pain 229
panoptic society 246, 247
paranoia 133
  and witchcraft 207, 212
participatory approach, to trauma 93, 96, 98, 100, 101
past: imcomplete character 233
pathological, the
  changing definitions 236
  delimitation of normal and the 253
  in 19th-century physiology 253–4
  relations between normality and 235, 238, 253–4
  as type of normal 237
  value-laden delimitation of normal and 254
pathological behaviour, patterns of 246
pathological behaviour of group 208
pathologisation of social category 235
pathologising discourses
  about female physiology/sexuality 188
  about homosexuality 186
  about STDs 188–91
pathologising gravity 49
pathology
  Canguilham on 252–8
  degree of permanency 236
  monstrosity and 252–3
  normalisation of 227
  and normality: inter-ralatedness of 223, 236
  (non)sosiological 260
  see also psychopathology(ies)
patient(s)
  agency of 35, 49, 113–18 passim
  assertion of personal reflexivity in 35, 49
  collaboration with clinician/researcher 116, 120
  compliance 46–8
  disenfranchised: damaging of 23
  efficacy, sense of: erosion of 23
  former: as consultants 120
  impact of interpellations on 41
  increasing independence 34
  internalisation of role/voice of therapist 49
  ostracism and depravation of rights and liberties 26

proactivity 43
problems attributed to 22
resistance to pathologising tendencies of experts 243
resistant 37
role-induction 42–3, 48
self-problematising/self-correcting tendencies 48
subjectivism/egocentrism/focus on self 33–35, 48
therapeutic subject positions 48, 49
see also entries beginning with self-
patriarchal culture/power
  anorexia as strategy against 113, 116
  and madness 159
patriotism and xenophobia 179
penal institutions/prisons 255, 257
penal policy 246
penal regimes 244
penology discourse 246
persecutory instrument, psychotherapy potentially a 25–6
persistent offenders: control of 246
personal details of narrative 37
personal reflexivity: therapy and 35
personal will, loss of, as legal defence 85
personality disorder 225
persuasion in psychotherapy 64
pharmacological management of mental disorders 55 (see also drug treatments)
philosophy: power and 258
phobias, psychological 178–9
PhotoVoice project 102–3
phrenology and criminality 244
physical causes and treatment: emphasis on 158
physiognomic typologies and psychopathology 142
physiology
  the normal and the pathological in 253–4, 260
  social sciences and: inter-relation 253
physique and criminal propensity 245
pluralist approach to social sciences 240
polemical biologism 69
police, and foreigners and xenophobia 170, 173–4, 176
political action: anorexic's chances at 118
political agenda: violence intervention and 76
  and xenophonia 175, 176, 177, 179
political allegiances and institutional power 225
political conflict: children affected by 87
political control: pathologies are problems of 182
political factors/problems 224
  and post-traumatic stress disorder 75
  reframed psychotherapeutically 22, 23
political ideology: dimension of social identity 139

political instrument: psychotherapy used as 23–6
political neutrality: of psychotherapy 24
political objects: served by psychological diagnosis 26
political repression: after-effects of 98
political science: object of 240
political strategies and species survival 262
political subjectivities, discourses of pathology and 222
political technologies: and construction of madness 159–60
politicisation of life: positive/negative aspects 262
poor, the
  subject position of 247–8
  surveilance of 248
possession (supernatural) 208
post-apartheid project: and xenophobia 176–7
post-disciplinary knowledge 249
post-disciplinary practices
  contextual dimension 242, 249
  discursive dimension 241, 248
  rethinking normality through 235–51
post-traumatic stress disorder 75–108
  categorisation 78, 79
  collective experience, PTSD as 80, 95
  community-based participatory research 93
  concept 77
  contextualising 94
  cross-cultural/community perspective 92–108
  DESNOS co-morbid with 133
  detainees issues 86
  diagnosis criteria 78–9, 88
  false-memory syndrome 83
  impact on family and significant others 80
  in homosexual males 135
  human rights issues/discourse and 88, 89
  individual life history in context with political movement and social trauma 95
  individualisation 79–80
  invoked in defence of victim and victimiser 86–7
  legalisation 84–5
  liberatory perspective 98–9
  literalisation 82–3
  mass-scale 80
  memory associated with 224
  mitigation in mass-action crime 85
  normative response to abnormal stimulus 84
  political ramifications of PTSD categorisation 85–8
  politically induced violence and repression and 95
  power-abuse implicated 79, 88
  pre-existing personality deficiencies 82–3
  refugee-status granted to victims 85

socio-political/medical perspectives 79
somatic symptoms 81
and state terrorism: drawing attention to 88
stressors 68, 75, 82, 83; as diagnostic entity 84, 134
transmission to future generations 95, 101
treatment 79
Westernisation 80–81
'potentially dangerous' behaviours and traits 246
power
  abuse of, and post-traumatic stress 88
  arbitrary 244
  hierarchy: and psychotherapies of damage 25
  knowledge and 247
  new economy of 247
  operation of: research on 240
  and philosophy 258
  and resistance 164–7
  secular networks of 257
  systems of, and production of pathology 29, 49, 51
  see also disempowerment
power relations 224
  and anorexia 110
  and psychopathology 146, 159
  relayed through subject 243–4
  and sexuality 258
  tied to social-scientific practices 238, 242
powerlessness converted into blame-worthiness 23
practice: relation between theory and 258
pre-frontal lobotomy 63, 64
prejudice, social, see social prejudice
pre-menstrual stress: construed as disease 192
Prichard, James 65
primary disorders 70
prisoners, male, 'at risk' to AIDS/STDs 186, 187
'Prisoners' Dilemma, The' 140–1
prisons/penal institutions 255, 257
pro-biopsychiatric position in theoretical approach 70
problematisation, interpersonal, in psychotherapy 20
procedures, therapeutic 29
  degree of failure 29
professional discourse, role in reproducing views of groups 141
professional institutions: madness and 160
professional power and madness 159, 160
projections and witchcraft 212
promiscuity
  double standards 191, 193
  gendered blameworthiness 202
  notions about AIDS and other STDs and 186, 188
  racist linking of 186
prompting of patient 36
prostitution, female 245

Prozac 27
psychiatric profession: stigma attached to 66
psychiatry, biological, see biological psychiatry
psychic harm, infliction of 84
psychic organisation 253
psychoanalysis 69, 257–8
  and neuroscience 68, 258
  opposition to fascism 257, 258
psychoanalytic culture 223
psychoanalytic culture/movement 62, 63, 223
psychodynamic psychiatry 67–8
  biological approaches reconciled/combined with 68–9
psychological/biological dualism 70
psychological defence detracts from protest 85
psychological distress: goal with regard to 29
psychological scars: legalisation 85
psychologist(s)
  effects of, within knowledge-generating contexts 99
  regarded as representative of oppressor 99
Psychologists Against Apartheid 76, 77, 87, 88
psychology: Canguilhem's critique of 260
psychopathology(ies)
  and biological psychiatry 55
  compulsion to diagnose 51
  construction of 38, 44–6
  of everyday life 222
  extra-therapeutic 20–1
  gravity to discover 31, 49, 52
  iatrogenic 23
  lack of adequate basis of refutation 51
  location points for indications of 37
  as myth 25
  nodes of 37, 49, 50
  problem areas 37
  production by therapy and discourse 20–54
  proliferation of categories of 27
  reconstructed out of narratives 39, 50
  recotextualised in socio-cultural milieu 135
  of social identity: 'race', ethnicity and 139–4
  socialisation of 223
  systematic generation of 28–9
  terminology 22
  vested interest of psychotherapist in 28, 51
  vulnerability of gays to 128–30
  see also pathological, the; pathologising; pathology(ies)
psychosocial stress: and neurological deficits 68
psychosocial trauma 98–100
psychotherapeutic alliance 119–22
psychotherapeutic narrative, see narrative

psychotherapeutic practices
  patient resistance to pathologising tendencies 243
  subject positions 243
psychotherapeutic relationships in anorexia 116–18
psychotherapeutic subject positions 48, 49
psychotherapist(s)
  answers/responses: prescribed, generic 34
  authoritative interpreter role 43
  avoids answering 34
  constructive/interpellative powers 38, 44–6, 48
  declarative powers 46–8
  detachment 34, 43
  economic imperative to find pathologies 28, 51
  emotional influence 41
  empowered by technical jargon/knowledge/discourse 28, 50, 51
  expanding jurisdiction of 27–8
  as iatrogenic process 51
  impulsion to discover pathology or dysfunction 28
  instructive powers 46–8
  neutrality of: and role-induction 43
  powers of control and intervention 28
  prescriptiveness of role 46–8, 50
  vested interest in psychopathology 28, 51
  ways of directing/structuring the session 34
psychotherapy 63
  of damage 25
  efficacy 50
  ethical problems 25
  failure rates 29
  goal of change, control and influence 29, 50
  problem-centric nature and structure of 51
  procedures: failure rates 29
  (and) production of pathology 20–54
  psychopathology as prime object of 51
  self-serving discourse 28
  state control of individual and 23–5
  technology 50–2
psychotics 59, 133
psychotropic medications 67
public protection and mental illness 225
public safety and criminality 246

qualitative judgement/criteria regarding abnormal 255
questioning, therapeutic 34, 35–9
  absence of control questions as couter/indications 38
  avoidance of therapist-directed 35
  indirect or oblique or rhetorical 38, 32
  and outflow of patient disclosure 36
  problem-centric 39

reconstruction of patient's words 38–9
soliciting accounts which support diagnosis 38–9

race
  conceptualisation and definitions 142
  and psychopathology of social identity 139–49
  diagnosis affected by 27
  inequalities of: lack of concern with 22
  raced and unraced categories 145
racial categories: attribution of qualities to 235
racial discrimination 22, 27, 142–7, 157
racial science 142, 143
racial typologies 143
racialised identities 143
racism
  endemic institutional 232
  new-nation discourse and 169
  as a pathology 232
  see also racial discrimination
racist notions about AIDS 186
racist values: unacknowledged conditions 238
rage 227–9
rape
  politicised perspective on 76
  and power imbalance and stress disorder 78
rape-crisis intervention 76
rape-trauma syndrome 93
  organisations 89
  refutes consensual sex 84
reason and unreason, separation of 160–1
recidivism: exterior signs attributed to 245
recidivist, chronic 246
reconstruction 167
recovery: psychological within social 104
recuperation 105
redistributive policies 147
reductionism
  in theoretical diveersity 70
  and victim-blaming 22–3, 49
refugees, post traumatic stress in 81
  (see also foreigner; xenophobia)
regulation: community-based treatment as device for 71
rehabilitation 246
reintegration 105
relational details of narrative 37
relative-deprivation theory: and xenophobia 172
relativism 69, 70
religion: dimension of social identity 139
religious/indigenous discourses: and madness 162–4
religious/indigenous taxonomies of madness 152
  incorporated as discourses 153
repression 83
research, participatory and community-based 93, 96, 98, 100, 116

reseptor science 68
reserpine 60
resistance:
  enacted: madness as 164
  lack of, in patients 46–8
  power and 164–5, 247
resources, limited: and xenophobia 171
restitution: colour-conscious policies invoked to exact 146
retributive principle 244
revenge: witchcraft and 216
revolutionary biology 140–41
rhetorical tricks/devices 38, 42, 50
ridiculing of the ideal in anorexia 111
role-induction 42–4, 48
ruptures to meaning 79

safer sex practices 187, 190, 203
  alternative 'precautions' and 'cures' 198–9
  sexworkers' constraints 197–8
  women's lack of power to negotiate 197–8
sangomas 162, 165, 209, 213
sanity; insanity in dialogue with 154
scapegoating
  and distancing 188
  hypothesis of xenophobia 171
  witchcraft persecutions 211
schizophrenia 64, 66
  biochemical treatment of 56, 59, 60, 61
  boundaries: variability of 154
  case history 161–2
  electroconvulsive treatment 59
  genetic findings 61, 67
  neurochemical findings 61
  proper 70
schizophrenics
  labelling and stigmatising 25
  trials of anti-psychotics vs other treatment 60
science: relative normativity 236
scientific discourse, role in reproducing views of groups 141
scientific progress: process of 56–7
seclusion 63
secondary disorders 70
self: care of 24, 262
self-assessment/-evaluation 32–3, 36
  validated by characterising of 'other' 141–2
self-attendance 33–5
self-blame feelings 131
  reframed by attribution of blame 76
self-concept, negative 131
self-correction 36
self-destructive behaviour in gays 131
self-esteem, erosion of 133
self-evaluation/-assessment 32–3, 49
self-examination and scrutiny 35–6
self-focus: outcome of therapy 34
self-harm symptoms, incidence in homosexuals 129
self-hate 131
self-images in advertising 231
self-interpretation: repositioning for new 233
self-monitoring 34

self-problematisation 29, 36, 49
self-representation, anorexic's chances at 118
selfhood, narratives of: and memory 231–2
selves, constructing and shaping: psychotherapy and 24
separatism 173
serendipitous discoveries in New Biological Psychiatry 59
sex and sexuality 257, 261
  as source of anxiety for women 114, 115, 116
sexual abuse 83, 113, 225, 226
  in anorexics 113
sexual dysfunction 133
sexual functions 261
sexual licentiousness label: AIDS and STDs and 188
sexual orientation 139 (see also homosexuality)
sexual pervert 29
sexual relationship, problematic: as cause of STD 194
sexuality
  female, see female sexuality
  identity and 157
  and law 258
  liberation of: regression of after AIDS emergence 187
  male, see male sexuality
  moralistic and punitive social construction 186
  power and 258
sexually transmitted diseases 185–206
  alternative 'precautions' and 'cures' 198–9
  construction of sexuality and 195–8
  cultural discourse 190
  female/male responsibility 203
  help-seeking behaviour inhibited 189
  labeling of sufferers 188, 189
  prevention inhibited by construction of 188, 204
  racialised discourse on causes 194–5
  secrecy surrounding 189
  social construction of 186–91
  stigma in construction of 185–206
  treatment inhibited by construction of 188, 204
sexworkers
  alcohol and drug dependence 198
  vulnerability to AIDS/STDs 186, 187, 197–8
shame 131
sharing experiences, understanding and vision 102
'shell shock' 92
sickness: absence of stability 235, 236
single parents: labelled and stigmatised 25
slimmers' disease: argument about anorexia being 117
social, the: as organism 236
social body: extensions to notions of pathology to 260
social capital 140

social comparison: and xenophobia 172
social conformity: therapy as means of advocating 23
social constructivism 100
social-contract theory 244
social control
  clinician role of agent of 118
  and psychological control 29
  therapy as instrument of 23
  see also control
social deviance
  contested boundaries of 158
  as pathology 254
  see also deviants
social discontent and xenophobia 171
social discriminations, see discrimination
social disharmony linked with witchcraft 208
social disorientation: and xenophobia 173
social dissent: therapy as means of suppressing 23
social distress: madness as symptom of 157
social environment problems in homosexuality 134
social expectations/practices: and madness 163–4
social identity/ies
  cultural categories 147
  discursive production 141
  evidence/explanations of origin and nature of 139, 140
  in-group and 139, 141, 142
  pluralist vision of 141
  in PTSD 104–5
  psychopathological appearance of: unpicking the 141–2
  psychopathology of 139–49
  'race', ethnicity, and the psychopathology of 139–49
  raced/unraced categories 145–6; potential solutions 146
  racial, and xenophobia 139
  racialising of 142–7
  relations between communities and 141
  role of 'race' and ethnicity in 142–4
  social tolerance/multiculturalism approach 140, 144
  see also identity
social ills: possibility of therapy/cure 259
social justice: and psychological recovery 104
social-medicine programme 262
social memory, disorder of 226
social pathology: witchcraft and 208
social policies: discourses and 247
social prejudice in social research 242 (see also gender; labelling; pathologising; racism; stigma)
social processes: and madness 156
social regulation discourses: deconstruction of 120
social relationships, traditional: and witchcraft 211

social reparation 104, 105
social sciences: concepts of norms and normal in 259–60
social-scientific practices: normalising and patholigising tendencies 243
social scientific research: as dialogue with readers 242
social setting: disruption of 95
social situations and illness experience 154
social stressors 68
social structures
  co-construction of new 105
  harm to 95, 98
social subjectivity 104
social transition: and xenophobia 169, 171, 173
social trauma 98
social utility and criminology 246
socialisation of psychopathology 223
  witchcraft and 216
societal reparation: psychological recovery and 104
society and mental illness 69
socio-cultural dimensions of psychiatry 70
socio-political advantage seen as inner strength 23
socio-political factors 49
  attention diverted from 22
  converted into individual pathology 23
socio-political power: asymmetrics reproduced 23, 49
socio-political values reflected by psychotherapy 24
sociology: analogy with physiology 253
solitary confinement 76
somatic explanations/aspects of mental disorders 55, 63, 156
somatic symptoms 131
sovereign power 256–7
Soweto 95
species, the
  health and 256
  political strategies and life of 262
  see also biological psychiatry
state
  control of individual, and psychotherapy 23–5, 49
  literature on terrorism of 88
  repression and violence 76
state-sponsored violence, limits of PTSD discourse 94
stereotyping
  anorexia 111
  as distancing strategy 188
  gender differences regarding 190–91
  of STDs 185
stigma 25, 66
  attached to psychiatric profession 66
  labelling and 25
  STDs discourse 198–202
stigmatic stress 133
stress see acute stress disorder; post-traumatic stress disorder
stress-deficit work 70

stressor(s) 68, 75, 82
  criterion 83, 84
  cumulative impact 131
  incidence in homosexuals 128, 131
  insidious: cumulative effect 131
  minority 130–1, 134
structural/funtional dualism 70
structure: contrast between normal/abnormal grounded in 254
subject positions 247, 249
subjection and objectification 247
subjective judgements on indicators of pathology 245
subjectivity(ies): 232, 233
  and discourses 21, 49, 100, 104, 162
  marketing of 233
  memory related to 223, 224
  secret or subjugated: memories and 224
  taxonomies incorporated into 153
subject(s)
  criminal, see criminal subject
  produced within and subjected to discourse 243–4
sub-populations, managing, and public safety 246
substance abuse 129
suggestion in psychotherapy 64
suicidality 133
  gay-related stress and 131
  incidence in homosexual men 129
supernatural forces
  and criminal responsibility 207
  harnessed for destruction and healing 213
  and madness 156
  see also witchcraft
superstition: science and 62
supervision 63
surveillance 246
'survivor syndrome' 92
survivors
  pathologising and medicalising of 104
  self-help groups 103
  see also war survivors
symbolic dimensions of terror 97–8
symbolic forms of language and culture and madness 156
symptomological details of narrative 37
symptoms: categorisation: and diagnostic power 26

talking, therapeutic 33–5
taxonomies of mental health/madness 152, 153, 163–6
teratology 254
terror 96–9
  conceptualising 97
  engendered nature of violence and 96–7
  indicators 97
  objectives of 97
  symbolic readings and strategies 97–8, 104
  women's perspective 96–7
theoretical diversity 70

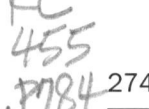

theories and concepts 236
theorising, psychological 62, 66
theorists: effects of, within knowledge-generating contexts 99
theory and practice 258
torture 76, 77, 83, 84, 86, 88, 92, 93
   judicial 244
tradition: construction of 231–2
traditional treatments/taxonomies of madness 152
traditional values: permissive sex threat to 187
tranquillisers 59
transcultural psychiatry 152, 207
transgenerational relations and witchcraft 216
trauma
   community and social dimensions 95
   constructing meanings 100–101
   continuing and chronic character 95
   deconstructing and reconstructing versions of 96
   intervention organisations 77
   medicalisation 78–9
   psychosocial 98–100
   reflexivity and 99–100
   social 98
traumatic neurosis 84
traumatic stress
   chronic 132
   conferences 77
   see also acute stress disorder; post-traumatic stress
treatment(s) 64, 65
   abandonment of unsuitable 60
   community-based 71
   harmful or useless 60
   motivating and guiding own 36
   see also drug treatments
trusting: difficulty in gays 131
Truth and Reconciliation Commission 87, 103, 226

ukuthwasa 157–8
unconscious, existence of the 68
underprivileged 145
United Nations Children's Fund 92
unjust, the: problems of adjusting to 22
'upperclass': exnomination of 145

valium 59
vested power 28

victim
   blaming: psychological reductionism and 22–3
   empowerment 84
   mentality 131
   pathologising of 94
   rights 85
   role: in anorexia 110, 115
victimisation 133
   of homosexuals 131
   and PTSD 77, 78, 84, 85–6
victimology: seeing beyond discourses of 104
vilified, the: constituted by talk about 223
violation of gays 131
violence
   against women 76, 78
   collective: and xenophobia 171
   gendered nature of 96
   impact: and post-traumatic stress 75, 77, 78
   intervention 76, 77
   linked with belief in witchcraft 208
   nationalism and 182–3
   South Africa's culture of 180
   see also xenophobia
violence against women movements 94
vital and social 256–7, 258–9, 262
vital norms and social norms 259–60
vitalism: Canguilhem's non-sociological 260
vulnerability, inherent 83, 125, 128–32, 225

war: effects on civilian populations 92
war neurosis 92
war survivors, limits of PTSD discourse 94
war trauma: contextualisation 94
'Whig' histories of psychiatry 57–8
whiteness
   as definitive national identity 145
   unraced/exnominated 144–6
witch persecutions 208–9
   fear of 216
   in the North 213–1
   targettir 215
   transgr 214

witchcraft-related practices 207–19
   consequences of belief in 208
   demographic/historical context 210–11
   exploitation of discursive frame of 216
   historical transition/social upheaval and 214
   interdisciplinary understandings 213–15
   origins of accusations and attacks 211–13
   as pathology 207–8
   power-relations and 21, 215
   in relation to underdevelopment 215–16
   STDs 192
   social tensions and frustrations and 216
'witches'
   as agents of supernatural forces 213
   smelling out 213–14
witness, wish to give 101
women
   ancestor possession 157
   blamed for STDs 190–4
   disempowerment 23
   focus towards institutional power 225
   generational conflicts between 225
   human rights violations of 97
   rape of, see rape
   reactions of therapists to 23
   repression: high rate of disorder caused by 157
   repression of normal bodily drives 114
   terror and violation of 96–8
   violence against 76
   witchcraft persecutions against elderly 209, 211–12, 215
   see also female; feminism; femininity
workshops 101, 102